Drug Hypersensitivity

Guest Editor

WERNER J. PICHLER, MD

IMMUNOLOGY AND ALLERGY CLINICS OF NORTH AMERICA

www.immunology.theclinics.com

Consulting Editor
RAFEUL ALAM, MD, PhD

August 2009 • Volume 29 • Number 3

SAUNDERS an imprint of ELSEVIER, Inc.

W.B. SAUNDERS COMPANY

A Division of Elsevier Inc.

1600 John F. Kennedy Blvd., ● Suite 1800 ● Philadelphia, PA 19103-2899.

http://www.theclinics.com

IMMUNOLOGY AND ALLERGY CLINICS OF NORTH AMERICA Volume 29, Number 3
August 2009 ISSN 0889–8561, ISBN-13: 978-1-4377-1229-2, ISBN-10: 1-4377-1229-0

Editor: Patrick Manley

Immunology and Allergy Clinics of North America (ISSN 0889–8561) is published quarterly by Elsevier Inc., 360 Park Avenue South, New York, NY 10010-1710. Months of issue are February, May, August, and November. Business and Editorial Offices: 1600 John F. Kennedy Blvd., Suite 1800, Philadelphia, PA 19103-2899. Customer Service Office: 11830 Westline Industrial Drive, St. Louis, MO 63146. Periodicals postage paid at New York, NY and additional mailing offices. Subscription prices are $233.00 per year for US individuals, $366.00 per year for US institutions, $113.00 per year for US students and residents, $286.00 per year for Canadian individuals, $163.00 per year for Canadian students, $454.00 per year for Canadian institutions, $325.00 per year for international individuals, $454.00 per year for international institutions, $163.00 per year for international students. To receive student/resident rate, orders must be accompanied by name of affiliated institution, date of term, and the *signature* of program/residency coordinator on institution letterhead. Orders will be billed at individual rate until proof of status is received. Foreign air speed delivery is included in all *Clinics* subscription prices. All prices are subject to change without notice. **POSTMASTER**: Send address changes to *Immunology and Allergy Clinics of North America,* Elsevier Journals Customer Service, 11830 Westline Industrial Drive, St. Louis, MO 63146. **Customer Service: 1-800-654-2452 (US and Canada). From outside of the United States and Canada, call 1-314-453-7041. Fax: 1-314-453-5170. For print support, e-mail: JournalsCustomerService-usa@ elsevier.com. For online support, e-mail: JournalsOnlineSupport-usa@elsevier.com.**

Reprints. For copies of 100 or more, of articles in this publication, please contact the Commercial Reprints Department, Elsevier Inc., 360 Park Avenue South, New York, New York 10010-1710. Tel. (212) 633-3812, Fax: (212) 462-1935, e-mail: reprints@elsevier.com.

Immunology and Allergy Clinics of North America is covered in *MEDLINE/PubMed (Index Medicus), Current Contents/Life Sciences, Science Citation Index, ISI/BIOMED, Chemical Abstracts,* and *EMBASE/Excerpta Medica.*

Printed and bound by CPI Group (UK) Ltd, Croydon, CR0 4YY
Transferred to Digital Print 2011

Contributors

CONSULTING EDITOR

RAFEUL ALAM, MD, PhD
Veda and Chauncey Ritter Chair in Immunology, Professor, and Director, Division
of Immunology and Allergy, National Jewish Health; and University of Colorado Health
Sciences Center, Denver, Colorado

GUEST EDITOR

WERNER J. PICHLER, MD
Division of Allergology, Clinic of Rheumatology and Clinical Immunology/Allergology,
Inselspital, Bern University Hospital and University of Bern, Bern, Switzerland

AUTHORS

WERNER ABERER, MD
Professor of Dermatology, Department of Dermatology and Venereology, Medical
University of Graz, Graz, Austria

I. AIMONE-GASTIN, MD, PhD
Laboratoire de Biochimie Biologie Moléculaire Nutrition Métabolisme, CHU de Brabois;
and Unité de Pathologie Cellulaire et Moléculaire en Nutrition, Inserm U724, Faculté de
Médecine, Vandoeuvre les Nancy, France

ANNICK BARBAUD, MD, PhD
Department of Dermatology, Fournier Hospital, University Hospital of Nancy, Nancy,
France

CHRIS H. BRIDTS, MLT
Laboratory Chief Technologist, Allergology Unit, Department of Immunology, Allergology
and Rheumatology, University Hospital Antwerp, University of Antwerp, Belgium

KNUT BROCKOW, MD
Department of Dermatology and Allergy Biederstein, Technische Universität München,
Munich, Germany

MARIANA CASTELLS, MD, PhD
Associate Professor, Harvard Medical School; Director, Desensitization Program;
Director, Allergy and Immunology Training Program, Brigham and Women's Hospital; and
Division of Rheumatology Allergy and Immunology, Department of Medicine, Brigham and
Women's Hospital, Harvard Medical School, Boston, Massachusetts

P. DEMOLY, MD, PhD
Exploration des Allergies-Maladies Respiratoires, INSERM U657, Hôpital Arnaud de
Villeneuve, CHU de Montpellier, Montpellier Cedex 5, France

DIDIER G. EBO, MD, PhD
Allergology Unit, Department of Immunology, Allergology and Rheumatology, University Hospital Antwerp, University of Antwerp, Belgium

E. FLORVAAG, MD
Senior Consultant, Laboratory of Clinical Biochemistry, Haukeland University Hospital; Section for Clinical Allergology, Department of Occupational Medicine, Haukeland University Hospital; and Professor, Institute of Internal Medicine, University of Bergen, Norway

THOMAS GENTINETTA, MSc
Research Scientist, Department of Allergology, Department of Rheumatology, Allergology and Clinical Immunology, Inselspital, University of Bern, Bern, Switzerland

J.L. GUÉANT, MD, PhD
Laboratoire de Biochimie Biologie Moléculaire Nutrition Métabolisme, CHU de Brabois; and Unité de Pathologie Cellulaire et Moléculaire en Nutrition, Inserm U724, Faculté de Médecine, Vandoeuvre les Nancy, France

R.M. GUÉANT-RODRIGUEZ, MD, PhD
Laboratoire de Biochimie Biologie Moléculaire Nutrition Métabolisme, CHU de Brabois; and Unité de Pathologie Cellulaire et Moléculaire en Nutrition, Inserm U724, Faculté de Médecine, Vandoeuvre les Nancy, France

OLIVER V. HAUSMANN, MD
Research fellow, Department of Allergology, Department of Rheumatology, Allergology and Clinical Immunology, Inselspital, University of Bern, Bern, Switzerland

S.G.O. JOHANSSON, MD
Professor, Department of Medicine, Clinical Immunology and Allergy Unit, Karolinska Institute; and Professor, Department of Clinical Immunology and Transfusion Medicine, Karolinska University Hospital, Solna, Stockholm, Sweden

YOKO KANO, MD, PhD
Department of Dermatology, Kyorin University School of Medicine, Tokyo, Japan

BIRGER KRÄNKE, MD
Associate Professor of Dermatology, Department of Dermatology and Venereology, Medical University of Graz, Graz, Austria

M. LAMBERT, MD
Service d'Anesthésie-Réanimation Chirurgicale, CHU de Nancy, Hôpital Central, Nancy Cedex; and Unité Inserm U684, Faculté de Médecine, Vandoeuvre les Nancy, France

PRISKA LOCHMATTER, MSc
Division of Allergology, Clinic of Rheumatology and Clinical Immunology/Allergology, Inselspital, Bern University Hospital and University of Bern, Bern, Switzerland

J.M. MALINOVSKY, MD, PhD
Service d'Anesthésie et Réanimation, CHU de Reims, Pôle URAD, Hôpital Maison Blanche, Reims, France

P.M. MERTES, MD, PhD
Service d'Anesthésie-Réanimation Chirurgicale, CHU de Nancy, Hôpital Central, Nancy Cedex; and Unité Inserm U684, Faculté de Médecine, Vandoeuvre les Nancy, France

D.A. MONERET-VAUTRIN, MD, PhD
Service de Médecine Interne, Immunologie Clinique et Allergologie, CHU de Nancy, Hôpital Central, Nancy Cedex, France

C. MOUTON-FAIVRE, MD
Service d'Anesthésie-Réanimation Chirurgicale, CHU de Nancy, Hôpital Central, Nancy Cedex, France

WERNER J. PICHLER, MD
Division of Allergology, Clinic of Rheumatology and Clinical Immunology/Allergology, Inselspital, Bern University Hospital and University of Bern, Bern, Switzerland

CORNELIA S. SEITZ, MD
Assistant Professor, Department of Dermatology, Venereology, and Allergology, University of Göttingen, Göttingen, Germany

BENNO SCHNYDER, MD
Division of Allergology, Clinic for Rheumatology and Clinical Immunology/Allergology, Inselspital, University of Bern, Bern, Switzerland

TETSUO SHIOHARA, MD, PhD
Department of Dermatology, Kyorin University School of Medicine, Tokyo, Japan

AXEL TRAUTMANN, MD
Associate Professor, Allergy Unit, Department of Dermatology, Venereology, and Allergology, University of Würzburg, Würzburg, Germany

ANNA ZAWODNIAK, MD
Division of Allergology, Clinic of Rheumatology and Clinical Immunology/Allergology, Inselspital, Bern University Hospital and University of Bern, Bern, Switzerland

Contents

Drug allergies are adverse drug reactions mediated by the specific immune system. Despite characteristic signs (eg, skin rash) that raise awareness for possible drug allergies, they are great imitators of disease and may hide behind unexpected symptoms. No single standardized diagnostic test can confirm the immune-mediated mechanism or identify the causative drug; therefore, immune-mediated drug hypersensitivity reactions and their causative drugs must be recognized by the constellation of exposure, timing, and clinical features including the pattern of organ manifestation. Additional allergologic investigations (skin tests, in vitro tests, provocation tests) may provide help in identifying the possible eliciting drug.

Anaphylactic reactions to neuromuscular blocking agents during general anesthesia constitute a major cause of concern and a great source of debate among anesthesiologists. The authors' recent investigations, taking the striking differences of incidence between Norway and Sweden as the point of departure, have provided valuable insights into the pathogenetic mechanisms and the highly uneven geographical distribution of these rare, but dramatic and notoriously unpredictable, events. Eventually, a cough syrup containing pholcodine emerged as the most likely suspect. This new knowledge led to the withdrawal of the drug from the Norwegian market and to the examination of the role of pholcodine-containing drugs in other countries. The present article is a brief summary of the research behind this development.

The incidence of immune-mediated anaphylaxis during anesthesia ranges from 1 in 10,000 to 1 in 20,000. Neuromuscular blocking agents represent the most frequently involved substances, followed by latex and antibiotics, but every drug or substance used may be involved. Diagnosis relies on tryptase measurements at the time of the reaction and skin tests and specific IgE or basophil activation assays.

Immediate and Delayed Reactions to Radiocontrast Media: Is There an Allergic Mechanism?

Knut Brockow

Radiocontrast media can cause immediate (1 hour) and nonimmediate (>1 hour) hypersensitivity reactions that remain unpredictable and a cause of concern for radiologists and cardiologists. Immediate hypersensitivity reactions resemble anaphylaxis, whereas nonimmediate ones clinically are predominated by exanthemas. Increasing evidence indicates that immediate reactions and nonimmediate skin exanthemas may be allergic reactions involving either contrast media–reactive IgE or T cells, respectively. Skin testing is a useful tool for the diagnosis of contrast media allergy. It may have an important role in the selection of a safe product in previous reactors, although validation data are still lacking. In vitro tests to search for contrast media–specific cell activation are currently under investigation.

Heparin Allergy: Delayed-Type Non–IgE-Mediated Allergic Hypersensitivity to Subcutaneous Heparin Injection

Axel Trautmann and Cornelia S. Seitz

Itching erythematous or eczematous plaques around injection sites are quite frequent side effects of heparin treatment and clinical symptoms of delayed-type non–IgE-mediated allergic hypersensitivity (DTH) to heparin. For diagnosis, intradermal, patch, and subcutaneous challenge tests with heparins are suitable. In most cases, changing the subcutaneous therapy from unfractionated to low molecular weight heparin or treatment with heparinoids does not provide improvement because of extensive cross-reactivity. Hirudin polypeptides, which exhibit a different chemical structure, are a safe therapeutic alternative for subcutaneous application, however. Importantly, despite DTH to subcutaneously injected heparins, most patients tolerate heparin intravenously. Moreover, in case of therapeutic necessity and DTH to heparins, the simple shift from subcutaneous to intravenous heparin administration without prior testing may be justified.

The Variable Clinical Picture of Drug-Induced Hypersensitivity Syndrome/Drug Rash with Eosinophilia and Systemic Symptoms in Relation to the Eliciting Drug

Yoko Kano and Tetsuo Shiohara

Drug-induced hypersensitivity syndrome (DIHS)/drug rash with eosinophilia and systemic symptoms (DRESS) is a life-threatening adverse reaction characterized by skin rashes, fever, leukocytosis with eosinophilia or atypical lymphocytosis, lymph node enlargement, and liver or renal dysfunction. The syndrome develops 2 to 6 weeks after initiation of administration of a specific drug. It has been demonstrated that various herpesvirus reactivations, in addition to human herpesvirus 6, contribute to internal organ involvement and the relapse of symptoms observed long after discontinuation of the causative drugs. A better understanding of the interplay in the development of DIHS/DRESS has implications for safer and more efficient treatment of this syndrome.

Skin tests with drugs help determine the cause and mechanism of drug hypersensitivity reactions. The diagnosis of adverse drug reactions is based primarily on history and clinical presentation. In type I, IgE-mediated allergic drug reactions, skin prick test and intradermal testing may provide rapid and supportive evidence for diagnosis or exclusion of IgE-mediated reactions. These tests often are more sensitive than laboratory assays for IgE antibodies to drug allergens, which are available only for a few drugs. Because intradermal skin tests occasionally induce adverse events, they should be performed by experienced personnel in an adequate environment.

Drug skin tests (eg, patch tests, prick tests with delayed readings, intradermal tests [IDT], especially with delayed readings) are used to investigate cutaneous adverse drug reactions (CADR) in delayed hypersensitivity reactions caused by a particular drug. Their value depends on the clinical features of the CADR and on the drug tested. In maculopapular rash (MPR), drug skin tests are of value, beginning with patch tests, and followed: 1) if negative by prick tests (with delayed readings at 24 hours); and, 2) if the injectable form of the drug is available, with IDT with immediate and delayed readings. This article discusses details of the use of patch tests as they apply to patients with various drug reactions. Drug skin tests are useful to study cross-reactivity between suspected drugs. False positive results can occur. The negative predictive value of drug skin tests is approximately 90%.

The diagnosis of a drug hypersensitivity reaction (DHR) is a challenging task because multiple and complex mechanisms are involved. Better understanding of immunologic pathomechanisms in DHRs and rapid progress in cellular-based in-vitro tests can help to adjust the correct diagnostic strategy to individual patients with different clinical manifestations of drug allergy. Thus, drug hypersensitivity diagnosis needs to rely on a combination of medical history and different in vivo and in vitro tests. In this article, the authors discuss current in vitro techniques, most recent findings, and new promising tools in the diagnosis of T-cell–mediated drug hypersensitivity.

Diagnosis of drug allergy involves first the recognition of sometimes unusual symptoms as drug allergy and, second, the identification of the eliciting drug. This is an often difficult task, as the clinical picture and underlying pathomechanisms are heterogeneous. In clinical routine, physicians frequently have to rely upon a suggestive history and eventual provocation tests, both having their specific limitations. For this reason both in vivo (skin tests) and in vitro tests are investigated intensively as tools to identify the disease-eliciting drug. One of the tests evaluated in drug allergy is the basophil activation test (BAT). Basophils with their high-affinity IgE receptors are easily accessible and therefore can be used as indicator cells for IgE-mediated reactions. Upon allergen challenge and cross-linking of membrane-bound IgE antibodies (via Fc-epsilon-RI) basophils up-regulate certain activation markers on their surface such as CD63 and CD203c, as well as intracellular markers (eg, phosphorylated p38MAPK). In BAT, these alterations can be detected rapidly on a single-cell basis by multicolor flow cytometry using specific monoclonal antibodies. Combining this technique with in vitro passive sensitization of donor basophils with patients' serum, one can prove the IgE dependence of a drug reaction. This article summarizes the authors' current experience with the BAT in the diagnostic management of immediate-type drug allergy mediated by drug-specific IgE antibodies.

Provocation tests are regarded as the "gold standard" to establish or exclude the presence of hypersensitivity to a certain drug because they reproduce not only allergy symptoms but other adverse manifestations, irrespective of their pathomechanism. Provocation testing is potentially harmful and should be considered only after balancing the risk-benefit ratio in the individual patient. The reasons for false-positive and false-negative results are numerous, including loss of sensitization, cofactors not being included in the diagnostic procedure, and the potential induction of tolerance during provocation. When conducted by experienced clinicians in a carefully monitored setting, however, drug provocation testing is a safe method to confirm or exclude drug hypersensitivity.

Drug desensitization is the induction of temporary clinical unresponsiveness to drug antigens to which patients have presented severe hypersensitivity reactions. It is typically achieved by gradual reintroduction of small doses of drug antigens at fixed time intervals, and it is aimed at providing increased safety and protection from side effects, including anaphylaxis. Delivery of full therapeutic doses is achieved during desensitization, allowing patients to receive firstline chemotherapy, antibiotics, or monoclonal antibodies, as well as other drugs such as insulin, aspirin, and iron. Desensitizations are high-risk interventions. Inhibition of cellular activation mechanisms occurs during drug desensitization, allowing for the protective clinical outcomes and lack of side effects in the majority of cases, but the cellular and molecular inhibitory mechanisms are incompletely understood. The indication for desensitization protocols can only be done by trained allergists and immunologists and should be implemented as standard of care because of their high success rates and outcomes-demonstrated safety profile.

THE CLINICS ARE NOW AVAILABLE ONLINE!

Access your subscription at:
www.theclinics.com

Foreword

Drug Allergy and Primum Non-nocere

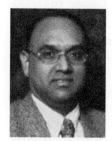

Rafeul Alam, MD, PhD
Consulting Editor

Drug-induced allergy is the moral equivalent of the primal sin for the medical profession. Arguably, the temptation here is not pleasure but a noble goal to help a sick patient. Nonetheless, we are in conflict with our first principle of *"primum non nocere"* whenever our patients experience an adverse event because of our intervention.

Drug allergy has always been a difficult subject because of poor understanding of the underlying mechanism. This was primarily a result of the difficulty in establishing a patient cohort, lack of appropriate study reagents, and inadequate knowledge about the immune response to small molecular-weight substances. Remarkable progress has been made in recent years in this very difficult area of science. Application of pharmacogenomic approaches led to identification of the role of HLA-B*1502, HLA-B58, and HLA-B57 for sensitivity to carmazepin, allopurinol, and abacavir, respectively.[1,2] The screening for these HLA genotypes now saves lives. HLA-B*1502 predisposes the Chinese Han population to Stevens-Johnson syndrome when taking carbamazepin.[3] Progress has also been made in understanding the immunologic basis for drug allergy. Precise binding of the offending drug to a particular HLA subtype leads to a productive CD8 T-cell immune response.[4] This type of research has allowed better classification of various drug allergies.[5] Better understanding has begun to result in newer diagnostic tests. Finally, drug desensitization protocols are beginning to be validated in a more systematic manner instead being presented as empirical experience.

Dr. Pichler has been performing pioneering studies in drug allergy and contributing to new knowledge in the field.[5] He has invited a distinguished group of investigators

Supported by NIH grants RO1 AI059719 and AI68088, PPG HL 36577 and N01 HHSN272200700048C

Immunol Allergy Clin N Am 29 (2009) xiii–xiv
doi:10.1016/j.iac.2009.06.002
0889-8561/09/$ – see front matter

and clinician-scholars, and in so doing has put together an outstanding update on drug allergy. This is a valuable asset for any practicing clinician.

Rafeul Alam, MD, PhD
Veda and Chauncey Ritter Chair in Immunology
Professor & Director, Division of Allergy & Immunology
National Jewish Health & University of Colorado Denver Health Sciences Center
1400 Jackson Street, Denver, CO 80206

E-mail address:
alamr@njc.org (R. Alam)

REFERENCES

1. Mallal S, Nolan D, Witt C, et al. Association between presence of HLA-B*5701, HLA-DR7, and HLA-DQ3 and hypersensitivity to HIV-1 reverse-transcriptase inhibitor abacavir. Lancet 2002;359:727–32.
2. Hetherington S, Hughes AR, Mosteller M, et al. Genetic variations in HLA-B region and hypersensitivity reactions to abacavir. Lancet 2002;359:1121–2.
3. Chung WH, Hung SI, Hong HS, et al. Medical genetics: a marker for Stevens-Johnson syndrome. Nature 2004;428:486.
4. Chessman D, Kostenko L, Lethborg T, et al. Human leukocyte antigen class I-restricted activation of CD8+ T cells provides the immunogenetic basis of a systemic drug hypersensitivity. Immunity 2008;28:822–32.
5. Posadas SJ, Pichler WJ. Delayed drug hypersensitivity reactions—new concepts. Clin Exp Allergy 2007;37:989–99.

Preface

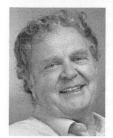

Werner J. Pichler, MD
Guest Editor

Most reviews on the topic of drug hypersensitivity start with the sentence: "Drug allergy is a difficult problem because…." Indeed, the multitude of drugs and clinical symptoms, and the variety of different mechanisms that underlie drug-induced diseases can promote a rather fatalistic attitude to drug hypersensitivity, as it seems just too complicated to address it well. Indeed, many physicians rely on history and experience alone, and do not test for drug allergy. As the tests are still not very sensitive, this approach is understandable. But will such an attitude improve this area of medicine?

The need for research in drug allergy in the United States has been strongly advocated by a task force of the Environmental Sciences Institute.[1] It is also our duty as physicians (or scientists of pharmaceutic industries) to tackle this problem with particular care, as it is an iatrogenic disease. However, the difficulties of research and translating that research to clinical practice are obvious. There is a lack of established animal models, each drug has unique features, and severe reactions with a single drug are still uncommon in a single center, so it remains a rare disease for a single drug, while it is a common disease with many features if all drugs are considered. As an iatrogenic disease, it is ethically problematic to perform provocation tests to prove a sensitization, which is, however, still considered to be the gold standard.[2] Consequently, we have a lack of well-standardized procedures to test for drug allergy.

The situation of drug-allergy research is somewhat better in Europe and Asia than in the United States. Why? In Europe and Asia, some clinical researchers have made drug allergy their own, proper topic. Young researchers from Japan, Taiwan, Australia, Great Britain, Spain, Italy, and Switzerland had the courage to take over the role of outsiders in clinical and scientific meetings, where a presentation on nonprotein antigens was and is still considered to be rather exotic. Early on, some of these outsiders met in small meetings and exchanged their knowledge and drug-allergy testing protocols. Thus, the limited experience of a single center was overcome and useful protocols elaborated. In Europe this group was called the European Network of Drug Allergy; in Japan it was the Japanese Research Committee on Severe Cutaneous Adverse Reactions (J-SCAR). Enormous input came also from the project EuroSCAR, a consortium of clinicians, researchers, and epidemiologists focusing on severe cutaneous drug reactions.

Immunol Allergy Clin N Am 29 (2009) xv–xvi
doi:10.1016/j.iac.2009.06.001
0889-8561/09/$ – see front matter

Progress in the clinic depends on progress in research. In spite of the above-mentioned limitations, there was progress in drug allergy research over the last years: A new classification of (type IV) drug hypersensitivity and a new concept of immune stimulation by drugs was developed; the important role of herpes virus coinfections in severe forms of drug hypersensitivity was described, and a baffling strong association of HLA-B alleles with certain drug hypersensitivity reactions was found for various drugs (for overview see Ref.).[3]

Now, can we transfer this novel knowledge to clinical practice? Yes. The most significant progress is the fact that in many countries the presence of the HLA-B5701-allele is already excluded before abacavir is given. It is one of the first widely used pharmacogenetic (actually immunogenetic) tests widely applied and also paid for by insurance companies. Our American colleagues have established very useful protocols for drug desensitizations, which enables one to continue life saving treatments in spite of IgE-mediated anaphylaxis to the drug. Our Japanese colleagues present their experience with the severe drug hypersensitivity reactions. From Europe come various skin testing protocols, which were standardized and are today widely used. They clearly help in the diagnosis and often allow clinicians to provide a less risky alternative. As a result, we have well-documented protocols not only for beta-lactam skin testing, but also for various drug classes. Three of them—namely for neuromuscular blocking agents—for allergies to anticoagulants and for contrast media (yes, there are true allergies to contrast media!) are presented in detail in this issue of The Clinics. In addition, an article in this issue addresses the fascinating role of a possibly harmless cough syrup containing pholcodin for the occurrence of perioperative anaphylaxis. These and overviews of immediate and delayed skin testing, provocation tests, and desensitization protocols are presented and supplemented by some in vitro tests for drug allergy diagnosis: namely basophil and lymphocyte activation tests.

I am aware that some important problems to this topic are not discussed in detail, but I purposely emphasized some "other" aspects in this issue, which are often overseen in reviews on drug allergy. So I hope the reader finds some new information in this issue of The Clinics and can use it in daily clinical practice.

I thank all of the contributors.

Werner J. Pichler, MD
University of Bern Inselspital
Allergology
Freiburgstrasse 10
Bern3010
Switzerland

E-mail address:
werner.pichler@insel.ch (W.J. Pichler)

REFERENCES

1. Adkinson NF Jr, Essayan D, Gruchalla R, et al. Health and Environmental Sciences Institute Task Force. Task force report: future research needs for the prevention and management of immune-mediated drug hypersensitivity reactions. J Allergy Clin Immunol 2002;109:S461–78.
2. Aberer W, Bircher A, Romano A, et al. European Network for Drug Allergy (ENDA); EAACI interest group on drug hypersensitivity. Drug provocation testing in the diagnosis of drug hypersensitivity reactions: general considerations. Allergy 2003;58:854–63.
3. Pichler WJ. Drug Hypersensitivity, Karger, Basel, Switzerland, 2007.

Approach to the Patient with Drug Allergy

Benno Schnyder, MD

KEYWORDS

- Drug allergy • Pseudoallergy • Immediate hypersensitivity
- Nonimmediate type hypersensitivity • Diagnosis • Therapy

Adverse drug reactions are frequent and occur in 10% to 20% of hospitalized patients and approximately 7% of the general population.[1] Whenever a patient treated with a drug develops an exacerbation or a new medical problem, an adverse drug reaction must be included in the differential diagnosis. The clinician should investigate whether one of the involved drugs is known to cause such a reaction and determine the temporal link between the onset of the reaction and drug administration. Adverse drug reactions have been classified by Rawlins and Thompson[2] in four types: (1) type A reactions that are common (approximately 80%) owing to the pharmacologic or toxic property of the causative drug and thus predictable that may occur in any individual; (2) type B reactions that are uncommon (approximately 10% to 15%), not predictable, and occur only in susceptible individuals; (3) type C reactions that are associated with long-term therapy (eg, benzodiazepine dependence); and (4) type D reactions that are carcinogenic and teratogenic effects.

Drug allergies are type B reactions that are mediated by the specific immune system (IgE- or T cell–mediated or, rarely, immune complex–mediated reactions). Other type B reactions without involvement of the specific immune system (5% to 10%) are classified as nonimmune-mediated (or nonallergic) hypersensitivity reactions[3,4]

MAKING THE DIAGNOSIS

Two questions are essential for the diagnosis of a drug allergy: (1) Is it a drug allergy? (2) Which drug has caused the disease? The most frequent manifestations of drug allergies are a skin rash, maculopapular exanthema, and anaphylactic reactions. Biologic agents may more often cause serum sickness and vasculitis; however, different conditions may mimic immune-mediated type B reactions and vice versa (**Table 1**). Sometimes blood eosinophilia may be helpful for the differential diagnosis. No single standardized diagnostic test is able to confirm a drug allergy; therefore, immune-mediated drug hypersensitivity reactions and their causative drugs must be

Division of Allergology, Clinic for Rheumatology and Clinical Immunology/Allergology, Inselspital, University of Bern, 3010 Bern, Switzerland
E-mail address: benno.schnyder@insel.ch

Immunol Allergy Clin N Am 29 (2009) 405–418
doi:10.1016/j.iac.2009.04.005
0889-8561/09/$ – see front matter © 2009 Elsevier Inc. All rights reserved.

Table 1
Signs of drug allergy/intolerance

	Symptoms	Examples
Guiding signs of frequent reactions	Urticaria, angioedema Skin rash (macular exanthema) Maculopapular exanthma (MPE) Eosinophilia	Urtikaria after acetylsalicylic acid After vancomycin infusion After 10 day amoxicillin treatment During MPE, DRESS
Guiding signs of rare reactions	Sharply localised pruritic erythematous reaction Symmetrical erythema in the flexural or intertriginous folds Disseminated, 1- to 3-mm sterile pustules in the skin Cytopenia	Fixed drug eruption Symmetrical drug related intertriginous and flexural exanthema (SDRIFE) Acute exanthematous pustulosis (AGEP) Thrombocytopenia after biologicals
Atypical signs mimicking other diseases	(Perioperative) cardial arrest Fever, malaise Lymphadenopathy Multiorgan failure Single organ involvement like nephritis, hepatitis or other Arthralgia Palpable purpuric papule of the legs	After muscle relaxants During Drug rash with eosinophilia and systemic symptoms (DRESS) DRESS (minocyclin) DRESS (allopurinol) Interstitial nephritis after floxapen Serum sickness Vasculitis after NSAID

recognized by the constellation of exposure, timing, and clinical features including the pattern of organ manifestation. For the assessment during a drug-induced type B reaction, a comprehensive investigation is important (including documentation of fever or lymphadenopathy, an examination of the skin including mucous membranes, and an assessment for blood eosinophilia or signs of liver involvement such as elevated transaminases and icterus). Initial questions on clinical assessment include the following:

Which active drug substances and xenobiotics are involved (including phytodrugs)?

What is the temporal relationship between the exposure of each drug and the onset of the reaction?

What is the nature of the reaction? Does it correspond to known adverse reactions to (one of) the involved drugs?

Were any other drugs administered concurrently that could have caused the reaction?

Are there any underlying conditions of the patient that could explain the reaction (eg, infections, food)?

If the reaction occurred in the past, did the reaction resolve after cessation of the drug (and, if so, how long did the recovery take)?

What is the genetic background of the patient? Recent findings show a strong genetic association between HLA alleles and the susceptibility to drug-specific immune-mediated hypersensitivity. HLAB*5701 is associated with abacavir hypersensitivity, HLA-B*5801 with allopurinol-induced severe cutaneous adverse reactions including drug-related eosinophilia with systemic symptoms

(DRESS), Stevens-Johnson syndrome induced (SJS), and toxic epidermal necrolysis (TEN), and HLA-B*1502 with carbamazepine-induced SJS and TEN but not with maculopapular exanthema. Carbamazepine induced SJS/TEN associated with B*1502 is seen in Southeast Asians but not in Caucasians.[5]

Sometimes the answers to these questions allow the classification of drug hypersensitivity into immediate and nonimmediate types of reactions (**Table 2**). This differentiation may narrow the differential diagnosis and be helpful for further management.

Various signs and symptoms of drug allergy listed in **Table 3** are described as potential early danger signals.[6] Even though the predictive value of these signs has not been investigated prospectively, it is prudent to take heed of them.

Immediate-type Hypersensitivity Reactions

Clinical aspects

Immediate-type hypersensitivity reactions manifest typically as urticaria (**Fig. 1**) with or without angioedema and anaphylaxis. Anaphylaxis is a severe allergic reaction involving multiple organs. The clinical presentation may be variable, and its definition is still a matter of debate.[7] The reaction may start with skin manifestations. Typical initial symptoms are a palmar or plantar itch with or without urticaria and angioedema. Additionally, there may be nausea, abdominal pain, vomiting, and diarrhea. There may be rhinoconjunctivitis, obstructive respiratory symptoms, cardiovascular events, altered mental state, and fainting.[7] Severe respiratory and cardiovascular manifestation such as arterial hypotension and cardiovascular collapse may be the primary manifestations, particularly in perioperative reactions.[8] Reactions typically follow a uniphasic course; however, 20% are biphasic in nature.[9]

Immediate-type hypersensitivity reactions may comprise type I allergies or poorly understood mechanisms such as so-called "pseudoallergic reactions" (nonimmune-mediated hypersensitivities).

IgE-mediated allergies (type I) usually occur within less than 1 hour after drug administration.[10] Sometimes, especially after oral drug intake, mild reactions may even appear after a few hours. It has been a dogma that allergic reactions to drugs are only those observed on re-exposure or longer lasting exposure (at least 3 days); however, more recent data show that a previous contact to the causative drug is

Table 2		
Classifying drug hypersensitivity: immediate versus nonimmediate reaction		
Parameter	**Immediate Reaction**	**Nonimmediate Reaction**
Time between exposure and onset of the reaction	≤1 h (in special conditions such as intolerance to acetylsalicylic acid ≤3 h)	≥6 h (in the case of strong T-cell sensitization earlier)
Time of recovery	Few hours	Several days to weeks
Clinical nature of the reaction	Urticaria, angioedema, anaphylaxis	Maculopapular exanthema and other skin manifestations including late appearing urticarial rash and angioedema, disorder of blood cells, systemic reactions such as drug rash with eosinophilia, and systemic symptoms (DRESS)

Table 3
Signs of severity

Type of Reaction	Signs of Severity
Immediate onset reactions	Involvement of extradermal organs, such as rhinconjunctivitis, obstructive respiratory symptoms, nausea, vomiting Sudden onset of generalized pruritus Itching of the perioral area, the inguina, palms, or soles Sudden flush if accompanied by conjunctivitis or rhinitis
Delayed onset reactions	Fever, malaise Prolonged clinical symptoms after discontinuation of the causative drug Lymphadenopathy Burning or painful skin Bullous lesions, epidermal detachment (Nikolsky's sign) Mucosal involvement Facial edema or diffuse erythematous swelling Confluent lesions of extended body surfaces Eosinophilia >1.5 × 10^9/L Liver involvement

not an obligatory prerequisite for immune-mediated drug hypersensitivity.[11–13] This paradox might be best explained by cross-reactivity between the involved drug and other xenobiotics to which the affected subject was previously exposed (see the article by Florwaag and Johansson elsewhere in this issue).

Pseudoallergic reactions tend to arise within 1 to 3 hours after drug administration. Often they require a higher dose than true IgE-mediated allergies. In susceptible persons, many active drug substances can elicit such reactions. Typical inducers are listed in **Table 4**.

Laboratory evaluations during the reaction
No optimal and readily available laboratory test can confirm the clinical diagnosis of an anaphylactic episode. Measurements of total tryptase in serum 60 to 240 minutes after the onset of symptoms may be helpful. A rise can be quantified as soon as 30 minutes after the onset of symptoms. The half-life of tryptase is about 120 minutes. To enable a comparison with baseline levels, a new sample should be collected more than 2 days after the reaction.[14] A transient increase of serum tryptase indicates an involvement of mast cells; however, the sensitivity of serum tryptase is low, and it does not allow differentiating between immunologic and nonimmunologic mast cell activation.

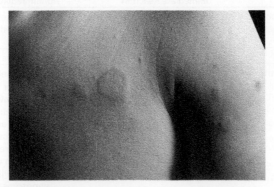

Fig. 1. Drug-induced urticaria.

Table 4 Immediate reactions and typically involved drugs	
Type of Reaction	**Involved Drugs**
IgE-mediated reaction	Beta-lactam antibiotics, quinolones, sulfonamide antibiotics, macrolides, pyrazolones, latex Neuromuscular blocking agents[a] Contrast medium[a]
Pseudoallergic reactions	Acetylsalicylic acid and other non-steroidal antirheumatics (NSAID) Plasma volume expander (colloids) Neuromuscular blocking agents[a] Contrast medium[a]

[a] Drugs that can induce IgE-mediated or pseudoallergic reactions.

Nonimmediate-type Hypersensitivity Reactions

Clinical aspects

Nonimmediate reactions occur more than 1 hour after drug administration; however, there is a certain overlap in the time of manifestations. Some IgE-mediated reactions occur after 1 hour, and some nonimmediate reactions may start prior to 1 hour. Nonimmediate drug allergies are most frequently T cell mediated, whereas IgG-mediated responses are rare. Nonimmediate drug allergies may be clinically manifested as a broad spectrum of diseases. Frequently involved drugs are listed in **Table 5**.

Maculopapular or morbilliform exanthema The most frequent type B reactions are maculopapular and morbilliform exanthemas, which are manifested as erythematous macules and infiltrated papules, particularly affecting the trunk and proximal extremities (**Fig. 2**). Typically, a more or less pronounced desquamation occurs after clearing of the lesions. Maculopapular exanthemas are observed in about 2% of hospitalized patients.[15] They usually appear more than 2 to 9 days after the drug has been started. A large body of experimental and clinical data indicates that these rashes correspond frequently to T cell–mediated (type IV) hypersensitivities.

Fixed drug eruption The most characteristic finding of a fixed drug eruption is the recurrence of similar lesions at the same sites, typically healing with residual hyperpigmentation. Rarely there are nonpigmenting forms. The validity of skin tests for identification of the causative drug is not known.[16] They may be positive only if performed in the affected area.

Symmetrical drug-related intertriginous and flexural exanthema (SDRIFE) Rarely, drug eruptions may present with a characteristic distribution pattern consisting of a sharply limited symmetrical erythema in the gluteal area and the flexural or intertriginous folds without any systemic symptoms and signs. This particular reaction was originally described as a special form of systemic contact-type dermatitis that occurs after ingestion or systemic absorption of a contact allergen in individuals previously sensitized by topical exposure to the same allergen in the same areas. Similar eruptions have been reported after systemic exposure to beta-lactam antibiotics and other drugs. Latency periods vary between a few hours and a few days after exposure.[17]

Acute generalized exanthematous pustulosis (AGEP) AGEP is a rare disease with disseminated, 1- to 3-mm sterile pustules in the skin that appear rather rapidly after 3 to 5 days of treatment. Patients have fever and massive leukocytosis in the blood,

Table 5
Nonimmediate reactions and typically involved drugs

Type of Reaction	Involved Drugs
Hemolytic anemia	Methyldopa, levodopa, interferon-alpha, cyclosporine, and fludarabine
Leucopenia	Aminopyrine and dipyrone, thyroid inhibitors, co-trimoxazole, sulfasalazine, clomipramine
Thrombopenia	Heparin, quinine, quinidine, therapeutic antibodies (biologics)
Serum sickness syndrome	Beta-lactam antibiotics
Drug-induced lupus	Hydralazine, procainamide, quinidine, minocycline, and anti–TNF-alpha agents
Vasculitis	Sulfonamide antibiotics and diuretics
Maculopapular exanthema (MPE)	Beta-lactam antibiotics, sulfonamide antibiotics, macrolides, diuretics
Fixed drug eruption	Phenytoin, sulfonamide antibiotics, tetracycline, barbiturates
Symmetrical drug-related intertriginous and flexural exanthema (SDRIFE)	Beta-lactam antibiotics, mercury
Acute generalized exanthematous pustulosis (AGEP)	Aminopenicillins, cephalosporins, macrolides, sulfonamide antibiotics, celecoxib, diltiazem, quinolone diltiazem, terbinafine, corticosteroids
Stevens-Johnson syndrome (SJS) and toxic epidermal necrolysis (TEN)	Nevirapine, allopurinol, phenytoin, carbamazepine, lamotrigine, co-trimoxazole, barbiturate, NSAID (oxicams), sertraline, pantoprazole, tramadol
Drug rash with eosinophilia and systemic symptoms (DRESS)	Carbamazepine, phenytoin, lamotrigine, minocycline, allopurinol, dapsone, sulfasalazine, co-trimoxazole, abacavir

sometimes with eosinophilia. Some pustules merge together and may form bullae. The lethality rate is about 4%, particularly in older people. Epicutaneous patch test reactions can cause a similar pustular reaction locally.[18,19]

Bullous exanthema Severe bullous exanthema may encompass different disorders. The most severe bullous skin diseases are SJS and TEN. These diseases differ solely in the extent of affected skin (<10% in SJS and >30% in TEN), with SJS/TEN overlap and skin detachment of 10% to 30% of the body surface. They are different from erythema exudativum multiforme, which is mainly caused by viral infections, is often recurrent, and affects younger persons.[20] SJS/TEN usually starts within the first 3 weeks of treatment with a macular, purple-red exanthema that can be painful. Within 12 hours, bullae may develop, even after stopping the drug. Mucous membranes (mouth, genitalia) are involved with blister formation. Lethality is dependent on age and the extent of skin detachment. The rate in SJS is approximately 10% and in TEN greater than 30%.[21] In the authors' experience, SJS/TEN may also evolve in patients despite concomitant high-dose prednisone treatment.

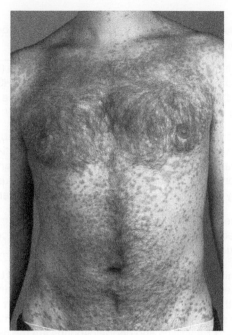

Fig. 2. Maculopapular or morbilliform exanthema.

Drug-hypersensitivity syndrome or drug-related eosinophilia with systemic symptoms Typical for this severe systemic disease are a macular exanthema, an erythematous centrofacial swelling, fever, general malaise, lymph node swelling, and involvement of other organs including hepatitis (50%), nephritis (10%), and more rarely pneumonitis, colitis, and pancreatitis.[22] The type of organ involvement depends on the type of drug causing it.[23] Minocyclin-induced DRESS is associated with lymphadenopathy, whereas allopurinol-induced DRESS has renal insufficiency. Over 70% of these cases have a marked eosinophilia (often >1 G/l), and activated T cells are often found in the circulation. Symptoms can start up to 12 weeks after the start of treatment, often after increasing the dose, and the condition may persist and recur for many weeks even after cessation of drug treatment. The lethality rate is about 10% and is mainly due to liver failure. A recurrence of symptoms, often in the third week, is typical. It is related to reactivation of herpes viruses, in particular human herpes virus 6, Epstein-Barr virus, or cytomegalovirus.

Japanese researchers have recently proposed diagnostic criteria for the diagnosis of this disease, which often remains unrecognized:[24]

1. Maculopapular rash developing more than 3 weeks after starting a limited number of drugs
2. Prolonged clinical symptoms after discontinuation of the causative drug
3. Fever (>38°C)
4. Liver abnormalities (alanine transanimase >100 U/L) or other organ involvement
5. Leukocyte abnormalities (at least one present):
   Leukocytosis (>11 x 10⁹/L)
   Atypical lymphocytosis (>5%)
   Eosinophilia (>1.5 x 10⁹/L)

6. Lymphadenopathy
7. Human herpes virus 6 reactivation (detected in the second to third week after the start of symptoms)

The diagnosis is confirmed by the presence of all seven criteria (typical drug induced hypersensitivity syndrome [DIHS]) or five[1–5] of them (atypical DIHS). The symptoms of DRESS/DIHS differ substantially depending on the drug (see the article by Kano and Shiohara elsewhere in this issue).

Interstitial nephritis Some drugs, in particular beta-lactam antibiotics, proton-pump inhibitors, sulfonamide antibiotics, disulfiram, non-steroidal anti-inflammatory drugs (NSAIDs), and others can cause an interstitial nephritis.[25] Some manifestations are associated with an exanthema, but, often, the symptoms start insidiously. Lower back pain and some malaise may be the only symptoms until renal insufficiency is discovered.

Cytopenia Drug-induced, IgG-mediated immune cytopenia may manifest as hemolytic anemia, an unexpected precipitous fall in peripheral leukocyte count. Drugs that are typically involved in such reactions are listed in **Table 5**.

Serum sickness syndrome Fever, arthralgias, macular and urticarial exanthemata, lymphadenopathy, and sometimes edema are the classical clinical manifestations of serum sickness. In the past, the widespread use of heterologous serum frequently produced the full serum sickness syndrome 1 to 3 weeks after antiserum administration. Currently, nonprotein drugs such as penicillins and cephalosporins are the most common causes of serum sickness, with a latency period of 6 to 8 hours. Drug-induced serum sickness is usually self-limited, with symptoms lasting 1 to 2 weeks before resolving.

Drug-induced lupus Typical clinical symptoms of drug-induced lupus erythematosus (DILE) are sudden onset of fever, malaise, myalgia, arthralgia, and arthritis several weeks after drug initiation. The skin is affected in about 25% of cases. Characteristic is an erythematous eruption, often on light-exposed surfaces. The average age of patients with DILE is nearly twice that of patients with idiopathic systemic lupus erythematosus (SLE). Approximately half the patients with drug-induced SLE are women compared with 90% of patients with idiopathic SLE. Similarly to idiopathic lupus, DILE can be divided into systemic, subacute cutaneous, and chronic cutaneous lupus. The clinical and laboratory manifestations of drug-induced SLE are similar to those of idiopathic SLE, but central nervous system and renal involvement are rare in DILE. Recognition of DILE is important because it usually reverts spontaneously within a few weeks after stopping the drug.[26]

Vasculitis Drugs may rarely elicit cutaneous or systemic vasculitis (incidence of 10 to 30 cases per 1 million people per year). Typical clinical manifestations are palpable purpuric papules predominantly of the legs; however, sometimes the condition manifests as a clinical syndrome indistinguishable from classical systemic forms of vasculitis such as Wegener's granulomatosis, polyarteritis nodosa, and Churg-Strauss syndrome. Withdrawal of the offending agent alone is often sufficient to induce prompt resolution of clinical manifestations, without the need for systemic therapy.[27]

Laboratory evaluations during the reaction
Laboratory tests during the acute phase may determine the severity and involvement of internal organs. The finding of an eosinophilia supports the diagnosis of an immune-mediated hypersensitivity reaction, and increased liver enzymes may indicate liver

involvement. For atypical skin lesions, a biopsy with histologic examination may help to recognize or exclude an important differential diagnosis.

In the rare cases with a presumed type II or III reaction, the IgG-mediated mechanism, the direct antiglobulin test (Coombs' test) helps diagnose immune hemolytic anemia, leading to further detailed analyses, often requiring the close collaboration of several disciplines.[28] Assessment of complement levels (C3, C4, CH50) and immune complexes (C1q binding or Raji cell assays) can support the diagnosis in cases with serum sickness syndrome, but negative values do not rule it out.

Allergologic Investigations

The clinical symptoms described previously are indicative of a drug reaction but do not in most instances provide sufficient evidence as to which drug has caused it. Allergologic tests with the suspected drugs may provide additional information and allow one to identify the causative agent.

Allergologic investigations in immediate-type hypersensitivity reactions

Skin tests are easy to perform and may provide some help in the identification of the causative drug. Most authors recommend performing these tests 1 to 6 months after the acute event, because effector cells may be exhausted and specific IgE antibodies may be temporarily depleted immediately after the reaction. Because the sensitivity of the tests might decrease over time, they should be performed in the first year after the reaction.[29]

In cases with severe or anaphylactic reactions, it is advisable to first perform skin tests with the presumably causative drugs only by prick. If responses are negative and the involved drug is available as a parenteral formulation, intradermal tests may than be carried out as described elsewhere;[29-31] however, negative skin tests do not have sufficient sensitivity to exclude an immune-mediated hypersensitivity in the case of a suggestive history.

In penicillin allergies, standardized preparations with penicilloylpolylysine and minor determinant mixture may be used. Although early American reports found a high sensitivity and specificity of skin tests using such standardized preparations, newer reports by Spanish researchers have detected a sensitivity of only 70%.[32] Currently, these preparations are not commercially available in the United States.

Penicillin allergy may also be evaluated by in vitro tests for specific IgEs; however, these tests have a low sensitivity. Additionally, assays for a few drugs such as suxamethonium, rocuronium, morphine, sulfamethoxazole, and chlorhexidine, are offered, some with potentially higher sensitivity.

A further in vitro test to identify the relevant drug may be the basophil activation test. This test is based on flow cytometric quantification of drug-induced CD63 expression or CD203c up-regulation or measurement of sulfo-leukotriene release by ELISA. The sensitivity in IgE-mediated reactions appears to be superior to CAP-based IgE determinations[33] and comparable with skin tests (see the article by Hausmann and colleagues elsewhere in this issue).

In pseudoallergic reactions, skin tests and determination of specific antibodies for identification of the causative drug are negative, because, by definition, such reactions are not based on specific immune reactions to the drug. A role of basophil activation testing in the diagnosis of pseudoallergic reactions could not be established, although some authors postulate some reactivity in NSAID-induced reactions.[34]

In selected cases with presumed pseudoallergic reactions, a diagnostic oral provocation test may be performed. More frequently, tests are carried out with alternative drugs to establish a safe substitution.

Allergologic investigations in nonimmediate-type hypersensitivity reactions
Skin tests (intradermal testing with readings at 24 hours and 48 hours and patch testing) with the suspected drugs may help to identify the causative agent; however, positive and negative predictive values of these tests are not known for most drugs. Skin tests are best performed after the complete clearing of clinical manifestations 1 to 6 months after the acute event. Patch tests are performed with the commercialized form of the involved drug diluted in petrolatum or water and intradermal tests with sterile sequential dilutions. The methods are described in more detail in guidelines for performing skins tests with drugs, which have been proposed by the Working Party of the European Society of Contact Dermatitis.[35]

The lymphocyte transformation test is an in vitro test. It is complex and requires skilled personnel; therefore, its availability is limited to specialized centers. Usually it is performed 1 to 6 months after the acute event; however, data from Japan suggest that in bullous skin diseases tests are more frequently positive in the first weeks of disease.[36]

Provocation tests in nonimmediate-type hypersensitivity reactions are not well standardized; neither the dose nor the time of treatment is established. No data on sensitivity or specificity are available. These tests cannot be recommended as a routine procedure for the identification of the culprit drug.

TREATMENT OF DRUG ALLERGY
Immediate-type Hypersensitivity Reactions

The causative or presumably causative drugs should immediately be withdrawn. In mild reactions with urticaria only, antihistamines are the primary recommended treatment; however, antihistamines cannot antagonize activated histamine that has already been released from mast cells.[37] In severe reactions with danger signals (see **Table 3**), angioedema, respiratory symptoms, or circulatory signs corresponding to an anaphylaxis, epinephrine (10 μg/kg) should be administered promptly via the intramuscular route in the anterolateral thigh. Glucocorticoids when given in pharmacologic quantities have an anti-inflammatory effect and may reduce the risk of late relapse;[38] however, the onset of action of glucocorticoids is late (>45 minutes) because it depends on new gene products.

Nonimmediate-type Hypersensitivity Reactions

During systemic T cell–mediated drug allergies, patients are more susceptible to react unspecifically to different xenobiotics. Withdrawal of the causative, potentially causative, or not urgently needed drug is prudent; however, there are some exceptions to this rule. In late occurring maculopapular exanthema in the absence of cutaneous danger signals (immediate-type hypersensitivity reactions), urgently required treatment may be continued. Such "treating through" requires monitoring for systemic involvement (fever, eosinophilia, lymphadenopathy, hepatitis) or involvement of mucosal surfaces.

Mild nonimmediate drug reactions are self-limited diseases, and treatment is symptomatic. In clinical praxis, corticosteroids (topical, sometimes systemic), antihistamines, or both are used to block or reduce prolonged or late phase reactions; however, there are no randomized trials for their use.

The management of SJS/TEN should best be undertaken in intensive care units with experience in the treatment of burns and involves warming of the environment, correction of electrolyte disturbances, administration of a high caloric enteral intake, and prevention of sepsis. The efficacy of drug treatment used in some case reports is difficult to evaluate; cyclosporine, cyclophosphamide, pentoxifylline, and thalidomide have all been tried.[39] Some recent data support corticosteroid use.[40] Intravenous immunoglobulins are widely used but their effectiveness is still debated.[41] Specific nursing care and adequate topical management reduce associated morbidity and allow a more rapid re-epithelialization of skin lesions. After healing, follow-up is needed for ophthalmologic and mucous membrane sequelae. Sun blocks are recommended. Avoidance of the responsible drug and chemically related compounds is essential not only for the patient but also for first-degree relatives.[39]

For DRESS, corticoids are used. Occasionally, liver transplantation is necessary.

Recommendation of Alternative Drugs

If a patient requires continued treatment, cross-reactivity among drugs should be taken into consideration. In choosing alternative compounds, skin testing may be helpful; however, the sensitivity of these tests remains limited. In patients who especially require one specific drug, a graded challenge with the alternative drug may be performed.

Beta-lactams
IgE-mediated allergy When a patient with immediate penicillin allergy requires an alternative β-lactam drug, consideration can be given to prescribing a cephalosporin of the second or higher generation. A review of several studies of cephalosporin administration to patients with a history of penicillin allergy found cephalosporin reactions in 4.4% of patients with positive skin tests for penicillin.[42] The incidence of cross-hypersensitivity reactions between penicillins and carbapenems is about 10%;[43] therefore, carbapenems may be used in penicillin-allergic patients.

T cell–mediated allergy In vitro data indicate that cross-reactivity of T cells between penicillins and cephalosporins is rare.[44] This finding is in agreement with clinical experience; however, clinical data on this topic in the literature are scarce.

Sulfonamides
A common clinical problem is the putative cross-reactivity among sulfonamides. Recent data have demonstrated that both IgE-mediated and T cell–mediated cross-reactivity between sulfonamide antibiotics and nonantibiotics are unlikely.[45,46] In patients allergic to sulfonamide antibiotics, other sulfonamide-derived drugs (eg, diuretics, sulfonylureas, celecoxib, and sumatriptan) have not been excluded; however, cross-reactions do occur with the anti-inflammatory compound sulfasalazine, which is metabolized to sulfapyridine. There is no relationship between sulfonamide allergy and intolerance to sulfite preservatives in food.

Radiocontrast media
There are both immediate-type and nonimmediate-type hypersensitivity reactions to radiocontrast media. In the specific immune-mediated reactions, iodide ions do not seem to be the causative moiety. Cross-reactivities occur predominantly in nonimmediate T cell–mediated reactions. Detailed intradermal skin testing might help identify non–cross-reactive contrast media.[47]

Desensitization

Desensitization may be a treatment option for drug-allergic patients for whom no alternative drug exists. Starting at a suballergenic dose with gradual increase may allow the application of full therapeutic doses with minimal risk for anaphylaxis.[48] The desensitized state is not permanent and is sustained only with a daily maintenance dose of the drug. Classically, the procedure is applied in IgE-mediated reactions, but its use has been extended to other drug reactions.[49] Drugs for which desensitization may be successful include allopurinol, co-trimoxazole, β-lactam antibiotics, and cisplatin. Patients with intolerance to acetylsalicylic acid can also be desensitized, with occasional beneficial effect in asthma and polyposis symptoms.[50] The mechanism of drug desensitization is not well understood (see the article by Castells elsewhere in this issue).

REFERENCES

1. Gomes ER, Demoly P. Epidemiology of hypersensitivity drug reactions. Curr Opin Allergy Clin Immunol 2005;5:309–16.
2. Rawlins M, Thompson W. Mechanisms of adverse drug reactions. In: Davies D, editor. Textbook of adverse drug reactions. New York: Oxford Press; 1991. p. 18–45.
3. Greenberger PA. Drug allergy. J Allergy Clin Immunol 2006;117(Suppl 2 Mini-Primer):464–70.
4. Johansson SG, Bieber T, Dahl R, et al. Revised nomenclature for allergy for global use: report of the Nomenclature Review Committee of the World Allergy Organization 2003. J Allergy Clin Immunol 2004;113:832–6.
5. Chung WH, Hung SI, Chen YT. Human leukocyte antigens and drug hypersensitivity. Curr Opin Allergy Clin Immunol 2007;7(4):317–23.
6. Bircher AJ. Symptoms and danger signs in acute drug hypersensitivity. Toxicology 2005;209:201–7.
7. El-Shanawany T, Williams PE, Jolles S. Clinical immunology review series: an approach to the patient with anaphylaxis. Clin Exp Immunol 2008;153:1–9.
8. Mertes PM, Laxenaire MC. Allergic reactions occurring during anaesthesia. Eur J Anaesthesiol 2002;19:240–62.
9. Ellis AK, Day JH. Diagnosis and management of anaphylaxis. Can Med Assoc J 2003;169:307–11.
10. Weiss ME, Adkinson NF. Immediate hypersensitivity reactions to beta-lactam antibiotics. Ann Intern Med 1987;107:204–15.
11. Chung CH, Mirakhur B, Chan E, et al. Cetuximab-induced anaphylaxis and IgE specific for galactose-alpha-1,3-galactose. N Engl J Med 2008;358(11):1109–17.
12. Harboe T, Johansson SG, Florvaag E, et al. Pholcodine exposure raises serum IgE in patients with previous anaphylaxis to neuromuscular blocking agents. Allergy 2007;62(12):1445–50.
13. Kvedariene V, Martins P, Rouanet L, et al. Diagnosis of iodinated contrast media hypersensitivity: results of a 6-year period. Clin Exp Allergy 2006;36(8):1072–7.
14. Ebo DG, Fisher MM, Hagendorens MM, et al. Anaphylaxis during anaesthesia: diagnostic approach. Allergy 2007;62:471–87.
15. Fiszenson-Albala F, Auzerie V, Mahe E, et al. 6-Month prospective survey of cutaneous drug reactions in a hospital setting. Br J Dermatol 2003;149(5):1018–22.
16. Lee AY. Fixed drug eruptions: incidence, recognition, and avoidance. Am J Clin Dermatol 2000;1(5):277–85.
17. Hausermann P, Harr T, Bircher AJ. Baboon syndrome resulting from systemic drugs: is there strife between SDRIFE and allergic contact dermatitis syndrome? Contact Dermatitis 2004;51:297–310.
18. Britschgi M, Steiner UC, Schmid S, et al. T-cell involvement in drug-induced acute generalized exanthematous pustulosis. J Clin Invest 2001;107:1433–41.

19. Roujeau J, Bioulac-Sage P, Bourseau C. Acute generalized exanthematous pustulosis: analysis of 63 cases. Arch Dermatol 1991;127:1333–8.
20. Roujeau JC, Stern RS. Severe adverse cutaneous reactions to drugs. N Engl J Med 1994;331:1272–85.
21. French LE. Toxic epidermal necrolysis and Stevens-Johnson syndrome: our current understanding. Allergol Int 2006;55:9–16.
22. Knowles SR, Shapiro LE, Shear NH. Anticonvulsant hypersensitivity syndrome: incidence, prevention and management. Drug Saf 1999;21:489–501.
23. Peyrière H, Dereure O, Breton H, et al. Network of the French Pharmacovigilance Centers. Variability in the clinical pattern of cutaneous side effects of drugs with systemic symptoms: does a DRESS syndrome really exist? Br J Dermatol 2006; 155(2):422–8.
24. Shiohara T, Inaoka M, Kano Y. Drug induced hypersensitivity syndrome (DIHS): a reaction induced by a complex interplay among herpesvirus and antiviral and antidrug immune responses. Allergol Int 2006;55:1–8.
25. Spanou Z, Keller M, Britschgi M, et al. Involvement of drug-specific T cells in acute drug-induced interstitial nephritis. J Am Soc Nephrol 2006;17(10):2919–27.
26. Sarzi-Puttini P, Atzeni F, Capsoni F, et al. Drug-induced lupus erythematosus. Autoimmunity 2005;38(7):507–18.
27. Doyle MK, Cuellar ML. Drug-induced vasculitis. Expert Opin Drug Saf 2003;2: 401–9.
28. Pruss A, Salama A, Ahrens N, et al. Immune hemolysis: serological and clinical aspects. Clin Exp Med 2003;3(2):55–64.
29. Brockow K, Romano A. Skin tests in the diagnosis of drug hypersensitivity reactions. Curr Pharm Des 2008;14(27):2778–91.
30. Torres J, Blanca M, Fernandez J, et al. Diagnosis of immediate allergic reactions to beta-lactam antibiotics. Allergy 2003;58(10):961–72.
31. Romano A, Blanca M, Torres MJ, et al. Diagnosis of nonimmediate reactions to β-lactam antibiotics. Allergy 2004;59(11):1153–60.
32. Torres MJ, Romano A, Mayorga C, et al. Diagnostic evaluation of a large group of patients with immediate allergy to penicillins: the role of skin testing. Allergy 2001; 56(9):850–6.
33. Sanz ML, Gamboa PM, Garcia-Aviles C, et al. Drug hypersensitivities: which room for biological tests? Eur Ann Allergy Clin Immunol 2005;37:230–5.
34. Nizankowska-Mogilnicka E, Bochenek G, Mastalerz L, et al. EAACI/GA2LEN guideline: aspirin provocation tests for diagnosis of aspirin hypersensitivity. Allergy 2007;62(10):1111–8.
35. Barbaud A, Concalo M, Bruynzeel D, et al. Guidelines for performing skin tests with drugs in the investigation of cutaneous adverse drug reactions. Contact Dermatitis 2001;45(6):321–8.
36. Kano Y, Hirahara K, Mitsuyama Y, et al. Utility of the lymphocyte transformation test in the diagnosis of drug sensitivity: dependence on its timing and the type of drug eruption. Allergy 2007;62:1439–44.
37. Evans C, Tippins E. Emergency treatment of anaphylaxis. Accid Emerg Nurs 2005;13(4):232–7.
38. Ewan PW. Anaphylaxis. Br Med J 1998;316:1442–5.
39. Ghislain PD, Roujeau JC. Treatment of severe drug reactions: Stevens-Johnson syndrome, toxic epidermal necrolysis and hypersensitivity syndrome. Dermatol Online J 2002;8:5.
40. Karaun SH, Jonkman MF. Dexamethasone pulse therapy for Stevens-Johnson syndrome/toxic epidermal necrolysis. Acta Derm Venereol 2007;87(2):144–8.

41. Mittmann N, Chan BC, Knowles S, et al. IVIG for the treatment of toxic epidermal necrolysis. Skin Therapy Lett 2007;12(1):7–9.
42. Kelkar PS, Li JT. Cephalosporin allergy. N Engl J Med 2001;345:804–9.
43. Sodhi M, Axtell SS, Callahan J, et al. Is it safe to use carbapenems in patients of allergy to penicillin? J Antimicrob Chemother 2004;54:1155–7.
44. Mauri-Hellweg D, Zann M, Frei E, et al. Cross-reactivity of T cell lines and clones to beta-lactam antibiotics. J Immunol 1996;157:1071–9.
45. Brackett CC. Likelihood and mechanisms of cross-allergenicity between sulfonamide antibiotics and other drugs containing a sulfonamide functional group. Pharmacotherapy 2004;24(7):856–70.
46. Strom BL, Schinnar R, Apter AJ, et al. Absence of cross-reactivity between sulfonamide antibiotics and sulfonamide nonantibiotics. N Engl J Med 2003; 349:1628–35.
47. Lerch M, Keller M, Britschgi M, et al. Cross-reactivity patterns of T cells specific for iodinated contrast media. J Allergy Clin Immunol 2007;119(6):1529–36.
48. Castells M. Desensitization for drug allergy. Curr Opin Allergy Clin Immunol 2006; 6:476–81.
49. Solensky R. Drug desensitization. Immunol Allergy Clin North Am 2004;24: 425–43.
50. Stevenson DD. Aspirin and NSAID sensitivity. Immunol Allergy Clin North Am 2004;24(3):491–505.

The Pholcodine Story

E. Florvaag, MD[a,b,c,*], S.G.O. Johansson, MD[d,e]

KEYWORDS

- Anaphylaxis • IgE antibodies • Neuromuscular blocking agents
- Pholcodine • Suxamethonium

Adverse reactions during general anesthesia in the form of anaphylaxis have been reported with increasing frequency during the past decades.[1] Although still rare in absolute numbers, they constitute a mounting threat to patient safety and a challenge to the diagnostic and therapeutic skills of anesthetists. Even when appropriately treated, mortality rates between 3.5% and 10% are reported.[2–4] Neuromuscular blocking agents (NMBAs) represent the most frequent cause, with suxamethonium (SUX) as the prominent culprit drug.

In most cases, the reactions appear IgE-mediated. Studies back in the 1980s identified the quaternary ammonium ion (QAI) as the most likely allergenic epitope for the specific binding of IgE to the NMBA.[5] Since up to half of the patients with NMBA-related anaphylactic reactions have not previously been exposed to anesthetic drugs,[1] IgE sensitization must have been initiated by some of the many other drugs such as morphine (MOR) derivatives or environmental chemicals known to contain the QAI epitope.

To screen for individuals IgE-sensitized to the QAI epitope, MOR has been suggested.[6] MOR has an unusual alkaloid structure with only one QAI epitope, which actually is a tertiary amine (**Fig. 1**). Therefore, it cannot by itself trigger mast cells or basophiles sensitized with IgE antibodies to QAI, but has been suggested for the detection of an IgE-sensitization to NMBA.

ANAPHYLAXIS TO NEUROMUSCULAR BLOCKING AGENTS IN NORWAY

During the 1990s, growing concern over the apparently increasing challenge of anaphylactic reactions during general anesthesia was voiced from anesthesiologists

---

[a] Laboratory of Clinical Biochemistry, Haukeland University Hospital, N-5021 Bergen, Norway
[b] Section for Clinical Allergology, Department of Occupational Medicine, Haukeland University Hospital, N-5021 Bergen, Norway
[c] Institute of Internal Medicine, University of Bergen, N-5021 Bergen, Norway
[d] Department of Medicine, Clinical Immunology and Allergy Unit, Karolinska Institute, S-171 76 Stockholm, Sweden
[e] Department of Clinical Immunology and Transfusion Medicine, Karolinska University Hospital, Solna, L2:04, S-171 76 Stockholm, Sweden
* Corresponding author. Laboratory of Clinical Biochemistry, Haukeland University Hospital, N-5021 Bergen, Norway.
E-mail address: erik.florvaag@helse-bergen.no (E. Florvaag).

Immunol Allergy Clin N Am 29 (2009) 419–427
doi:10.1016/j.iac.2009.04.002
0889-8561/09/$ – see front matter © 2009 Published by Elsevier Inc.
immunology.theclinics.com

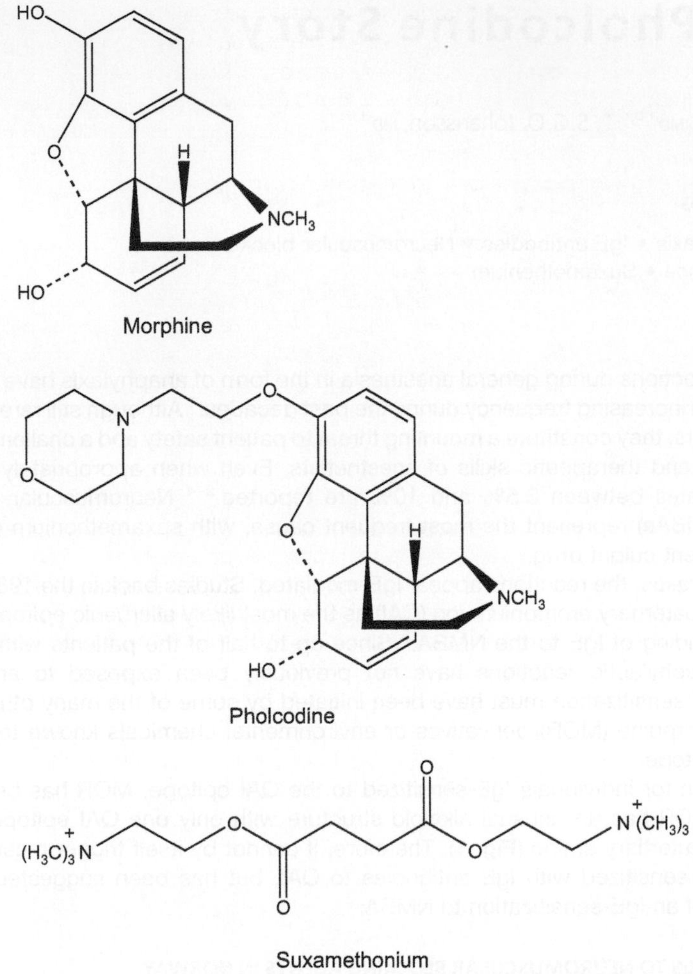

Morphine

Pholcodine

Suxamethonium

Fig. 1. The structures of MOR, PHO, and SUX. (*From* Florvaag E, Johansson SGO, Öman H, et al. Prevalence of IgE antibodies to morphine. Relation to the high and low incidence of NMBA anaphylaxis in Norway and Sweden, respectively. Acta Anaesthesiol Scand 2005;49:442; with permission.)

and the Norwegian Medicines Agency.[7] Some key issues were the uncertainties in estimating prevalences and calculating the anaphylactic risk of individual NMBAs relative to their market shares. Several of the controversies were related to the statistical challenge posed by the rarity of reactions and the drawbacks of the spontaneous reporting systems on which the official strategies were based. In addition, criticism was pointed at the validity of the diagnostic methods applied in follow-up examinations. In a cooperation between anesthesiologists and allergy-competent specialists (allergology is not a medical specialty in Norway), the Norwegian Network for Anaphylactic Reactions during Anaesthesia (NARA) was started in 1998. It established and better standardized national routines for immediate and follow-up diagnostic investigations.

Based on a standardized follow-up protocol and 83 cases of anaphylaxis during anesthesia referred to the Section for Clinical Allergology, Department of Occupational Medicine, Bergen, Norway during a 6-year period, the first Norwegian clinical report was published.[8] An in-hospital frequency of one anaphylactic reaction per 5,200 general anesthesias, where NMBAs were administered, was found. Further, 71.1% of the reactions were classified as IgE-mediated, of which 93.2% were related to NMBAs, primarily SUX and rocuronium. Only 3.6% were caused by latex and the few remaining cases by other exposures. It could also be very carefully estimated from the in-hospital data that if, at the time of a SUX-induced anesthesia, a patient was IgE-sensitized to SUX, the risk of anaphylaxis would be around 1:20.[9]

THE COMPARATIVE RESEARCH MODEL FOR THE DIFFERENCES BETWEEN NORWAY AND SWEDEN

The prevalence data for Norway based partly on official spontaneous reports and partly on the 6-year single center study showed that anaphylactic reactions to NMBAs were on the order of 10 times higher in Norway than in Sweden. Such differences between these nations could have a number of reasons. One clearly had to consider the biases inherent in spontaneous reporting systems, different anesthetic practices, and the fact that in Norway a specialized diagnostic service was established through NARA. Finally, one had to consider the possibility that the two populations were differently exposed to an unknown environmental factor that gave rise to production of IgE-antibodies with specificities relevant for the QAI-epitope.

To our surprise, while establishing a radioimmunoassay for morphine at our laboratory we observed that in a control group of allergic subjects with serum IgE-levels of 1,000 kU/L or more about 30% had IgE-antibodies to MOR. The bindings were completely inhibited by MOR, indicating that they were immunologic and epitope specific and not caused by any unspecific mechanism. The data (unpublished) naturally gave rise to the somewhat intriguing question of why so many allergic Norwegians were IgE-sensitized to MOR. At that time, the best answer we could come up with was that it probably had to do with exposure to an unknown environmental factor.

Against this background, we decided to use the socially and geographically closely related countries Norway and Sweden as a research model. The authors considered that the genetics would be similar and knew that the anesthetic practices were largely identical. Studies were primarily set up to look for any significant differences in exposure to QAI-containing substances between the two countries and, if such a difference was identified, whether it would give rise to differences in IgE-sensitization.

ENVIRONMENTAL EXPOSURE STUDIES

To look for the proposed unknown exposure factor, 84 household and other environmental chemicals (skin care ointments, hair care products, cough syrups, lozenges, toothpastes, cleansers, and motor oils) were collected from the homes of both MOR- and SUX-sensitized and nonsensitized individuals in Bergen and Stockholm. Several of these chemical products inhibited IgE binding to SUX and MOR, thus confirming a sensitizing potential. However, Swedes and Norwegians seemed to be equally exposed to the same household chemicals and no definite differences in exposures was found.

Examining the other main group of exposures to the QAI structure, namely drugs, the populations in the two countries, although to different degrees, were exposed to the same compounds. However, there was one decisive exception: the use in Norway, but not in Sweden, of a cough mixture that, in contrast to all other drugs, contained pholcodine (PHO).

To explore this intriguing discrepancy in exposure, the authors decided to perform a comparative study with the aim of documenting the prevalence of IgE-sensitization to PHO in comparative populations in Norway and Sweden. Sera from allergic patients with known or suspected IgE-mediated airway or skin allergy, and healthy controls (blood donors), were tested for IgE antibodies to PHO, MOR, and SUX using Immuno-CAP (Phadia AB, Uppsala, Sweden), and compared to sera from patients with a documented IgE-mediated, NMBA-initiated anaphylactic reaction.

Serum samples were obtained from the allergy diagnostic laboratories at Haukeland University Hospital, Bergen, Norway, and Karolinska University Hospital, Stockholm, Sweden. Three hundred samples from each laboratory were collected consecutively during the period from March to April 2002, from volumes left after analyses for IgE antibodies requested by referring physicians. In addition, serum samples from 500 and 1000 blood donors in Bergen and Stockholm, respectively, were included. For comparison, serum samples from 65 Norwegian patients with a documented IgE-mediated, NMBA-induced anaphylactic reaction during anesthesia were analyzed.

The results showed that in Norway 0.4% of blood donors, 3.7% of allergic patients, and 38.5% of patients with anaphylactic reaction to NMBAs were sensitized to SUX; as were 5%, 10%, and 66.7%, respectively, to MOR.[10] Among blood donors and allergic patients from Stockholm, none with IgE antibodies to SUX or MOR was found. IgE antibodies to PHO, were found in 6% of blood donors from Bergen, but in none from Stockholm.

Thus, since more than 10 times as many blood donors and 3 times as many allergic patients had IgE antibodies to MOR than to SUX, the former is not ideal for screening of sera for IgE-sensitization to QAI in a country like Norway.

THE PHOLCODINE HYPOTHESIS

Pholcodine (3-(2-morpholinoethyl)morphine) was originally synthesized in France in the 1950s. In principle, it is a morphine molecule with a morpholino side chain (see **Fig. 1**). This modification changes its pharmacological effects in that it does not cause depression of respiration, pain relief, and central nervous system (CNS) excitation, and thus is void of euphorizing properties and risk of addiction. PHO is a cough suppressant acting directly on the cough center of the CNS, and has become a widely used cough medicine in numerous formulations. After single doses, it is rapidly absorbed from the gastrointestinal tract ($t_{max} = 1.6 \pm 1.2$ h), but eliminated much more slowly than other opiates with a mean half-life of 50.1 ± 4.1 h. It freely crosses the blood-brain barrier. The concentration in saliva becomes 3.6 times higher than in plasma.[11]

There are several producers of PHO and the international sales are monitored by the United Nations International Narcotics Control Board (www.incb.org). Purchases of PHO vary considerably between countries. Australia, United Kingdom, France, and Norway are among the highest consumers, whereas Denmark, Sweden, Germany, and the United States are examples of nonconsuming nations.

As an allergen, the authors' studies have shown PHO to contain one QAI epitope in addition to being monovalent for another allergenic epitope it shares with MOR.[10] NMBAs, like SUX, are structurally bivalent for the QAI epitope (see **Fig. 1**).

In Norway, PHO has been available in the cough mixture Tuxi from one producer (Weifa AS, Oslo, Norway). It has been on the market since 1966 in varying formulations and was largely purchased over the counter, but has not been available in Sweden. Estimates based on sales data indicate that approximately 40% of the Norwegian population has been exposed.

These findings provided the basis for the authors' "pholcodine hypothesis," suggesting that a high consumption of PHO-containing cough mixtures could be related to a high prevalence of IgE-sensitization to PHO, MOR, and, in part, to SUX (ie, QAI);

and, as a consequence, higher frequencies of IgE-mediated, NMBA-induced anaphylaxis.

THE EFFECT OF PHOLCODINE EXPOSURE ON IGE PRODUCTION

A pilot study aimed at exploring the effect on IgE production, in IgE-sensitized and nonsensitized individuals, of exposure to cough syrup and environmental chemicals containing PHO-, MOR-, and SUX-related allergen structures was performed. The Tuxi cough mixture was chosen since it contains PHO and was consumed in great quantities in Norway.

Two participants, found to have IgE antibodies to PHO, MOR, and SUX considered related to the previous use of PHO-containing cough mixtures, were recruited from the Section for Clinical Allergology, Department of Occupational Medicine at Haukeland University Hospital in Bergen, Norway. Two other, scientists, one atopic and one non-atopic, who had not used PHO-containing cough syrups and did not have IgE anti-bodies to PHO, served as controls.

The first week, the subjects took a PHO-free drug (noscapine and codeine, respec-tively). After a two-week interval, a PHO-containing drug (Tuxi cough mixture) was taken, at a dose corresponding to 20 mg of PHO, once daily for 7 consecutive days. Serum was collected before the start and 2 weeks after the end of each expo-sure period. In addition, IgE levels of the two sensitized individuals were followed for a few months.

None of the subjects developed any clinical symptoms or changes in serum levels of IgE or IgE antibodies to the monitored substances during the first control week. However, after 7 days with the PHO-containing cough syrup, the sensitized individuals experienced some clinical symptoms (pruritus and mild localized urticaria), and large increases in the concentration of IgE (60- to 105-fold) (**Fig. 2**) and IgE antibodies to

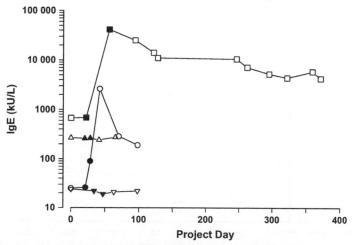

Fig. 2. Serum levels of IgE (kU/L) of person EF (*open square*), HE (*open circle*), HÖ (*open triangle*), and TH (*open diamond*) before and after oral intake (between *filled symbols*) of cough syrup containing PHO. (*From* Florvaag E, Johansson SGO, Öman H, et al. Pholco-dine stimulates a dramatic increase of IgE in IgE-sensitized individuals. A pilot study. Allergy 2006;61:51; with permission.)

PHO, MOR, and SUX (30- to 80-fold). In contrast, the IgE concentrations of the two nonsensitized controls did not change during noscapine, codeine, or PHO exposure.

Three individuals IgE-sensitized to PHO were exposed to household chemicals selected for containing or lacking PHO, MOR, and SUX allergenic epitopes. They had the questionable pleasure of exposing themselves to PHO-allergens by eating four daily doses of licorice candy totaling 256 g for a week; eating 6 times daily salmiak lozenges, totaling 42 lozenges for another week; and, during the same week, washing their hair three times with L'Oreal Professional Vitamino Color shampoo. As a reference, for a week they enjoyed four daily tablets of Dekadin menthol, which does not contain PHO-allergens. In both cases no increase or significant drop in the concentrations of IgE and IgE antibodies to PHO, MOR, or SUX was seen (**Fig. 3**). However, compared to other persons who were IgE-sensitized to PHO but had not been this extremely exposed, their IgE levels remained remarkably stable. Thus, it seems as if household chemicals sharing PHO-allergens, including the QAI-epitope, but lacking the unique PHO structure, cannot initiate an IgE-sensitization but can, to some minor degree, stimulate and maintain such an IgE-antibody production.

The results indicated, however, that if an individual IgE-sensitized to PHO is exposed to even small amounts of cough syrups containing PHO, the IgE system is very strongly stimulated.[12] Thus it appeared possible that such cough syrups, by sensitizing and boosting, could put people at risk for developing an allergic anaphylaxis to NMBA.

PHOLCODINE EXPOSURE OF INDIVIDUALS WITH PREVIOUS IGE-MEDIATED NEUROMUSCULAR BLOCKING AGENT ANAPHYLAXIS

A controlled, randomized clinical trial on a population with previously diagnosed IgE-mediated anaphylaxis towards NMBAs was then initiated. The primary aim was to study whether PHO exposure caused changes in serum levels of IgE and IgE antibodies to PHO, MOR, and SUX in a larger number of individuals, thereby corroborating the results from the pilot study.

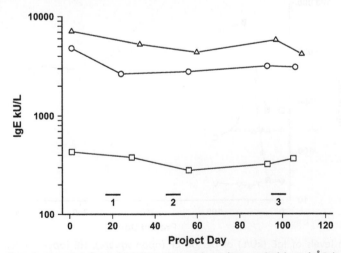

Fig. 3. IgE values in samples from EF (*open triangle*), LF (*open circle*) and ÅS (*open square*) taken before and after the three 1-week household chemical exposure sessions (1, 2, and 3). (*From* Florvaag E, Johansson SGO, Öman H, et al. Pholcodine stimulates a dramatic increase of IgE in IgE-sensitized individuals. A pilot study. Allergy 2006;61:52; with permission.)

Seventeen patients from a previous clinical study on anaphylaxis during general anaesthesia[8] were recruited at the Haukeland University Hospital in Bergen, Norway. The patients were randomized to ingest one single daily dose, about one-third of that recommended, of the cough syrup Tuxi or guaifenesin (Solvipect, Nycomed Pharma, Asker, Norway). IgE and IgE antibodies to SUX, MOR, PHO, and inhalant and food allergen mixes, were quantified before and 4 and 8 weeks after start of exposure.

There were no significant differences in the concentrations of IgE or IgE antibodies to PHO, MOR, or SUX between the study groups before cough syrup exposure. At 4 weeks after start of exposures, there was a large increase in IgE concentrations in the pholcodine group. No changes were seen in the guaifenesin group. The highest increase occurred with antibodies to SUX, MOR, and PHO; whereas the rise in IgE levels was intermediate. IgE antibodies to inhalant and food allergens also showed some, but only slight elevation.

This study demonstrated that individuals who have suffered anaphylaxis during general anesthesia and are IgE-sensitized to an NMBA respond with a remarkable and statistically highly significant increase in IgE production when exposed to small doses of cough syrup containing pholcodine.[9]

PHOLCODINE-CONTAINING COUGH MIXTURE WITHDRAWN FROM THE MARKET

Based on the result of the authors' studies, the Norwegian producer decided not to renew the marketing license for the PHO-containing cough syrup Tuxi, which was taken off the market in March 2007. This decision was strongly supported by the Norwegian Medicines Agency. The immunologic and clinical consequences of taking PHO off the market are now being studied, although reaching a statistically significant decrease of the low number of NMBA-related anaphylaxis will probably take some time.

However, there are already some indications of what happens when PHO exposure is reduced. Today, after one year without Tuxi, the percentage of sera sent to Haukeland University Hospital allergy laboratory found to have IgE antibodies (>0.35 kU_A/L) to PHO, MOR, and SUX are about half as many as when Tuxi was on the market (E. Florvaag, personal communication, 2008).

It was recently brought to the authors' attention that, during the 1970s and 1980s, a PHO-containing cough syrup, Tussokon, (Pharmacia AB, Uppsala, Sweden) was available in Sweden. It was phased out of the market from 1987 to 1989 because of "changes in recommendations for treatment of cough and because other, more efficient pharmacological preparations had become available" according to the producer. Nothing is mentioned about any possible relation to anaphylaxis during anesthesia. We have managed to find some allergic patients' sera from these years in our freezers. As many as 5% to 6% of the Swedish sera from the 1970s and 1980s have IgE antibodies to PHO.[13] However, from the 1990s, just 2% positive sera were found; and among 300 sera from 2002[10] and approximately 200 sera from 2005 (Johansson, S.G.O., unpublished data) no PHO-positive sample was found.

INTERNATIONAL STUDY IN PROGRESS

The Norwegian findings prompted continued studies in other countries. Reports of NMBA-induced anaphylaxis are more prevalent in countries like Australia, France, and United Kingdom, which, like Norway, represent high consumers of PHO; than reports from low- or nonconsuming countries like Germany, United States, and Finland. Accordingly, an international study on the connection between PHO consumption and IgE-sensitization in nine countries is presently undertaken and preliminary data seem to support the PHO hypothesis (Johansson, S.G.O., unpublished data).

NEW OPPORTUNITIES TO PREVENT ANAPHYLAXIS

The accumulating data on the connection between PHO consumption, IgE-sensitization to PHO and SUX, and the prevalence of IgE-mediated anaphylaxis to NMBAs present new opportunities for preventing these dreaded adverse events. Strategies would primarily need to include, as in Norway, the removal of PHO-containing drugs from the many national markets where they are still available. However, according to the broad spectrum of chemicals in the environment causing exposure to the QAI-structure, through the use of drugs, household, or occupational products, it is to be expected that other substances may exist that have similar IgE-stimulating properties. If so, these also need be identified and similarly removed.

OTHER CLINICAL CONSEQUENCES OF IGE-SENSITIZATION TO PHO

From recent years of clinical practice at the Center for Clinical Allergology in Bergen, Norway, the authors have been confronted with two types of diagnostic challenges now looked upon as typical consequences of PHO-sensitization. The first is referrals for high serum levels of "total IgE" from about 1,000 kU/L and above. These IgE levels, which could not be explained by severe clinical allergy or other causes (eg, active atopic eczema, parasitic infestations), are associated with a high frequency of IgE antibodies to PHO.

Likewise are referrals of patients without any significant clinical symptoms, but where the GP has requested and found a number of low-level serum IgE-antibodies to airway and food allergens. Serological exploration of such cases often end up with finding considerable elevated "total IgE" and IgE-antibodies to PHO. Based on the PHO hypothesis the correct approach in these two situations is to clarify whether PHO-containing medicines have been used, to stop further exposure, and to follow up with serological normalization. A third challenge in PHO-sensitized individuals is related to the treatment options in severe allergic asthma. The decision whether anti-IgE treatment is indicated, and the calculation of the correct dose is partly based upon the measured levels of serum IgE. The effect of PHO on this variable may therefore influence decision outcomes in such cases.

SUMMARY

Considerable support for the PHO hypothesis has been established and several studies with new and complementary data are under way. The hypothesis carries promising prospects for the prevention of IgE-mediated anaphylaxis to NMBAs.

PHO works in rare and subtle ways, and the mechanism of effect on IgE-synthesis is not known. As a MOR-analogous antitussive, and structurally a monovalent hapten with two independent allergenic epitopes, it only very rarely gives rise to severe IgE-mediated allergic reactions towards itself. However, it does so considerably more often to quite a different group of drugs—the NMBAs, which are bivalent to the QAI-containing epitope and, thus, structurally complete allergens. The use as a cough depressant and cold medicine, which to a considerable degree is sold over the counter, allows its distribution and potential sensitization to become widespread in populations.

Alarmingly, IgE-sensitization and extremely high levels of IgE-antibodies can virtually go clinically unnoticed until the unfortunate individual suddenly needs an, often immediate, surgical intervention. The rapid induction of general anesthesia under such circumstances, to avoid aspiration of gastric contents during intubation, is often done by the use of a quick acting NMBA such as SUX. By intravenous injection, the allergenic drug rapidly gains a general distribution in the unknowingly sensitized victim. This is an extremely unfortunate situation and one that, within minutes, may dramatically challenge the qualifications of the responsible anesthetist and threaten patient safety.

Following such adverse events considerable uncertainty may exist as how to safely administer a successive general anesthesia to the patient if needed at a later time in life. Good advice can only be obtained after thorough examinations. First, analysis of serum drawn in close relationship to the reaction documented by an increased serum tryptase should be followed by a standardized, allergological follow-up investigation. It is important to examine carefully all the drugs used during induction and maintaining of anesthesia, as well as other drugs administered and additional exposures that may take place in the operating theater.

REFERENCES

1. Mertes P-M, Laxenaire MC. Adverse reactions to neuromuscular blocking agents. Curr Allergy Asthma Rep 2004;4:7–17.
2. Currie M, Webb RK, Williamson JA, et al. The Australian Incident Monitoring Study. Clinical anaphylaxis: an analysis of 2000 incident reports. Anaesth Intensive Care 1993;21:621–5.
3. Mitsuhata H, Matsumoto S, Hasegawa J. The epidemiology and clinical features of anaphylactic and anaphylactoid reactions in the perioperative period in Japan. Masui 1992;41:1664–9.
4. Axon AD, Hunter JM. Editorial III: anaphylaxis and anaesthesia— all clear now? Br J Anaesth 2004;93:501–4.
5. Baldo BA, Fisher MM. Substituted ammonium ions as allergenic determinants in drug allergy. Nature 1983;306:262–4.
6. Fisher MM, Baldo BA. Immunoassays for the diagnosis of anaphylaxis to neuromuscular blocking drugs: the value of morphine for the detection of IgE antibodies in allergic subjects. Anaesth Intensive Care 2000;28:167–70.
7. Laake JH, Røttingen J-A. Rocoronium and anaphylaxis—a statistical challenge. Acta Anaesthesiol Scand 2001;45:1196–203.
8. Harboe T, Guttormsen AB, Irgens Å, et al. Anaphylaxis during anaesthesia in Norway. A six-year single centre study. Anesthesiology 2005;102:897–903.
9. Harboe T, Johansson SGO, Florvaag E, et al. Pholcodine exposure raises serum IgE in patients with previous anaphylaxis to neuromuscular blocking agents. Allergy 2007;62:1445–50.
10. Florvaag E, Johansson SGO, Öman H, et al. Prevalence of IgE antibodies to morphine. Relation to the high and low incidence of NMBA anaphylaxis in Norway and Sweden, respectively. Acta Anaesthesiol Scand 2005;49:437–44.
11. Chen ZR, Bochner F, Somogyi A. Pharmacokinetics of pholcodine in healthy volunteers: single and chronic dosing studies. Br J clin Pharmacol 1988;26:445–53.
12. Florvaag E, Johansson SGO, Öman H, et al. Pholcodine stimulates a dramatic increase of IgE in IgE-sensitized individuals. A pilot study. Allergy 2006;61:49–55.
13. Johansson SGO, Öman H, Nopp A, et al. Pholcodine caused anaphylaxis in Sweden 30-years ago. Allergy 2009;64:820–1.

Perioperative Anaphylaxis

P.M. Mertes, MD, PhD[a,b],*, M. Lambert, MD[a,b],
R.M. Guéant-Rodriguez, MD, PhD[c,d], I. Aimone-Gastin, MD, PhD[c,d],
C. Mouton-Faivre, MD[a], D.A. Moneret-Vautrin, MD, PhD[e],
J.L. Guéant, MD, PhD[c,d], J.M. Malinovsky, MD, PhD[f], P. Demoly, MD, PhD[g]

KEYWORDS

- Anesthesia • Allergy • Anaphylaxis • IgE • Skin test
- Neuromuscular blocking agent

Anesthesia is commonly regarded as a high-risk activity. Many experts acknowledge that "very impressive" safety improvements have been made in this field, leading some investigators to conclude that anesthesia-related mortality has decreased in the previous 2 decades.[1] Nevertheless, anaphylaxis remains a major cause of concern for anesthetists who routinely give many potentially causative agents and who are the medical practitioners most likely to see severe anaphylactic reactions.

Virtually every drug used in anesthesia has been reported to cause a reaction, and no premedication has proven to be able to prevent anaphylactic reactions.[2] On the other hand, the incidence of anesthetic anaphylaxis can be reduced by preventing second reactions in patients with a history of anaphylaxis. Most patients who have experienced anaphylaxis should be evaluated by a specialist in allergy-immunology.

[a] Service d'Anesthésie-Réanimation Chirurgicale, CHU de Nancy, Hôpital Central, 29 Avenue de Lattre de Tassigny, 54035 Nancy Cedex, France
[b] Unité Inserm U684, Faculté de Médecine, 9 Avenue de la Forêt de Haye, 54505 Vandoeuvre les Nancy, France
[c] Laboratoire de Biochimie Biologie Moléculaire Nutrition Métabolisme, CHU de Brabois, Avenue du Morvan, 54511 Vandoeuvre les Nancy, France
[d] Unité de Pathologie Cellulaire et Moléculaire en Nutrition, Inserm U724, Faculté de Médecine, 9 Avenue de la Forêt de Haye, 54505 Vandoeuvre les Nancy, France
[e] Service de Médecine Interne, Immunologie Clinique et Allergologie, CHU de Nancy, Hôpital Central, 29 Avenue de Lattre de Tassigny, 54035 Nancy Cedex, France
[f] Service d'Anesthésie et Réanimation, CHU de Reims, Pôle URAD, Hôpital Maison Blanche, 45 rue Cognacq-Jay, 51092 Reims, France
[g] Exploration des Allergies-Maladies Respiratoires, INSERM U657, Hôpital Arnaud de Villeneuve, CHU de Montpellier, 371 Avenue du Doyen Gaston Giraud, 34295 Montpellier Cedex 5, France
* Corresponding author. Service d'Anesthésie-Réanimation, CHU de Nancy, Hôpital Central, 29 Avenue de Lattre de Tassigny, 54035 Nancy Cedex, France.
E-mail address: pm.mertes@chu-nancy.fr (P. M. Mertes).

Immunol Allergy Clin N Am 29 (2009) 429–451
doi:10.1016/j.iac.2009.04.004
0889-8561/09/$ – see front matter © 2009 Published by Elsevier Inc.

immunology.theclinics.com

Determining the cause of these adverse events and the drug responsible, and adequately communicating those findings, can reduce second reactions.

EPIDEMIOLOGY

Perioperative anaphylactic reactions are potential life-threatening immediate hypersensitivity reactions that are unrelated to the drug's pharmacologic characteristics and correspond to immune-mediated allergic and nonimmune-mediated so-called "pseudo-allergic or anaphylactoid" reactions.[3] They result from the release of preformed and newly synthesized mediators from mast cell and basophils.

The reality of the risk of an allergic reaction occurring during anesthesia is established on the basis of the more than 15,000 cases of perioperative hypersensitivity reactions published in the literature during the last 20 years.[4] Despite increasing awareness about anaphylactic reactions to drugs and compounds used in anesthesia, their incidence remains poorly defined owing to uncertainties over the accuracy and completeness of reporting.

Most reports on the incidence of anaphylaxis originate in France, Australia, New Zealand, the United Kingdom, Thailand, Spain, and Norway. They reflect an active policy of systematic clinical or laboratory investigation of hypersensitivity reactions, or result from the analysis of drug-related adverse event databases. Based on these reports, the estimated incidence of all immune- and nonimmune-mediated immediate anesthetic hypersensitivity reactions was 1 in 5000 to 1 in 13,000 in Australia, 1 in 5000 in Thailand, 1 in 4600 in France, 1 in 1250 to 1 in 5000 in New Zealand, 1 in 3500 in England.[4-8]

The estimated incidence of immune-mediated reactions was 1 in 10,000 to 1 in 20,000 in Australia,[9] 1 in 13,000 in France,[10] 1 in 10,263 in Spain,[11] 1 in 5500 in Thailand,[8] and 1 in 1700 to 1 in 20,000 in Norway.[12] In most series, they represent at least 60% of all hypersensitivity reactions observed within the perioperative period.[11,13-16] Wide variations are reported concerning the expected mortality rate, ranging from 3% to 9%;[17,18] the overall morbidity is unknown.

CAUSAL AGENTS

The overall distribution of the various causal agents incriminated in anaphylaxis during anesthesia is similar in most reported series. Neuromuscular blocking agents (NMBAs)

Table 1
Substances responsible for IgE-mediated hypersensitivity reactions in France: results from seven consecutive surveys

Substance	1984–1989 (n = 821) (%)	1990–1991 (n = 813) (%)	1992–1994 (n = 1030) (%)	1994–1996 (n = 734) (%)	1997–1998 (n = 486) (%)	1999–2000 (n = 518) (%)	2001–2002 (n = 502) (%)
NMBAs	81.0	70.2	59.2	61.6	69.2	58.2	54
Latex	0.5	12.5	19.0	16.6	12.1	16.7	22.3
Hypnotics	11.0	5.6	8.0	5.1	3.7	3.4	0.8
Opioids	3.0	1.7	3.5	2.7	1.4	1.3	2.4
Colloids	0.5	4.6	5.0	3.1	2.7	4.0	2 .8
Antibiotics	2.0	2.6	3.1	8.3	8.0	15.1	14.7
Other	2.0	2.8	2.2	2.6	2.9	1.3	3.0
Total	100	100	100	100	100	100	100

represent the most frequently involved substances, with a range of 50% to 70%, followed by latex (12% to 16.7%) and, in recent reports, antibiotics (15%) (**Table 1**).

NEUROMUSCULAR BLOCKING AGENTS
Immune-Mediated Hypersensitivity Reactions

Most hypersensitivity reactions to NMBAs are acute IgE-dependent allergic reactions. Of all the drugs studied so far that elicit immediate allergic reactions, NMBAs demonstrate several intriguing departures from the currently accepted explanations of the mechanisms underlying the allergic immune response to "small" molecules such as drugs and simple chemicals.[19] Until recently, low molecular weight molecules were considered as haptens incapable of inducing the production of drug-specific antibodies by themselves. Consequently, prior covalent binding of the drug or of one of its degradation products to a protein carrier and processing by professional antigen-presenting cells before presentation of peptides on the cell surface in close association with a class I or II histocompatibility molecule were regarded as the initial steps of sensitization. Recent reports have challenged this dogma. At least some muscle relaxants bind loosely to plasma proteins; however, there appears to be no conclusive evidence that covalent conjugation to endogenous proteins to form sensitizing antigenic drug-protein complexes occurs with any of the NMBAs or their degradation products. A possible direct interaction with proteins present on the surface of antigen-presenting cells (class II histocompatibility molecules), as reported for sensitizing metal and some antibiotics, should also be given consideration.[20] In this regard, the capacity of dendritic cells, which are considered to be the most powerful antigen-presenting cells, to present NMBA-related epitopes that are recognized by T cells has been demonstrated in vitro.[21]

The elicitation of an IgE-mediated reaction is influenced by different immunochemical requirements. In immediate allergic reactions, mast cells and basophils are activated by cross-linking of FcεRI molecules, which is thought to occur by binding of multivalent antigens to the attached molecules. In 1983, Baldo and Fisher demonstrated the role of alcuronium-reactive antibodies in some life-threatening reactions elicited by this NMBA.[22] Structure-activity studies designed to explore the molecular basis of the antibody binding have established that quaternary and tertiary ammonium ions were the main component of the allergenic sites on the reactive drugs. Because the structure of NMBAs includes two substituted ammonium ions per molecule, this divalency could explain allergen-induced mediator release in a sensitized subject even in the absence of protein binding.[23] The IgE recognition site of the molecule depends also on the molecular environment of the ammonium ion and on the hydrophobicity and distance to polar groups such as hydroxyls.[24] This factor may explain the heterogeneity of the cross-reactivity among patients.

Cross-sensitization among the different agents has been reported to be frequent, ranging from 60% to 70% of patients allergic to NMBAs, but it is not constant.[10,15,16] Indeed, the patterns of cross-reactivity vary considerably among patients. Cross-reactivity to all NMBAs is relatively unusual but seems to be more frequent with aminosteroid NMBAs than with benzylisoquinoline-derived NMBAs.[25] In addition to the previously mentioned steric considerations, which could explain why two muscle relaxants do not necessarily behave similarly, further hypotheses have been proposed. In some cases, the antigenic determinant may correspond to the tertiary or quaternary ammonium epitope or extend to the adjacent part of the molecule. The relative affinities of the various muscle relaxants to their corresponding IgEs may also have a role.[26]

In 15% to 50% of cases, IgE-mediated anaphylaxis to an NMBA has been reported at the first known contact with an NMBA.[6,13,15,27] This observation suggests a possible cross-reaction with IgE antibodies generated by previous contact with apparently unrelated chemicals. This hypothesis is particularly attractive in cases in which patients react to relatively small and ubiquitous epitopes such as a substituted ammonium group. Indeed, these structures occur widely in many drugs but also in foods, cosmetics, disinfectants, and industrial materials. There would seem to be ample opportunity for sensitive individuals to come into contact with and synthesize IgE antibodies to these unusual, and previously unsuspected, antigenic determinants. Recently, Florvaag and colleagues hypothesized that the striking difference in the rate of allergic reactions to NMBAs, which is more than six times as common in Norway as in Sweden, could be due to differences in preoperative sensitization. They demonstrated a higher prevalence of IgE antibodies to quaternary or tertiary ammonium ion among blood donors and atopic patients from Norway when compared with those from Sweden.[28] This study also pointed out that, among common environmental household chemicals with quarternary/tertiary ammonium ions able to bind antibodies, the only difference between Norway and Sweden was in the use of cough mixtures containing pholcodine. The later elaborated finding that pholcodine exposure in sensitized individuals, particularly in patients having experienced an allergic reaction to an NMBA,[29] was responsible for a significant increase in specific IgEs to NMBAs led to the hypothesis that pholcodine exposure could lead to IgE sensitization to pholcodine and other quaternary ammonium ions, thereby increasing the risk of allergic reaction to NMBAs. The pholcodine hypothesis is under further investigation in a collaborative study involving several countries across Europe and the United States in an attempt to establish a possible relation between the prevalence of IgE against substituted (quaternary or tertiary) ammonium ions and pholcodine consumption, a parameter that varies considerably between countries (for a more detailed discussion, see the article by Florvaag and Johannson elsewhere in this issue).

Differences regarding the relative risk of allergic reactions between NMBAs have been recognized in large epidemiologic surveys.[10,12–15,27] In most reports, suxamethonium appears to be more frequently involved, with some differences reflecting variations in anesthetic practices from one country to another.[12–15,18] In contrast, pancuronium and cis-atracurium are the NMBAs associated with the lowest incidence of anesthetic anaphylaxis in large series.[13–16] Some controversy has arisen concerning a potential increased prevalence of immediate hypersensitivity reactions to rocuronium. A trend concerning an increased frequency of allergic reactions to rocuronium was initially reported in Norway and France,[26,30] but not in Australia,[31] the United Kingdom,[32] and the United States.[33] Because of statistical limitations, an analysis of epidemiologic data from Norway was unable to confirm whether rocuronium represented an increased risk.[12] In the same time period, surveys conducted in France by the GERAP (Groupe d'Etudes des Réactions Anaphylactoïdes Peranesthésiques), a network of 40 French allergo-anesthesia outpatient clinics whose aim is to promote the survey of allergic and nonimmune-mediated reactions occurring during anesthesia, seemed to indicate a trend toward an increased risk when the respective market shares of the different NMBAs were taken into account.[14–16] Further large epidemiologic studies will be necessary to elucidate this problem.

To explain the possible differences observed regarding the risk of allergic reactions with the different NMBAs, it has been suggested that the flexibility of the chain between the ammonium ions as well as the distance between the substituted ammonium ions might be of importance during the elicitation phase of IgE-mediated reactions.[34] Flexible molecules, such as suxamethonium, are considered more potent in stimulating sensitized cells than rigid molecules like pancuronium. This hypothesis would be contradicted if a higher risk of sensitization associated with rocuronium were to be confirmed. Interestingly, in the past, as for rocuronium, alcuronium has been claimed to be associated with a high risk for anaphylaxis. If an increased risk with rocuronium is further confirmed by epidemiologic surveys, propenyl ammonium groups present in both NMBAs might be involved in this apparent increased allergenicity. These considerations represent an important issue in the design of an ideal NMBA with a reduced risk of allergic reactions.

Nonimmune-Mediated Hypersensitivity Reactions

The rate of non–IgE-mediated immediate hypersensitivity reactions usually varies between one-fifth and one-third of the reported cases in most large series.[12,14–16] In a recent report based on spontaneous reporting to the Yellow Card Scheme, the main reporting system for adverse drug reactions in the United Kingdom, nonallergic suspected reactions to NMBAs occurred with almost the same frequency as those with an allergic component.[18] Although the precise mechanisms of the non–IgE-mediated reactions remain difficult to establish, they are assumed to result from direct nonspecific mast cell and basophil activation, which causes direct histamine release.[35] Reactions resulting from direct histamine release are usually less severe than IgE-mediated reactions,[15,16] with the exception of a subset of patients who have been considered as "superresponders" to the histamine-releasing effect of NMBAs. Histamine release is predominantly found with the use of the benzylisoquinolines d-tubocurarine, atracurium, and mivacurium, and the aminosteroid rapacuronium.[36]

Recently, severe bronchospasm resulting from the administration of rapacuronium has been reported in children. Increased airway resistance related to rapacuronium administration has been reported in children and adults. It has been suggested that the higher affinity of rapacuronium for M2 versus M3 muscarinic receptors could account for the high incidence of bronchospasm observed in clinical practice.[37] As a result of these adverse reactions, rapacuronium has been withdrawn from the market in the United States.

LATEX

Allergy to natural rubber latex is the second most common cause of anaphylaxis during anesthesia in the general population. In children who are subjected to numerous operations, particularly those sustaining spina bifida, it is the primary cause of anaphylaxis.[38–41] The relative frequency of allergy to latex has rapidly increased, rising from 0.5% before 1980 to 20% in France in 2002.[16] Thirty percent of these patients had a history of symptoms suggestive of latex sensitization which could have been detected before the reaction.[16] Nevertheless, a low rate of allergic reactions to latex has been reported in countries where a strategy aimed to reduce latex exposure has been implemented.[12]

ANTIBIOTICS

Antibiotics are commonly administered perioperatively and can cause allergic reactions. A discussion of allergic reactions to antibiotics is beyond the scope of this review; however, their frequency has increased over the last 20 years. Currently, allergy to β-lactams represents 12% to 15% of the perioperative reactions observed in France.[15,16] Vancomycin, which is increasingly used for prophylaxis, has also been incriminated in some cases; however, in most cases, the adverse reactions observed are related to the nonimmune-mediated red-man syndrome associated with rapid vancomycin administration.[42]

HYPNOTICS

Hypnotics commonly used in anesthesia are thiopental, propofol, midazolam, etomidate, ketamine, and inhaled anesthetics. Allergic reactions involving these drugs appear to be relatively rare. The estimated incidence of hypersensitivity reactions with thiopental has been estimated to be 1 in 30,000.[43] Most of the generalized reactions are thought to be related to its ability to elicit direct leukocyte histamine release; however, there is evidence for IgE-mediated anaphylactic reactions based on skin tests and specific IgE assays.[44,45] Recently, thiopental has been involved in less than 1% of allergic reactions in France.[16]

Ever since Cremophor EL, used as a solvent for some nonbarbiturate hypnotics, has been avoided, many previously reported hypersensitivity reactions have disappeared. In the last French surveys, reactions to propofol accounted for less than 2.5% of allergic reactions, and reactions to midazolam, etomidate, or ketamine appeared to be rare.[15,16] No immune-mediated immediate hypersensitivity reaction involving isoflurane, desflurane, or sevoflurane has been reported despite their wide use.

OPIOIDS

Reactions to morphine, codeine phosphate, meperidine, fentanyl, and its derivatives are uncommon. Because of their direct histamine-releasing properties, especially regarding morphine, distinction between anaphylaxis and nonimmune-mediated histamine release is not always easy. Only 12 cases were recorded in the last 2 years of an epidemiologic survey in France, nine of them being related to morphine administration.[16]

LOCAL ANESTHETICS

Local anesthetics include amine (lidocaine, mepivacaine, prilocaine, bupivacaine, levobupivacaine, ropivacaine) and ester derivatives of benzoic acid (eg, chloroprocaine, procaine, tetracaine). Allergic reactions to local anesthetics are rare despite their frequent use. It is estimated that less than 1% of all reactions to local anesthetics have an allergic mechanism.[14,46] Inadvertent intravascular injection leading to excessive blood concentrations of the local anesthetic, or systemic absorption of epinephrine combined with the local anesthetic are by far the most common causes of adverse reactions produced by these drugs. Although severe anaphylactic reactions have been reported with both types of local anesthetics, ester local anesthetics, having the capability of producing metabolites related to para-aminobenzoic acid, are more likely than amide local anesthetics to provoke an allergic reaction. Amide local anesthetics have been involved in less than 0.6% of the perioperative reactions.[16]

COLLOIDS

All synthetic colloids used to restore intravascular fluid volume have been shown to produce clinical anaphylaxis. The overall incidence of reactions has been estimated to range from 0.033%[47] to 0.22%.[48] Gelatins and dextrans are more frequently incriminated than albumin or hetastarch. Direct release of histamine has been reported with urea-linked gelatin, with antihistamine being efficient for the prevention of these reactions.[49] Evidence for IgE-mediated adverse reactions to gelatin have also been reported.[48] In addition, adverse reactions to urea-linked gelatin (0.852%) seem to be more frequent than with modified fluid gelatin (0.338%),[48] whereas IgG-mediated adverse reactions to hydroxyethyl starch are less frequent. The rate of adverse reactions has been estimated to be 0.275% for dextrans, 0.099% for albumin, and 0.058% for hydroxyethyl starch solutions.[48]

DYE

Vital dyes have been used for many years in a variety of clinical situations and have long been considered a rare cause of anaphylaxis. This association may be due, in part, to misleading nomenclature.[50] Patent blue V (also called E131, acid blue 3, disulfine blue) and isosulfan blue (also called patent blue violet or lymphazurine), which belong to the group of triarylmethan dyes and share the same formula, are the most commonly used. A recent literature review that included various names of these dyes revealed an impressive number of case reports of hypersensitivity reactions,[51] and it has been suggested that sensitization occurs using everyday products containing blue dyes. In view of the increasing use of blue dyes for lymphatic mapping for sentinel lymph node biopsy, the incidence of anaphylaxis to these drugs can be expected to increase. The mechanism underlying the allergic reaction to patent blue remains unclear. Both direct mast cell and basophil activation and cross-linking of specific IgE antibodies are possible causative factors. Evidence supporting an IgE-mediated mechanism, at least in some patients, comes from two clinical reports, one demonstrating an immune-mediated mechanism by a passive transfer test[52] and the second demonstrating the presence of specific IgE detected by an ELISA test.[53]

Methylene blue has also been shown to be an effective dye for sentinel lymph node localization, with only a limited number of complications reported. Anaphylactic reactions involving methylene blue seem to be rare, perhaps because this small molecule does not bind to plasma proteins, reducing the risk of sensitization via a hapten-protein complex. This dye differs structurally from isosulfan blue and patent blue V; therefore, cross-reactivity is not expected. Nevertheless, several reports of sensitization to both patent blue and methylene blue have been reported.[54,55] These reports support the systematic investigation of a possible cross-reactivity before the use of an alternate dye. A negative skin test with methylene blue in the case of a hypersensitivity reaction to patent blue V or isosulfan blue might be an argument in favor of using methylene blue for future sentinel lymph node mapping.

The clinical diagnosis of reactions elicited by dyes is difficult. Reactions are usually relatively delayed (ie, 30 minutes following injection), long lasting, and justify a prolonged survey in an intensive care unit when prolonged epinephrine administration is necessary.[54]

APROTININ

Aprotinin is a naturally occurring serine protease inhibitor that has found widespread application either by the intravenous route or as a component of biologic sealants because of its ability to decrease blood loss and, as a consequence, transfusion requirements. Anaphylactic reactions are mediated by IgG and IgE antibodies. The risk of anaphylactic reactions has been estimated to range from 0.5% to 5.8% when used intravenously during cardiac surgery; 5 in 100,000 applications are affected when it is used as a biologic sealant.[56,57] Patients previously treated with this drug present an increased risk, and any new administration should be avoided for at least 6 months following an initial exposure.[58] Aprotinin used to reduce blood loss has recently been withdrawn from the market.

OTHER AGENTS

Several cases of allergic reactions to antiseptics have been reported in the literature. They mainly concern allergic reactions to chlorhexidine after insertion of central catheters impregnated with this antiseptic, or after intraurethral use or topical application.[59] Rare cases of anaphylaxis following topical use of povidone-iodine have been reported.[16]

Protamine, whose use to reverse heparin anticoagulation has increased over the last 2 decades, has also been incriminated. Reactions may involve a number of mechanisms including IgE, IgG, and complement. In a recent systematic literature review analyzing 9 retrospective studies and 16 prospective studies, the incidence of anaphylactic reactions was estimated to be 0.19% (retrospective studies) and 0.69% (prospective studies), respectively.[60]

A large number of clinical cases involving many other substances have been published in the literature. These reports underline the importance of a careful and systematic investigation of all substances used during the procedure in the event of perioperative anaphylaxis.

CLINICAL FEATURES

Anaphylaxis is generally an unanticipated reaction. The signs of anaphylaxis occurring during anesthesia differ to some extent from the signs and symptoms that occur during anaphylaxis not associated with anesthesia. All early symptoms usually observed in the awaken patient, such as malaise, pruritus, dizziness, and dyspnea, are absent in the anesthetized patient. In addition, cutaneous signs may be difficult to notice in a completely draped patient, and many signs, such as an increase in heart rate, a decrease in blood pressure, or an increase in airway resistance, may be initially misinterpreted as a result of an interaction between the clinical status of the patient and the drugs administered during the procedure, dose-related site effects of the drugs, or excessively light anesthesia. Reactions may be well established before they are noticed; therefore, vigilance is essential and is the first step toward the diagnosis, successful management, and further investigation of anesthetic anaphylaxis.

The difference between IgE and non–IgE-mediated anaphylactic reactions cannot be made on clinical grounds alone because clinical symptoms and signs can be very similar. Every hypersensitivity reaction occurring during the perioperative period should be investigated to identify the mechanism of the reaction as well as the responsible substance.[6,61,62] Other differential diagnoses are shown in **Table 2**.

Clinical manifestations show striking variations of intensity in different patients, ranging from mild hypersensitivity reactions to severe anaphylactic shock and death.[6,13] When a classification based on symptom severity is applied, IgE-mediated reactions are usually more severe than non–IgE-mediated reactions.[15,16] In addition, for an as yet unexplained reason, IgE-mediated reactions to NMBAs have been shown to be more severe than reactions to other substances like latex in some series.[14–16]

Anaphylaxis may occur at any time during anesthesia and may progress slowly or rapidly. Ninety percent of reactions appear at anesthesia induction within minutes after the intravenous injection of the offending agent, such as in cases of allergy to an NMBA or antibiotic.[6,61] If the signs appear later during the maintenance of anesthesia, they suggest an allergy to latex, volume expanders, or dyes. Latex allergy should also be considered when gynecologic procedures are performed. Particles from obstetricians' gloves, which accumulate in the uterus during obstetric

Table 2
Differential diagnosis of anaphylaxis during the perioperative period

All Substances	Succinylcholine
Overdose of vasoreactive substance	Malignant hyperthermia
Asthma	Myotonias and masseter spasm
Arrhythmia	Hyperkalemia
Myocardial infarction	—
Pericardial tamponade	—
Pulmonary edema	—
Pulmonary embolism	—
Tension pneumothorax	—
Venous embolism	—
Sepsis	—
Hereditary angioedema	—
Mastocytosis	—

maneuvers, could suddenly be released into the systemic blood flow following oxytocin injection.[10] Anaphylactic reactions to antibiotics have also been reported following removal of a tourniquet during orthopedic surgery.[63]

The most commonly reported initial features are pulselessness, difficulty in ventilation, and desaturation.[9] In the authors' experience, a decreased end-tidal CO_2 is also of diagnostic value. In our most recent series, cutaneous symptoms were observed in 66% to 70% of patients in cases of IgE-mediated reactions, whereas they were present in more than 90% of patients in non–IgE-mediated reactions.[15,16] On the contrary, cardiovascular collapse and bronchospasm were present in more than 50% and 39% of IgE-mediated reactions but only in 11% and 19% of non–IgE-mediated reactions, respectively.[15,16] The absence of cutaneous symptoms does not exclude the diagnosis of anaphylaxis. In addition, clinical features may occur in isolation, such as a sudden cardiac arrest without any other clinical signs, as was true in 29 of 491 IgE-mediated reactions in our last published survey.[16] A comparison of the clinical signs observed in IgE-mediated reactions versus non–IgE-mediated reactions based on the results extracted from the French database of the GERAP is detailed in **Table 3**. These results concur with previously published data.[9,10,13] An anaphylactic

Table 3
Clinical signs observed in IgE-mediated reactions compared with non–IgE-mediated reactions

Clinical Signs	IgE-Mediated Reactions (%)	Non–IgE-Mediated Reactions (%)
Cutaneous symptoms	326 (66.4)	206 (93.6)
Erythema	209	151
Urticaria	101	177
Edema	50	60
Cardiovascular symptoms	386 (78.6)	70 (31.7)
Hypotension	127	50
Cardiovascular collapse	249	12
Cardiac arrest	29	—
Bronchospasm	129 (39.9)	43 (19.5)

reaction restricted to a single clinical symptom (eg, bronchospasm, tachycardia with hypotension) can easily be misdiagnosed because many other pathologic conditions may have an identical clinical presentation. In mild cases restricted to a single symptom, spontaneous recovery may be observed even in the absence of any specific treatment; however, under such circumstances, the lack of a proper diagnosis and appropriate allergy assessment can lead to fatal re-exposure.

In most cases, after adequate treatment, clinical signs regress within an hour without sequelae. In some cases, bronchospasm can be particularly severe and resistant to treatment, with a risk of cerebral anoxia or death. Treatment mainly depends on early adrenaline administration and volume expansion. Adrenaline administration should be tailored to the severity of symptoms (**Table 4**) (ie, initial dose of 10 to 20 µg intravenously in grade II reactions and 100 to 200 µg in grade III reactions, repeated every 1 to 2 minutes as necessary).[2] Rapid but goal-oriented administration of adrenaline is mandatory to ensure treatment efficacy but also to minimize potential side effects of treatment.[16] Prolonged inotropic support may also be required in some patients. Moreover, prior treatment with beta blockers is a potential risk factor explaining an absence of tachycardia as well as resistance of arterial hypotension to adrenaline.[64] In cases resistant to adrenaline, the use of vasoactive drugs such as noradrenaline, glucagons, or even vasopressin or vasopressin analogues has been advocated.

POPULATION AT RISK

The potential severity of anaphylaxis during anesthesia underscores the interest of developing a rational approach to reduce its incidence by identifying potential risk factors before surgery. Although several risk factors occur more frequently in patients with anaphylaxis during anesthesia, their prevalence in the general population is such that few would benefit in terms of preoperative screening for a potential sensitization toward anesthetics.[65]

Recently, recommendations have been proposed concerning the identification of a population at risk for perioperative anaphylaxis who would benefit from preoperative investigation.[2] Indeed, false-negative results or false-positive results of preoperative investigation could have disastrous consequences in regard to anesthesia by leading to a change to a maladapted anesthesia technique. Patients at risk have been defined as follows:

> Patients who are allergic to one of the drugs or products likely to be administered or used during the anesthesia procedure and for whom the diagnosis has been established by a previous allergy investigation

Table 4	
Grade of severity for quantification of immediate hypersensitivity reactions	
Grade	**Symptoms**
I	Cutaneous signs: generalized erythma, urticaria, angioedema
II	Measurable but not life-threatening symptoms Cutaneous signs, hypotension, tachycardia Respiratory disturbance: cough, difficulty to inflate
III	Life-threatening symptoms: collapse, tachycardia or bradycardia, arrhythmias, bronchospasm
IV	Cardiac and/or respiratory arrest

Patients who have shown clinical signs suggesting an allergic reaction during a previous anesthesia

Patients who have presented with the clinical manifestations of allergy when exposed to latex, regardless of the circumstances in which this occurred

Children who have had multiple operations, especially those with spina bifida, because of the high frequency of sensitization to latex and the high incidence of anaphylactic shock caused by latex in such patients

Patients who have experienced clinical manifestations of allergy to avocado, kiwi, banana, chestnut, and buckwheat because of the high frequency of cross-reactivity with latex

In contrast, according to this recommendation, patients who are allergic to a drug or other product that is not likely to be used during the course of the anesthesia or who are atopic (eg, those with asthma or hay fever) should not be considered at risk for perioperative anaphylaxis.[2] Other recommendations consider patients with a history of hay fever, rhinitis, asthma, or eczema (atopy) as being at risk for latex allergy.[66]

INVESTIGATION OF AN ALLERGIC REACTION

Any suspected hypersensitivity reaction during anesthesia must be extensively investigated using combined perioperative and postoperative testing to confirm the nature of the reaction, to identify the responsible drug, to detect possible cross-reactivity in cases of anaphylaxis to an NMBA, and to provide recommendations for future anesthetic procedures.[2,67] Although serious attempts have been made to standardize and validate in vitro and in vivo techniques for the diagnosis of drug allergy,[2,65,67–69] none of the available diagnostic tests demonstrate absolute accuracy. False-positive test results may merely cause an inconvenience (unnecessary avoidance of a safe drug), whereas false-negative or equivocal results may be extremely dangerous and severely undermine correct secondary prevention. The problem in the assessment of the reliability of tests is that, when a single diagnostic test is negative, it is impossible to determine whether it is a false-negative test or whether the patient is tolerant to the tested agent unless the agent is administered. Whenever possible, confirmation of the incriminated allergen should be based on immunologic assessment using more than one test. In the event of discrepancies between different tests, an alternative compound that was completely negative in tests is advocated.

The diagnostic strategy is based on a detailed history including concurrent morbidity, previous anesthetic history, and any known allergies, and a combination of investigations performed both immediately and days to weeks later. Biologic investigations include mediator release assays at the time of the reaction,[70] quantification of specific IgE immediately or 6 weeks later,[70,71] skin tests,[68] and other biologic assays such as histamine release tests or basophil activation assays.[69,72] Early tests are essentially designed to determine whether an immunologic mechanism is involved. Delayed skin tests attempt to identify the responsible drug.

HISTAMINE AND TRYPTASE

During an IgE-mediated reaction, basophils and mast cells are activated and then degranulate and release mediators in intracellular fluids. These mediators can be measured in the patient's serum and have proved to be useful for the diagnosis of anaphylaxis during anesthesia.[15,62,70,73,74] Histamine concentrations are maximal almost immediately and decrease thereafter with a half-life of about 20 minutes; therefore, circulating levels should be assayed within the first hour of a reaction, and, in mild cases, only the early measurements may be increased.[73] Histamine assay should be avoided during pregnancy (particularly near term) and in patients receiving high doses of heparin because of a high rate of false negativity due to accelerated histamine degradation. When increased, histamine circulating levels confirm basophil cell activation which can result from direct or IgE-mediated activation. In our most recent study, the sensitivity of this test for the diagnosis of anaphylaxis was estimated to be 75%, the specificity 51%, the positive predictive value 75%, and the negative predictive value 51%. Urinary methylhistamine assays are no longer available.

Tryptase reaches a peak in the patient's serum 30 minutes after the first clinical manifestations. Its half-life is 90 minutes. The levels usually decrease over time, but in some cases, elevated levels can still be detected for up to 6 hours or more after the onset of anaphylaxis.[70] Basophils and mast cells highly differ in the amount of tryptase contained in their granules; mast cells contain high tryptase levels (12–35 pg/cell) and basophils very low levels (<0.05 pg/cell). Although elevated tryptase levels can be observed in different situations, an elevated tryptase concentration greater than 25 μg.L^{-1} is usually regarded as specific for mast cell activation and differentiates between an IgE-mediated and alternative effector cell activation.[70,72] The absence of increased serum tryptase does not rule out an allergic reaction.[72] In our last series, using tryptase measurements for the diagnosis of anaphylaxis, the sensitivity was estimated at 64%, specificity at 89.3%, positive predictive value at 92.6%, and negative predictive value at 54.3%.[15]

SPECIFIC IgE ASSAY

In vitro tests are available to detect the presence of serum-specific IgE antibodies. Baldo and Fisher were the first to demonstrate that drug-reactive IgEs were involved in anaphylactic reactions using NMBAs coupled to epoxy Sepharose in a radioimmunoassay.[75] The detection of antidrug-specific IgE assays in serum is performed by a sandwich-type immunoassay in which the serum IgE is first adsorbed to a reactive phase and subsequently quantified via the binding of an anti-IgE tracer. The reactive phase is prepared by covalently coupling a drug derivative to a solid phase such as nitrocellulose membrane or a polymer.

IgE binding to different NMBAs bound to solid phases and competitive inhibition assays with several muscle relaxants, other drugs, and chemicals including morphine demonstrate a cross-reactivity of specific IgE.[22,75,76] Nevertheless, some patients do not react with all NMBAs, showing that the substituted ammonium ion is not always the only part of the epitope. Gueant and colleagues[77] improved a radioimmunoassay method for detecting NMBA-specific IgE in serum using a quaternary ammonium compound coupled to Sepharose (QAS-RIA). The sensitivity of this test was estimated at 88%. An inhibition step in the presence of 130 nmol of soluble drug is performed, and in most cases, the highest inhibition is observed with the incriminated drug (83.3%). Guilloux and colleagues[78] have developed a radioimmunoassay test by coupling p-aminophenyl phosphoryl choline on agarose (PAPPC-RIA). P-aminophenyl phosphoryl choline contains a larger choline derivative (quaternary ammonium ion), including a secondary ammonium group, an aromatic ring, and a phosphate group. Both methods were found to have similar sensitivity and specificity. Recently, Fisher and Baldo[76] supported the use of a morphine-based immunoassay for the detection of specific IgE to ammonium ions in the sera of sensitized subjects. More recently, Ebo and colleagues[79] investigated the diagnostic value of quantification of IgE by the ImmunoCAP method (Phadia AB, Uppsala, Sweden) in the diagnosis of rocuronium allergy. They also studied whether IgE inhibition tests can predict clinical cross-reactivity between NMBAs. They concluded that the rocuronium ImmunoCAP constitutes a reliable technique to diagnose rocuronium allergy provided an assay-specific decision threshold is applied, because these assays reach a sensitivity of more than 85% and absolute specificity.

Specific IgEs against thiopental, morphine, phenoperidine, and propofol have also been detected in the serum of sensitized patients using IgE radioimmunoassays.[80,81] The presence of hydrophobic IgE reacting nonspecifically with propofol has been reported.[82] With respect to latex, a radioallergosorbent test is available. Although it is considered to be less sensitive than the skin prick test, a 92.8% sensitivity has been reported.[83]

These findings have recently led to limiting the indications for specific IgE assays to the diagnosis of anaphylaxis to NMBA, thiopental, and latex.[2] These tests are usually performed several weeks after the reaction but also can be performed at the time of the reaction.[2,70,71]

SKIN TESTING

In most reports, skin tests in association with history remain the mainstay of the diagnosis of an IgE-mediated reaction. Intradermal skin or prick tests are usually performed 4 to 6 weeks after a reaction, because, before 4 weeks, the intracellular stocks of histamine and other mediators are still lower than normal.[84] Skin tests to NMBAs may remain positive for years later. Ideally, testing should be performed by a professional experienced in performing and interpreting tests with anesthetic agents (**Table 5**).[2]

Prick tests and intradermal reactions with dilutions of commercially available drug preparations are advised. Although highly reliable, skin tests are not infallible.[85] Standardized procedures and dilutions must be precisely defined for each agent tested to avoid false-positive results. Control tests using saline (negative control) and codeine (positive control) must accompany skin tests to determine whether the skin is apt to release histamine and react to it.

A certain degree of controversy remains as to the maximal concentrations to be used when sensitization to NMBAs is investigated.[86,87] Detailed recommendations for skin and intradermal test dilutions of anesthetic drugs including NMBAs have been proposed by the SFAR and the French Society of Allergology (Société Française d'Allergologie et d'Immunologie Clinique) (**Table 5**).[2] The accuracy of these recommended maximal concentrations has been confirmed in a prospective study conducted in 120 healthy volunteers tested with all NMBAs available at increasing concentration both on the anterior part of the forearm and the back. Results were similar on both injection sites.[68] Skin tests are interpreted after 15 to 20 minutes. A prick test is considered positive when the diameter of the wheal is at least equal to half of that produced by the positive control test and at least 3 mm greater than the negative control. Intradermal tests are considered positive when the diameter of the wheal is twice or more the diameter of the injection wheal.

Any drug administered during the perioperative period should be considered as a potential cause.[61] In addition, because of the frequent but not systematic cross-reactivity observed with muscle relaxants, all available NMBAs should be tested.[2,13,64,72] In most cases, patients allergic to one muscle relaxant can be given another agent chosen on the basis of skin test screening. In our experience, we suggest that the concentration of muscle relaxant used for skin testing be increased to a dilution of 10^{-1} of the commercially available substance tested to reduce false-negative results. Furthermore, we recommend leukocyte histamine release or

Table 5
Concentrations of anesthetic agents normally nonreactive in practice of skin tests

Available Agents			Prick Tests		Intradermal Tests	
INN	Concentration $(mg \cdot mL^{-1})$	Dilution	Maximal Concentration $(mg \cdot mL^{-1})$	Dilution	Maximal Concentration $(\mu g \cdot mL^{-1})$	
Atracurium	10	1/10	1	1/1000	10	
Cis-atracurium	2	Undiluted	2	1/100	20	
Mivacurium	2	Undiluted	0.2	1/1000	2	
Pancuronium	2	Undiluted	2	1/10	200	
Rocuronium	10	Undiluted	10	1/100	100	
Suxamethonium	50	1/5	10	1/500	100	
Vecuronium	4	Undiluted	4	1/10	400	
Etomidate	2	Undiluted	2	1/10	200	
Midazolam	5	Undiluted	5	1/10	500	
Propofol	10	Undiluted	10	1/10	1000	
Thiopental	25	Undiluted	25	1/10	2500	
Alfentanil	0.5	Undiluted	0.5	1/10	50	
Fentanyl	0.05	Undiluted	0.05	1/10	5	
Morphine	10	1/10	1	1/1000	10	
Remifentanil	0.05	Undiluted	0.05	1/10	5	
Sufentanil	0.005	Undiluted	0.005	1/10	0.5	
Bupivacaine	2.5	Undiluted	2.5	1/10	250	
Lidocaine	10	Undiluted	10	1/10	1000	
Mepivacaine	10	Undiluted	10	1/10	1000	
Ropivacaine	2	Undiluted	2	1/10	200	

Abbreviation: INN, International Nonproprietary Name.
Data from Mertes PM, Laxenaire MC. [Anaphylactic and anaphylactoid reactions occurring during anaesthesia in France: seventh epidemiologic survey (January 2001–December 2002)]. Ann Fr Anesth Reanim 2004;23(12):1133–43 [in French].

basophil activation testing of the muscle relaxant selected on the basis of a negative skin test to ensure an absence of an in vitro basophil activation release. This testing should help avoid future adverse reactions and provide documented advice for the future administration of anesthesia.[2,13] No diagnostic procedure can be devoid of false-positive or false-negative results. Although rare, some cases have been reported of renewed allergic reactions following exposure to an NMBA considered to be safe.[85,88] When administering an NMBA to a sensitized patient with a negative skin test, one should bear in mind the risk-benefit ratio. In addition, any new muscle relaxant should be routinely tested in patients known to be allergic to this class of agents to detect possible cross-reactivity.[2]

The estimated sensitivity of skin tests for muscle relaxants is approximately 94% to 97%.[89] The sensitivity for other substances varies. It is good for synthetic gelatins and β-lactams but poor for barbiturates, opioids, and benzodiazepines.[13] There has been some controversy concerning the advantages of prick versus intradermal testing. Studies comparing both techniques show little differences between them;[90,91] however, reliability over time concerning prick testing has not been assessed, and the reliability of prick tests alone in the individual patient has been questioned by some authorities.[92] Consequently, prick testing is advised for the diagnosis of the muscle relaxant responsible for an anaphylactic reaction, but intradermal testing should be preferred when investigating cross-reaction.[93] Latex sensitization must be investigated by prick tests using two different commercial extracts.[94] Both prick and intradermal tests have been proposed in the literature for the diagnosis of sensitization to blue dyes; however, false-negative prick tests have been occasionally reported in the literature. These reports strongly suggest favoring intradermal tests using up to a 1:100 dilution for the diagnosis of sensitization to blue dyes in patients with a history of a possible immediate hypersensitivity reaction to dyes.[54]

MEDIATOR RELEASE TESTS
Basophil Activation Evaluation by Secreted Mediator Assays

Allergen-induced mediator release tests quantify mediators released during effector cell degranulation, mainly peripheral blood basophils, following stimulation with specific antigen. There are two categories of mediator release tests: histamine release tests and sulphidoleukotriene release tests (cellular allergen stimulation test). Mata and colleagues[95] evaluated in vitro leukocyte histamine release tests for the diagnosis of allergy to muscle relaxant drugs in 40 patients and a control group of 44 subjects with negative leukocyte histamine release. The tests were positive in 65% of the allergic patients, for a threshold corresponding to specificity at 100%. The concordance between the leukocyte histamine release test and QAS-RIA was 64%.[95,96] Despite good specificity, the diagnostic application of these tests remains limited because of the heavy experimental conditions and insufficient sensitivity; therefore, they are not used as routine diagnostic tests.[2] They could be useful when cross-reactivity among muscle relaxants is investigated with a view to future anesthesia in sensitized patients. Similarly, reports concerning the monitoring of serotonin,[97] eosinophil cationic protein,[98] or LTC4[99] release have also been published; however, these assays cannot be recommended in routine clinical practice at the present time.

Flow Cytometry

The basis of flow-assisted allergy diagnosis relies on quantification of shifts in the expression of basophilic activation markers after challenge with a specific allergen using specific antibodies conjugated with a fluorochrome or dye. Activated basophils not only secrete quantifiable bioactive mediators but also up-regulate the expression of different markers which can be detected efficiently by flow cytometry using specific monoclonal antibodies.[69,100–103] Currently, the most commonly used antibody in allergy diagnosis is anti-CD63 and, to a lesser extent, anti-CD203c. This technique has been clinically validated for several classical IgE-mediated allergies, including indoor and outdoor inhalant allergies, primary and secondary food allergies, natural rubber latex allergy, Hymenoptera venom allergy, and some drug allergies.[69] Although it does not allow differentiating between IgE-dependent and IgE-independent basophil activation, it is anticipated that it might constitute a unique tool in the diagnosis of IgE-independent hypersensitivity reactions as well as the diagnosis of IgE-mediated anaphylaxis when a specific IgE assay is unavailable.[69,104] Several methodologic issues remain to be addressed, including realization of the test on whole blood or isolated basophils, the need for preactivation with IL-3, the choice of appropriate dose for different allergens, positive and negative controls, characterization and activation markers, and the appropriate diagnostic threshold for different allergens.[69] Nevertheless, once fully validated, the basophil activation test using flow cytometry will probably represent an interesting diagnostic tool for NMBA anaphylaxis and cross-sensitization studies.

Challenge Tests

Indications for these tests are limited. They are restricted to local anesthetics, β-lactams, and latex.[105] They should only be performed in the situation of negative skin tests. Local anesthetics can be tested by subcutaneously injecting 0.5 to 2 mL of undiluted anesthetic solution (without epinephrine). The test is considered negative if no any adverse reaction occurs within 30 minutes after injection.[106]

PREVENTION
Primary Prevention

Prevention of anaphylaxis has two major objectives: (1) preventing the sensitization of a patient to a particular allergen, or (2) preventing the occurrence of an anaphylactic reaction to a reintroduced allergen in a presensitized patient. In this regard, prevention of latex allergy in spina bifida or multioperated children by primary prevention, which consists of avoiding latex during medical and surgical care of these patients, has been found to be very effective.[107] Similarly, the wearing of powderless, low-latex-allergen gloves by health care workers has been proposed as a possible means to reduce the levels of latex aeroallergen in the operating room and the rate of sensitization to latex in health care workers.

Secondary Prevention

Avoidance of causal agent
Prevention of anaphylactic reactions relies mainly on accurate documentation of previous reactions and avoidance of the incriminated drug. During the preanesthetic consultation, a detailed history should be taken with special emphasis on atopy, drug allergy, and allergy to latex and tropical fruits. The use of a specific questionnaire is particularly helpful.[64,105]

Latex-sensitive patients should be managed by complete avoidance of potential latex exposure.[105,108] This avoidance is most easily achieved if a comprehensive institutional policy exists. Patient care must be carefully coordinated among all professionals, including pre- and postoperative nursing and operating teams. Whenever possible, the patient should be scheduled for elective surgery as the first case of the day to reduce exposure to aerosolized latex particles. Warnings identifying a risk for latex allergy should be posted inside and outside the operating room and in perioperative care areas, and the patient should wear a medical alert bracelet or necklace. A checklist of recommendations should accompany the patient throughout his or her hospital stay. In addition, a list of readily available non-latex alternatives should be established in collaboration with the facility's central supply service and should be prominently displayed in patient care locations.

Steroids and Antihistamines

Pretreatment with corticosteroids or histamine receptor antagonists, by either H_1 or H_1 and H_2 receptor antagonists, remains controversial. It has been proposed as an efficient way to reduce anaphylaxis due to chymopapaine administration.[109] Prophylaxis has also been found to reduce the severity but not the overall incidence of adverse reactions to dye.[110]

Pretreatment with H_1 and H_2 receptor antagonists has been found to reduce histamine-mediated adverse effects in various studies.[42,49] Antihistamine administration was effective in reducing the adverse effects of nonimmune histamine release following muscle relaxant, gelatin,[49] or vancomycin[42] administration.

Histamine detected during alarming immune-mediated reactions is merely a marker of the co-release of more dangerous mediators. Allergic reactions to anesthetic drugs have been documented in several epidemiologic surveys even when H_1 and H_2 receptor antagonists and steroids were applied preoperatively.[14–16] No evidence of beneficial effects of the prophylactic administration of corticosteroids in allergic reactions to anesthetic drugs have been shown. Many authorities believe that pretreatment with corticosteroids, antihistamines, or both does not reliably prevent immune-mediated reactions.[92]

Monovalent Hapten Inhibition

Monovalent hapten inhibition with hapten dextran has been shown to significantly reduce but not completely abolish adverse reactions to dextran.[111] The use of monovalent haptens, which can occupy antibody sites without bridging specific IgE fixed on sensitized cells, has also been proposed for muscle relaxants. In this respect, any molecule presenting a substituted tertiary or quaternary ammonium ion could be considered as a potential monovalent hapten. Although choline and tiemonium were initially used, clinical tolerance of the highest doses was poor. As a result, the concentrations obtained were too low to be effective.[23] Moneret-Vautrin and colleagues[112] demonstrated inhibition of skin mast-cell reactivity to muscle relaxants by mixing them with the monovalent haptens cytidylcholine and ethamsylate. Furthermore, they obtained an inhibition of leukocyte histamine release for up to 3 hours following the infusion of these monovalent haptens in patients allergic to muscle relaxants. Morphine, with its high affinity to reactive muscle relaxant antibodies, has also been proposed as a possible preventive hapten;[13] however, large doses of morphine would be necessary, and H_1 and H_2 receptor antagonists would be required to counteract the cardiovascular effects of such high doses. This possibility has not yet been evaluated, and prevention of NMBA-induced anaphylaxis by monovalent haptens cannot be recommended at present in standard clinical practice.[2]

SUMMARY

Perioperative anaphylaxis remains a significant adverse event during anesthesia that remains underestimated because it is underreported. NMBAs, latex, and antibiotics are the most frequently involved drugs, but any drug used during the perioperative period might be involved. Because no premedication can effectively prevent an allergic reaction, any suspected hypersensitivity reaction must be investigated to confirm the anaphylaxis and to identify the eliciting drug. Patients must be fully informed about the investigations and advised to provide a detailed report before future anesthesia. The wearing of a warning bracelet or possession of a warning card is mandatory.

With the exception of high-risk patients, systematic preoperative screening for sensitization against anesthetic drugs is not justified at this time. A thorough pre-anesthetic history is the most important tool for screening at-risk subjects. Particular attention must be paid to patients who have already experienced such a reaction during anesthesia, those alleging an allergy to muscle relaxants, or those at risk of latex sensitization. In these patients, the choice of the safest possible anesthetic agents should be based on the result of a rigorously performed allergologic assessment.

In view of the relative complexity of allergy investigation, an active policy to identify patients at risk and to provide all necessary support from providing expert advice to anesthetists and allergologists to the constitution of allergo-anesthesia centers should be promoted.

REFERENCES

1. Lienhart A, Auroy Y, Pequignot F, et al. Survey of anesthesia-related mortality in France. Anesthesiology 2006;105(6):1087–97.
2. Mertes PM, Laxenaire MC, Lienhart A, et al. Reducing the risk of anaphylaxis during anaesthesia: guidelines for clinical practice. J Investig Allergol Clin Immunol 2005;15(2):91–101.
3. Johansson SG, Bieber T, Dahl R, et al. Revised nomenclature for allergy for global use: report of the Nomenclature Review Committee of the World Allergy Organization, 2003. J Allergy Clin Immunol 2004;113(5):832–6.
4. Laxenaire MC. [What is the real risk of drug hypersensitivity in anesthesia? Incidence. Clinical aspects. Morbidity-mortality. Substances responsible]. Ann Fr Anesth Reanim 2002;21(Suppl 1):38s–54s [in French].
5. Fisher MM, More DG. The epidemiology and clinical features of anaphylactic reactions in anaesthesia. Anaesth Intensive Care 1981;9(3):226–34.
6. Mertes PM, Laxenaire MC. Allergic reactions occurring during anaesthesia. Eur J Anaesthesiol 2002;19:240–62.
7. Watkins J. Adverse anaesthetic reactions: an update from a proposed national reporting and advisory service. Anaesthesia 1985;40(8):797–800.
8. Thienthong S, Hintong T, Pulnitiporn A. The Thai Anesthesia Incidents Study (THAI Study) of perioperative allergic reactions. J Med Assoc Thai 2005; 88(Suppl 7):S128–33.
9. Whittington T, Fisher MM. Anaphylactic and anaphylactoid reactions: clinical anaesthesiology. Baillieres Clin Anaesthesiol 1998;12:301–23.
10. Laxenaire MC. Epidémiologie des réactions anaphylactoïdes peranesthésiques. Quatrième enquête multicentrique (juillet 1994–décembre 1996). Ann Fr Anesth Reanim 1999;18:796–809 [in French].
11. Escolano F, Valero A, Huguet J, et al. [Prospective epidemiologic study of perioperative anaphylactoid reactions occurring in Catalonia (1996–7)]. Rev Esp Anestesiol Reanim 2002;49(6):286–93 [in Spanish].
12. Harboe T, Guttormsen AB, Irgens A, et al. Anaphylaxis during anesthesia in Norway: a 6-year single-center follow-up study. Anesthesiology 2005;102(5): 897–903.
13. Fisher M, Baldo BA. Anaphylaxis during anaesthesia: current aspects of diagnosis and prevention. Eur J Anaesthesiol 1994;11(4):263–84.
14. Laxenaire M, Mertes PM, GERAP. Anaphylaxis during anaesthesia: results of a 2 year survey in France. Br J Anaesth 2001;21(1):549–58.
15. Mertes PM, Alla F, Laxenaire MC. Anaphylactic and anaphylactoid reactions occurring during anesthesia in France in 1999–2000. Anesthesiology 2003;99:536–45.
16. Mertes PM, Laxenaire MC. [Anaphylactic and anaphylactoid reactions occurring during anaesthesia in France: seventh epidemiologic survey (January 2001–December 2002)]. Ann Fr Anesth Reanim 2004;23(12):1133–43 [in French].
17. Mitsuhata H, Matsumoto S, Hasegawa J. [The epidemiology and clinical features of anaphylactic and anaphylactoid reactions in the perioperative period in Japan]. Masui 1992;41:1664–9 [in Japanese].
18. Light KP, Lovell AT, Butt H, et al. Adverse effects of neuromuscular blocking agents based on yellow card reporting in the UK: are there differences between males and females? Pharmacoepidemiol Drug Saf 2006;15(3):151–60.
19. Baldo B, Fisher M, Pham N. On the origin and specificity of antibodies to neuromuscular blocking (muscle relaxant) drugs. An immunochemical perspective. Clin Exp Allergy 2009;39(3):325–44.

20. Pichler WJ. T cells in drug allergy. Curr Allergy Asthma Rep 2002;2(1):9–15.
21. Aubert N, Mertes PM, Janaszak M, et al. Dendritic cells present neuromuscular blocking agent-related epitopes to T cells from allergic patients. Allergy 2004; 59(9):1022–3.
22. Baldo BA, Fisher MM. Substituted ammonium ions as allergenic determinants in drug allergy. Nature 1983;306(5940):262–4.
23. Vervloet D, Arnaud A, Senft M, et al. Anaphylactic reactions to suxamethonium: prevention of mediator release by choline. J Allergy Clin Immunol 1985;76: 222–5.
24. Didier A, Cador D, Bongrand P, et al. Role of the quaternary ammonium ion determinants in allergy to muscle relaxants. J Allergy Clin Immunol 1987; 79(4):578–84.
25. Mertes PM, Aimone-Gastin I, Gueant-Rodriguez RM, et al. Hypersensitivity reactions to neuromuscular blocking agents. Curr Pharm Des 2008;14(27):2809–25.
26. Laxenaire MC, Gastin I, Moneret-Vautrin DA, et al. Cross-reactivity of rocuronium with other neuromuscular blocking agents. Eur J Anaesthesiol Suppl 1995;11: 55–64.
27. Galletly DC, Treuren BC. Anaphylactoid reactions during anaesthesia: seven years' experience of intradermal testing. Anaesthesia 1985;40(4):329–33.
28. Florvaag E, Johansson SG, Oman H, et al. Prevalence of IgE antibodies to morphine: relation to the high and low incidences of NMBA anaphylaxis in Norway and Sweden, respectively. Acta Anaesthesiol Scand 2005;49(4):437–44.
29. Harboe T, Johansson SG, Florvaag E, et al. Pholcodine exposure raises serum IgE in patients with previous anaphylaxis to neuromuscular blocking agents. Allergy 2007;62(12):1445–50.
30. Heier T, Guttormsen AB. Anaphylactic reactions during induction of anaesthesia using rocuronium for muscle relaxation: a report including 3 cases. Acta Anaesthesiol Scand 2000;44(7):775–81.
31. Rose M, Fisher M. Rocuronium: high risk for anaphylaxis? Br J Anaesth 2001; 86(5):678–82.
32. Watkins J. Incidence of UK reactions involving rocuronium may simply reflect market use. Br J Anaesth 2001;87(3):522.
33. Bhananker SM, O'Donnell JT, Salemi JR, et al. The risk of anaphylactic reactions to rocuronium in the United States is comparable to that of vecuronium: an analysis of Food and Drug Administration reporting of adverse events. Anesth Analg 2005;101(3):819–22.
34. Birnbaum J, Vervloet D. Allergy to muscle relaxants. Clin Rev Allergy 1991; 9(3–4):281–93.
35. Moss J. Muscle relaxants and histamine release. Acta Anaesthesiol Scand Suppl 1995;106:7–12.
36. Doenicke AW, Czeslick E, Moss J, et al. Onset time, endotracheal intubating conditions, and plasma histamine after cis-atracurium and vecuronium administration. Anesth Analg 1998;87(2):434–8.
37. Jooste E, Klafter F, Hirshman CA, et al. A mechanism for rapacuronium-induced bronchospasm: M2 muscarinic receptor antagonism. Anesthesiology 2003; 98(4):906–11.
38. Karila C, Brunet-Langot D, Labbez F, et al. Anaphylaxis during anesthesia: results of a 12-year survey at a French pediatric center. Allergy 2005;60(6): 828–34.
39. Niggemann B, Breiteneder H. Latex allergy in children. Int Arch Allergy Immunol 2000;121(2):98–107.

40. Hourihane JO, Allard JM, Wade AM, et al. Impact of repeated surgical procedures on the incidence and prevalence of latex allergy: a prospective study of 1263 children. J Pediatr 2002;140(4):479–82.

41. Moneret-Vautrin DA, Laxenaire MC, Bavoux F. Allergic shock to latex and ethylene oxide during surgery for spinal bifida. Anesthesiology 1990;73(3): 556–8.

42. Renz CL, Thurn JD, Finn HA, et al. Antihistamine prophylaxis permits rapid vancomycin infusion. Crit Care Med 1999;27(9):1732–7.

43. Clarke RS. Epidemiology of adverse reactions in anaesthesia in the United Kingdom. Klin Wochenschr 1982;60(17):1003–5.

44. Harle D, Baldo B, Fisher M. The molecular basis of IgE antibody binding to thiopentone: binding of IgE from thiopentone-allergic and non-allergic subjects. Mol Immunol 1990;27:853–8.

45. Fisher M, Ross J, Harle D, et al. Anaphylaxis to thiopentone: an unusual outbreak in a single hospital. Anaesth Intensive Care 1989;17(3):361–5.

46. Fisher MM, Bowey CJ. Alleged allergy to local anaesthetics. Anaesth Intensive Care 1997;25(6):611–4.

47. Ring J, Messmer K. Incidence and severity of anaphylactoid reactions to colloid volume substitutes. Lancet 1977;1(8009):466–9.

48. Laxenaire MC, Charpentier C, Feldman L. Anaphylactoid reactions to colloid plasma substitutes: incidence, risk factors, mechanisms. A French multicenter prospective study. Ann Fr Anesth Reanim 1994;13(3):301–10.

49. Lorenz W, Duda D, Dick W, et al. Incidence and clinical importance of perioperative histamine release: randomised study of volume loading and antihistamines after induction of anaesthesia. Trial Group Mainz/Marburg. Lancet 1994; 343(8903):933–40.

50. Scherer K, Bircher AJ, Figueiredo V. Blue dyes in medicine–a confusing terminology. Contact Dermatitis 2006;54(4):231–2.

51. Cimmino VM, Brown AC, Szocik JF, et al. Allergic reactions to isosulfan blue during sentinel node biopsy–a common event. Surgery 2001;130(3):439–42.

52. Pevny I, Bohndorf W. [Group allergy due to patent blue sensitization]. Med Klin 1972;67(20):698–702 [in German].

53. Wohrl S, Focke M, Hinterhuber G, et al. Near-fatal anaphylaxis to patent blue V. Br J Dermatol 2004;150(5):1037–8.

54. Mertes PM, Malinovsky JM, Mouton-Faivre C, et al. Anaphylaxis to dyes during the perioperative period: reports of 14 clinical cases. J Allergy Clin Immunol 2008;122(2):348–52.

55. Keller B, Yawalkar N, Pichler C, et al. Hypersensitivity reaction against patent blue during sentinel lymph node removal in three melanoma patients. Am J Surg 2007;193(1):122–4.

56. Kober BJ, Scheule AM, Voth V, et al. Anaphylactic reaction after systemic application of aprotinin triggered by aprotinin-containing fibrin sealant. Anesth Analg 2008;107(2):406–9.

57. Levy JH, Adkinson NF Jr. Anaphylaxis during cardiac surgery: implications for clinicians. Anesth Analg 2008;106(2):392–403.

58. Dietrich W, Ebell A, Busley R, et al. Aprotinin and anaphylaxis: analysis of 12,403 exposures to aprotinin in cardiac surgery. Ann Thorac Surg 2007;84(4):1144–50.

59. Garvey LH, Kroigaard M, Poulsen LK, et al. IgE-mediated allergy to chlorhexidine. J Allergy Clin Immunol 2007;120(2):409–15.

60. Nybo M, Madsen JS. Serious anaphylactic reactions due to protamine sulfate: a systematic literature review. Basic Clin Pharmacol Toxicol 2008;103(2):192–6.

61. Kroigaard M, Garvey LH, Menne T, et al. Allergic reactions in anaesthesia: are suspected causes confirmed on subsequent testing? Br J Anaesth 2005; 95(4):468–71.
62. Malinovsky JM, Decagny S, Wessel F, et al. Systematic follow-up increases incidence of anaphylaxis during adverse reactions in anesthetized patients. Acta Anaesthesiol Scand 2008;52(2):175–81.
63. Laxenaire MC, Mouton C, Frederic A, et al. Anaphylactic shock after tourniquet removal in orthopedic surgery. Ann Fr Anesth Reanim 1996;15(2):179–84.
64. Mertes PM, Laxenaire M. Anaphylaxis during general anaesthesia: prevention and management. CNS Drugs 2000;14(2):115–33.
65. Fisher MM. The preoperative detection of risk of anaphylaxis during anaesthesia. Anaesth Intensive Care 2007;35(6):899–902.
66. Task Force on Allergic Reaction to Latex. American Academy of Allergy and Immunology committee report. J Allergy Clin Immunol 1993;92:16–8.
67. Kroigaard M, Garvey LH, Gillberg L, et al. Scandinavian clinical practice guidelines on the diagnosis, management and follow-up of anaphylaxis during anaesthesia. Acta Anaesthesiol Scand 2007;51(6):655–70.
68. Mertes PM, Moneret-Vautrin DA, Leynadier F, et al. Skin reactions to intradermal neuromuscular blocking agent injections: a randomized multicenter trial in healthy volunteers. Anesthesiology 2007;107(2):245–52.
69. Ebo DG, Bridts CH, Hagendorens MM, et al. Basophil activation test by flow cytometry: present and future applications in allergology. Cytometry B Clin Cytom 2008;74B(4):201–10.
70. Laroche D, Lefrancois C, Gerard JL, et al. Early diagnosis of anaphylactic reactions to neuromuscular blocking drugs. Br J Anaesth 1992;69(6):611–4.
71. Guttormsen AB, Johansson SG, Oman H, et al. No consumption of IgE antibody in serum during allergic drug anaphylaxis. Allergy 2007;62(11):1326–30.
72. Mertes PM, Laxenaire MC. Allergy and anaphylaxis in anaesthesia. Minerva Anestesiol 2004;70(5):285–91.
73. Laroche D, Dubois F, Gérard J, et al. Radioimmunoassy for plasma histamine: a study of false positive and false negative values. Br J Anaesth 1995;74:430–7.
74. Fisher MM, Baldo BA. Mast cell tryptase in anaesthetic anaphylactoid reactions. Br J Anaesth 1998;80(1):26–9.
75. Baldo BA, Fisher MM. Anaphylaxis to muscle relaxant drugs: cross-reactivity and molecular basis of binding of IgE antibodies detected by radioimmunoassay. Mol Immunol 1983;20(12):1393–400.
76. Fisher MM, Baldo BA. Immunoassays in the diagnosis of anaphylaxis to neuromuscular blocking drugs: the value of morphine for the detection of IgE antibodies in allergic subjects. Anaesth Intensive Care 2000;28:167–70.
77. Gueant JL, Mata E, Monin B, et al. Evaluation of a new reactive solid phase for radioimmunoassay of serum specific IgE against muscle relaxant drugs. Allergy 1991;46(6):452–8.
78. Guilloux L, Ricard-Blum S, Ville G, et al. A new radioimmunoassay using a commercially available solid support for the detection of IgE antibodies against muscle relaxants. J Allergy Clin Immunol 1992;90(2):153–9.
79. Ebo DG, Venemalm L, Bridts CH, et al. Immunoglobulin E antibodies to rocuronium: a new diagnostic tool. Anesthesiology 2007;107(2):253–9.
80. Baldo BA, Fisher MM, Harle DG. Allergy to thiopentone. Clin Rev Allergy 1991; 9(3–4):295–308.
81. Fisher MM, Harle DG, Baldo BA. Anaphylactoid reactions to narcotic analgesics. Clin Rev Allergy 1991;9(3–4):309–18.

82. Gueant JL, Mata E, Masson C, et al. Non-specific cross-reactivity of hydrophobic serum IgE to hydrophobic drugs. Mol Immunol 1995;32(4):259–66.

83. Hemery ML, Arnoux B, Rongier M, et al. Correlation between former and new assays of latex IgE-specific determination using the K82 and K82 recombinant allergens from the Pharmacia Diagnostics laboratory. Allergy 2005;60(1):131–2.

84. Soetens FM. Anaphylaxis during anaesthesia: diagnosis and treatment. Acta Anaesthesiol Belg 2004;55(3):229–37.

85. Fisher MM, Merefield D, Baldo B. Failure to prevent an anaphylactic reaction to a second neuromuscular blocking drug during anaesthesia. Br J Anaesth 1999; 82(5):770–3.

86. Levy JH, Gottge M, Szlam F, et al. Weal and flare responses to intradermal rocuronium and cis-atracurium in humans. Br J Anaesth 2000;85:844–9.

87. Berg CM, Heier T, Wilhelmsen V, et al. Rocuronium and cisatracurium-positive skin tests in non-allergic volunteers: determination of drug concentration thresholds using a dilution titration technique. Acta Anaesthesiol Scand 2003;47(5): 576–82.

88. Thacker MA, Davis FM. Subsequent general anaesthesia in patients with a history of previous anaphylactoid/anaphylactic reaction to muscle relaxant. Anaesth Intensive Care 1999;27(2):190–3.

89. Laxenaire MC, Moneret-Vautrin DA. Allergy and anaesthesia. Curr Opin Anaesthesiol 1992;5:436–41.

90. Leynadier F, Sansarricq M, Didier JM, et al. Prick tests in the diagnosis of anaphylaxis to general anaesthetics. Br J Anaesth 1987;59(6):683–9.

91. Fisher MM, Bowey CJ. Intradermal compared with prick testing in the diagnosis of anaesthetic allergy. Br J Anaesth 1997;79(1):59–63.

92. McKinnon RP. Allergic reactions during anaesthesia. Curr Opin Anaesthesiol 1996;9:267–70.

93. Moneret-Vautrin DA, Laxenaire MC. Skin tests in diagnosis of allergy to muscle relaxants and other anaesthetic drugs. In: Assem ES, editor. Allergic reactions to anaesthetics: clinical and basic aspects, vol. 30. Basel: Karger; 1992. p. 145–55.

94. Turjanmaa K, Palosuo T, Alenius H, et al. Latex allergy diagnosis: in vivo and in vitro standardization of a natural rubber latex extract. Allergy 1997;52(1):41–50.

95. Mata E, Gueant JL, Moneret-Vautrin DA, et al. Clinical evaluation of in vitro leukocyte histamine release in allergy to muscle relaxant drugs. Allergy 1992;47(5): 471–6.

96. Gueant JL, Masson C, Laxenaire MC. Biological tests for diagnosing the IgE-mediate allergy to anaesthetic drugs. In: Assem K, editor. Monographs in allergy. Basel: Karger; 1992. p. 94–107.

97. Bermejo N, Guéant J, Mata E, et al. Platelet serotonin is a mediator potentially involved in anaphylactic reaction to neuromuscular blocking drugs. Br J Anaesth 1993;70(3):322–5.

98. Assem E. Release of eosinophil cationic protein (ECP) in anaphylactoid anaesthetic reactions in vivo and in vitro. Agents Actions 1994;41:C11–3.

99. Assem E. Leukotriene C4 release from blood cells in vitro in patients with anaphylactoid reactions to neuromuscular blockers. Agents Actions 1993;38: C242–4.

100. Abuaf N, Rajoely B, Ghazouani E, et al. Validation of a flow cytometric assay detecting in vitro basophil activation for the diagnosis of muscle relaxant allergy. J Allergy Clin Immunol 1999;104(2 Pt 1):411–8.

101. Sabbah A, Drouet M, Sainte-Laudry J, et al. [Contribution of flow cytometry to allergologic diagnosis]. Allerg Immunol (Paris) 1997;29(1):15–21 [in French].

102. Sainte-Laudy J, Vallon C, Guerin JC. Analysis of membrane expression of the CD63 human basophil activation marker: applications to allergologic diagnosis. Allerg Immunol (Paris) 1994;26(6):211–4.
103. Monneret G, Benoit Y, Gutowski M, et al. Detection of basophil activation by flow cytométrie in patients with allergy to muscle-relaxant drugs. Anesthesiology 2000;92(1):275–7.
104. De Week AL, Sanz ML, Gamboa PM, et al. Diagnostic tests based on human basophils: more potentials and perspectives than pitfalls. II. Technical issues. J Investig Allergol Clin Immunol 2008;18(3):143–55.
105. [Prévention du risque allergique peranesthésique: recommandations pour la pratique clinique]. Available at: www.sfar.org. Accessed April 15, 2004 [in French].
106. Allombert-Marechal G, Vervloet D, Arnaud A, et al. [Provocation tests to local anesthetics]. Presse Med 1984;13(31):1903–4 [in French].
107. Cremer R, Lorbacher M, Hering F, et al. Natural rubber latex sensitisation and allergy in patients with spina bifida, urogenital disorders and oesophageal atresia compared with a normal paediatric population. Eur J Pediatr Surg 2007;17(3):194–8.
108. Task Force on Latex Sensitivity. Natural rubber latex allergy: considerations for anesthesiologists. Park Ridge (IL): American Society of Anesthesiologists; 1999.
109. Moss J, Roizen MF, Nordby EJ, et al. Decreased incidence and mortality of anaphylaxis to chymopapain. Anesth Analg 1985;64(12):1197–201.
110. Raut CP, Hunt KK, Akins JS, et al. Incidence of anaphylactoid reactions to iso-sulfan blue dye during breast carcinoma lymphatic mapping in patients treated with preoperative prophylaxis: results of a surgical prospective clinical practice protocol. Cancer 2005;104(4):692–9.
111. Hedin H, Ljungstrom KG. Prevention of dextran anaphylaxis: ten years experience with hapten dextran. Int Arch Allergy Immunol 1997;113(1–3):358–9.
112. Moneret-Vautrin DA, Kanny G, Gueant JL, et al. Prevention by monovalent haptens of IgE-dependent leucocyte histamine release to muscle relaxants. Int Arch Allergy Immunol 1995;107(1–3):172–5.

Immediate and Delayed Reactions to Radiocontrast Media: Is There an Allergic Mechanism?

Knut Brockow, MD

KEYWORDS

- Radiocontrast media • Hypersensitivity • Skin test
- Diagnosis • Immediate • Non-immediate • Mechanism

Radiocontrast media (RCM) are administered more than 75 million times per year for performing diagnosis and treatment of vascular disease and enhancement of radiographic contrast.[1] Adverse reactions after RCM administration are common.[2] Symptoms after RCM exposure may be regarded as hypersensitivity reactions or toxic reactions related to the well-defined toxicity of the compounds, or may be caused by factors unrelated to RCM, such as chronic idiopathic urticaria (**Fig. 1**).[2] Hypersensitivity reactions to RCM may present clinically as anaphylaxis with the potential to result in fatalities or as delayed occurring exanthemas, not unlike those to other drugs. They have been classified in regard to the time interval between administration and the first appearance of symptoms as immediate when they occur within 1 hour after RCM administration or nonimmediate when they occur 1 hour to 10 days after iodinated RCM injection.[2] Recently, positive skin tests have been described in case reports and in a multicenter study in patients with RCM hypersensitivity.[3–12] In addition, laboratory data in favor of an allergic mechanism have been published.[9,13–15] This review is focused on the current understanding of the mechanisms of immediate and nonimmediate hypersensitivity reactions to RCM and how this translates into recommendations concerning diagnostic procedures.

RADIOCONTRAST MEDIA

All RCM are highly concentrated solutions of tri-iodinated benzene derivatives.[16] There are currently four types of contrast media commercially available: ionic monomers, nonionic monomers, ionic dimers, and nonionic dimers.[17] The ionic contrast media are highly water soluble by means of their carboxylate group. The nonionic

Department of Dermatology and Allergy Biederstein, Technische Universität München, Biedersteiner Strasse 29, 80802 Munich, Germany
E-mail address: knut.brockow@lrz.tum.de

Immunol Allergy Clin N Am 29 (2009) 453–468
doi:10.1016/j.iac.2009.04.001
0889-8561/09/$ – see front matter © 2009 Published by Elsevier Inc.

immunology.theclinics.com

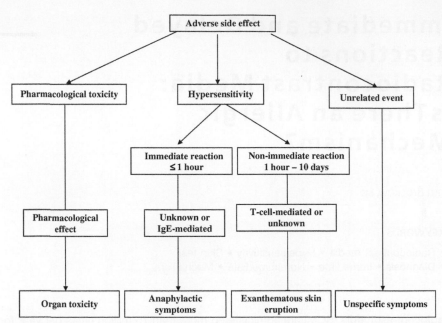

Fig. 1. Classification of adverse side effects after RCM administration. (*Adapted from* Brockow K, Christiansen C, Kanny G, et al. Management of hypersensitivity reactions to iodinated contrast media. Allergy 2005;60:157; with permission.)

products are made water soluble by introducing long side chains rich in hydroxyl groups. The majority of RCM marketed are nonionic monomers, whereas ionic monomers have been continuously withdrawn in most countries, at least for intravenous use. All compounds are nonreactive, have low protein-binding capacity, and are excreted unmetabolized in urine within 24 hours after injection.

EPIDEMIOLOGY

The frequency and mechanisms of hypersensitivity reactions differ between the different types of RCM. Mild immediate reactions have been reported in 3.8% to 12.7% of patients receiving intravenous injections of ionic monomeric RCM and in 0.7% to 3.1% of patients receiving nonionic RCM.[18–20] Severe immediate adverse reactions to ionic RCM have been reported in 0.1% to 0.4% of intravenous procedures, whereas reactions to nonionic RCM are less frequent (0.02% to 0.04%).[18–21] Fatal hypersensitivity reactions may occur in 1 to 3 persons per 100,000 contrast media administrations and are not related to one particular type of RCM.[21]

The frequency of nonimmediate reactions varies from 0.5% to 23.0%.[22] This large variation may be due to the difficulty in verifying whether symptoms occurring days after exposure are, in fact, caused by the RCM. Various types of exanthema account for the majority of RCM-induced nonimmediate hypersensitivity reactions. Such exanthemas have been reported to affect 1% to 3% of RCM-exposed patients.[23–25] Unlike immediate reactions, there seems to be a higher incidence of nonimmediate exanthemas associated with dimeric nonionic RCM but not to other types of RCM.[26]

The main risk factor for immediate as well as nonimmediate hypersensitivity reactions is a previous reaction. Previous reactors have a 21% to 60% risk of a repeat immediate reaction when re-exposed to ionic RCM.[2,22–24] When patients with a previous reaction to an ionic RCM are subsequently given a nonionic RCM, the incidence of a severe immediate repeat reaction is reduced up to tenfold.[2] Predisposing factors for nonimmediate skin reactions are a previous hypersensitivity reaction, as well as interleukin-2 treatment and a history of drug and contact allergy.[25,27,28] The occurrence of an immediate reaction is not a risk factor for developing a nonimmediate reaction and vice versa.

CLINICAL PRESENTATION OF RADIOCONTRAST MEDIA HYPERSENSITIVITY

Immediate RCM reactions resemble anaphylaxis. Pruritus and urticaria, sometimes accompanied with angioedema, occurs in 65% to 85% of patients with immediate reaction.[18,27,29] Other frequent reactions are heat sensation, nausea, and vomiting; however, whether these represent real hypersensitivity or toxic reactions remains more unclear.[2] Gastrointestinal symptoms such as abdominal pain and diarrhea also occur. More severe reactions involve the respiratory and cardiovascular systems, with dyspnea, bronchospasm, or a sudden drop in blood pressure. Hypotension is associated with a loss of consciousness (anaphylactic shock) and with reflex tachycardia.[18] The onset of immediate hypersensitivity reactions is very rapid, with about 70% occurring within 5 minutes after injection[3,18] and 96% of severe or fatal reactions within 20 minutes after injection.[30] Several grading systems for the severity of hypersensitivity reactions have been published, with the classification system published by Ring and Messmer most widely used.[31]

The most frequent clinical manifestation of nonimmediate RCM reactions is a maculopapular exanthema occurring hours to several days after the RCM administration (**Table 1**).[3,25] Other descriptions of the skin reaction include erythema, urticaria, angioedema, fixed drug eruption, macular exanthema, erythema exsudativum multiforme, scaling skin eruption, pruritus, or pompholyx.[16,25] More untypical presentations, such as a graft-versus-host reaction,[32] a symmetrical drug-related intertriginous and flexural exanthema (SDRIFE),[10] or a drug-related eosinophilia with systemic symptoms (DRESS), have been described.[33] RCM are not different from other drugs such as penicillins in their ability to cause a wide spectrum of nonimmediate drug reactions. Nonimmediate RCM reactions are usually mild to moderate in

Table 1
Clinical manifestations of immediate and nonimmediate hypersensitivity reactions to radiocontrast media (most frequent reactions in bold)

Immediate Reactions	Nonimmediate Reactions
Pruritus	**Pruritus**
Urticaria	**Exanthema (mostly macular or maculopapular drug eruption)**
Angioedema/facial edema	Urticaria, angioedema
Abdominal pain, nausea, diarrhea	Erythema multiforme minor
Rhinitis (sneezing, rhinorrhea)	Fixed drug eruption
Hoarseness, cough	Stevens-Johnson syndrome
Dyspnea (bronchospasm, laryngeal edema)	Toxic epidermal necrolysis
Respiratory arrest	Graft-versus-host reaction
Hypotension, cardiovascular shock	Drug-related eosinophilia with systemic symptoms (DRESS)
Cardiac arrest	Symmetrical drug-related intertriginous and flexural exanthema (SDRIFE)
	Vasculitis

severity and self-limiting.[3] Rare cases of severe reactions have been reported, such as cutaneous vasculitis, Stevens-Johnson syndrome, toxic epidermal necrolysis, and papulopustular eruptions[34–40] Systemic symptoms with more immediate-type manifestations such as hypotension, fever, abdominal pain, dyspnea, and biphasic reactions have been reported occasionally.[12,41,42]

PATHOPHYSIOLOGY OF IMMEDIATE REACTIONS TO RADIOCONTRAST MEDIA

The mechanisms of the allergy-like reactions to RCM have been a matter of speculation for decades (**Table 2**). Anaphylaxis to RCM may be theoretically due to (1) a direct membrane effect possibly related to the osmolality of the contrast media solution or the chemical structure of the contrast media molecule (pseudo-allergy),[17] (2) an activation of the complement system,[43] (3) direct bradykinin formation,[43] or (4) an IgE-mediated mechanism.

A higher histamine release after incubation of high osmolal ionic monomeric RCM in comparison with low osmolal nonionic RCM has been reported for rat and human mast cells[44,45] and for human basophils.[46] On the other hand, Stellato and colleagues reported heterogeneity of human basophils and human mast cells isolated from lung, skin, and heart concerning their ability to release histamine and tryptase after incubation with RCM. For mast cells, they found no correlation between the osmolality of RCM and histamine release.[46] Similarly, an activation of the complement system has been described, with a decrease of CH50 in the presence of RCM in vitro.[44] In vivo, the anaphylatoxins C3a and C4a were reported to be increased in a fraction of patients with immediate life-threatening reactions to RCM, without significant differences between RCM-intolerant and tolerant patients.[47] The increase has been attributed to a secondary activation of the complement system by tryptase. In other studies, complement activation has also been demonstrated in patients who did not develop immediate reactions.[48] All of these concepts regarding direct histamine release, complement activation, or bradykinin formation remain controversial as long as pathologic changes are reported for reactors as well as for nonreactors.[49,50] Factors for a patient-specific predisposition explaining why some patients react and others do not must still be elucidated.

Increasing evidence suggests that immediate hypersensitivity reactions may indeed be caused by an IgE-mediated allergic mechanism. The following data support this concept:

Immediate hypersensitivity reactions to contrast media are associated with histamine release from basophils and mast cells.[43,47] Extensive mast cell activation as the cause of the clinical symptoms has been convincingly demonstrated by Krause and Niehues.[45] They demonstrated that patients with hypersensitivity reactions after contrast medium exposure had increased plasma levels of both histamine and tryptase, and that the levels correlated with the severity of the reaction. Other investigators have reported high levels of tryptase in connection with severe or fatal reactions.[11,51,52]

Especially in Japan, pretesting with an intravenous injection of a small amount (usually 0.5–1 mL) of RCM as a means of predicting severe or fatal reactions was performed in the 1970s and 1980s. This approach was abandoned after it was found that it was not useful in predicting severe reactions to ionic or nonionic contrast media, and after severe cardiovascular reactions to these minute amounts of RCM were described.[53,54] The possibility of reacting to low amounts is typical for an IgE-mediated reaction.

Table 2
Arguments for and against radiocontrast media allergy

Reaction Type	Con	Pro
Immediate hypersensitivity reactions	No sensitization phase	Preclinical sensitization to cross-reactive substance possible
	Repeated reactions do not always recur and do not always increase in severity	Previous reaction highest risk factor for subsequent reaction, case reports with increasing severity
	No increase of plasma leukotrienes after RCM administration	Mast cell mediator release correlates with severity of reaction, positive basophil activation test to RCM in patients
	Only anecdotal reports of RCM-specific IgE antibodies	Low levels of IgE antibodies to ioxaglic acid in one study
	Low affinity of IgE to RCM	Specific IgE to RCM higher in reactors than in controls in one study
	RCM are not able to form haptens	Positive skin tests in patients but not in controls in optimal concentrations
Nonimmediate hypersensitivity reactions	No sensitization phase	Preclinical sensitization to cross-reactive substance possible
	RCM are not able to form haptens	PI concept
	Not all patients show positive skin tests	Positive skin tests in patients but not in controls in optimal concentrations, skin test positivity may be lost over time
	Atypical manifestations reported	Maculopapular exanthema and time course resembles drug allergy
	Repeated reactions do not always recur or increase in severity	Previous reaction highest risk factor for subsequent reaction, case reports with breakthrough reactions
	—	Histopathology shows T-cell pathology and T-cell activation in acute reaction and in skin test
	—	Enhanced frequency in interleukin-2 treated patients
	—	Positive lymphocyte transformation test and lymphocyte activation test
	—	Demonstration of RCM-specific T cells
	—	Generation of RCM-specific T-cell lines and T-cell clones

Further indirect evidence for an IgE-mediated reaction has been reported in rare cases with severe reactions. Several groups have reported positive skin test results for patients with severe immediate reactions to either ionic or nonionic RCM.[47,52,58–61] Some of these patients were shown to react not only to the culprit contrast medium but also to other contrast media.[47,55,56] Recently, the frequency of positive skin tests was investigated in more than 200 patients with RCM hypersensitivity and in 82 controls in a European multicenter study.[3] When a nonirritative skin test concentration was used, the intradermal test (IDT) was positive in 26% of patients but remained negative in 96.3% of controls. The relatively high percentage of skin test–positive patients may be influenced by the selective inclusion of patients with typical features of RCM hypersensitivity and involvement of allergy departments experienced in drug hypersensitivity. One patient with a severe anaphylaxis to an unknown ionic RCM experienced urticaria, rhinoconjunctivitis, and glottis edema 5 minutes after an IDT with a nonionic CM. The percentage of positive skin test results was even 50% in the 28 patients who could be tested within 2 to 6 months after the reaction. At later time points, the frequency of positive tests decreased significantly, possibly owing to loss of sensitization over time as reported for other drug allergies.[62]

Basophil activation tests were found to be positive in patients with immediate hypersensitivity reactions as another indirect indication for an IgE-mediated allergy.[63]

Two groups have performed immunoassays to search for contrast medium–specific IgE to ionic RCM in the sera from patients with moderate-to-severe immediate reactions after exposure to RCM.[15,48] Laroche and colleagues studied specific IgE to ionic RCM in 20 patients with immediate reactions. Significantly higher levels of specific IgE against ioxaglate and ioxitalamate were reported in a comparison with control patients. Mita and colleagues reported ioxaglate-specific IgE in 43% of patients (16/34) with a history of reaction to this RCM and in 20.6% of patients (14/68) who reacted to this RCM and in whom serum was sampled in the next 24 hours, but in none of the 10 RCM-tolerant control patients. These RCM-specific IgE levels were not much higher when compared with the levels in controls (usually less than twofold higher than the cut-off level), and the dissociation constant KD (18.7 mM) was very low, which has been regarded as an argument against specificity. These studies were performed with ionic RCM coupled to a solid phase. Contemporary assays for nonionic RCM used today have not been described, because it is extremely difficult to bind nonionic RCM to a solid phase, limiting research in this field.

This evidence collectively challenges the dogma that all immediate hypersensitivity reactions to RCM are pseudo-allergic reactions, and that diagnostic testing is of no value. The fact that as many as 50% of patients had a positive skin test when tested 2 to 6 months after the reaction indicates that in a subgroup of contrast media–induced immediate hypersensitivity reactions may be immunologic reactions involving contrast media–reactive IgE antibodies. In patients with negative skin tests, the mechanism involved remains speculative. An important argument against an allergic mechanism is that patients can react to a contrast media on first exposure, and the reaction does not always recur. This lack of a clear sensitization phase is similar to the situation described in anaphylaxis to muscle relaxants,[63] in which it has been proposed that previously nonexposed patients may have already been sensitized. The chemical structures responsible for the sensitization remain unknown. On the other hand, the positive immediate skin tests reported by several investigators, the detection of contrast media–specific IgE antibodies in sera from immediate reactors to ionic contrast media, as well as the positive basophil activation test in immediate reactors with positive IDTs to the implicated nonionic contrast media strongly support the concept of an IgE-mediated mechanism, at least in a fraction of patients (see **Table 2**).

PATHOPHYSIOLOGY OF NONIMMEDIATE REACTIONS TO RADIOCONTRAST MEDIA

During the past decade, much information on the pathogenesis of nonimmediate reactions induced by RCM has become available. These data indicated that the majority of these reactions are T cell mediated (see **Table 2**). The current evidence for an allergic mechanism in many of these patients is summarized as follows:

The clinical presentation of the majority of nonimmediate RCM reactions is a maculopapular exanthema and is comparable with other drug-induced, T cell–mediated hypersensitivity reactions, such as to penicillins. The reported onset of skin eruptions 2 to 10 days after the first exposure to a contrast medium and 1 to 2 days after re-exposure to the same substance is typical for nonimmediate allergic drug reactions.

The histopathology of exanthematous reactions to RCM and positive skin test sites provides evidence for a T cell–mediated mechanism.[9,14] The histopathologic findings are identical to those reported for other drugs known to cause T cell–mediated allergic skin reactions. A dermal lymphocyte-rich infiltrate is accompanied by intraepidermal spongiosis and sometimes hydropic degeneration of the basal cell layer.[28] Immunohistologic studies of positive skin test sites have shown that the perivascular infiltrate consists mainly of CD4+ and CD8+ (CD45RO+) T cells.[9,14] The dermal perivascular mononuclear cell infiltrate in most patients with maculopapular exanthemas shows higher levels of CD4 lymphocytes than CD8 T lymphocytes, with moderate expression of CD25 and a higher expression of HLA-DR and CLA.[14] There is a high presence of eosinophils. Skin biopsies obtained at the site of positive skin tests to the culprit RCM showed similar results to those seen in the initial acute phase biopsy, with higher expression of CD69 in lymphocytes.[8,14,64]

The enhanced frequency of RCM-related side effects in interleukin-2–treated patients is indicative of a T cell–mediated pathology,[65] because interleukin-2 has been reported to reduce the threshold for T-cell activation and to increase the possibility for clinical symptoms.

The observation that previous reactors are at high risk for a new reaction is typical for an allergic reaction. In the majority of cases reported, readministration of the culprit contrast medium to patients with a previous nonimmediate exanthema results in a repeat reaction.[37,38,66–68] In most (but not all) cases, a more severe reaction with subsequent RCM exposure has been reported. After provocation tests, a reappearance of the exanthemas after intravenous administration of the culprit contrast medium has been reported in patients with previous contrast medium–induced eruptions.[69,70]

A large number of studies on patients with contrast medium–induced nonimmediate skin reactions have reported positive delayed skin tests when the patients were tested with the culprit contrast medium.[16] In the large European multicenter study, 37% of patients with nonimmediate reactions were positive in delayed IDTs or patch tests.[3] The majority of the patients reacted not only to the culprit contrast medium but also to other structurally similar contrast media. More than 30% of the skin test–positive patients in the study had been administered an RCM for the first time; therefore, there is a lack of a sensitization phase, which can again only be explained by the fact that these previously nonexposed patients may have already been sensitized. Different patterns of RCM cross-reactivity indicate that several chemical entities might be involved. No positive skin tests have been obtained with the contrast medium excipients tris(hydroxymethyl)aminomethane (trometamol) and ethylenediaminetetraacetic acid (EDTA), and only rare patients have been reported to react to inorganic iodide.[71]

The presence of contrast medium–specific T cells in patients with nonimmediate exanthematous skin eruptions was confirmed in recent in vitro and ex vivo findings. Peripheral blood mononuclear cells (PBMCs) from patients showed an enhanced in vitro proliferation in the presence of the culprit contrast medium when added to the culture (mainly in the range of 10–100 mg iodide/mL).[9] Flow cytometric analysis showed an increase in the different T-lymphocyte activation markers (CD69, CD25, and human leukocyte antigen D-related) and in the skin homing receptor (cutaneous lymphocyte-associated antigen) in CD4+ lymphocytes, whereas perforin expression was increased in the CD8+ cytotoxic lymphocytes.[14] Approximately 0.5% to 3% of T cells expressed the early T-cell activation marker CD69 after incubation with contrast media.[13] On the other hand, the precursor frequency of peripheral T cells specific for RCM was estimated to range from 0.05% to 0.6% by CFSE staining assays in PBMCs.[13] It has been speculated that the reactive cell population consisted of a minority of drug-specific T cells and a higher number of cytokine-activated bystander T cells amplifying the reaction.[72] A high level of cross-reactivity between different RCM was confirmed by CD69 up-regulation and lymphocyte proliferation, as well as in generated T-cell lines and T-cell clones from patients with RCM hypersensitivity.[13] When analyzing different T-cell clones, different patterns of cross-reactivity were identified, with broad, more restricted, or no cross-reactivity depending on the clone. These in vitro experiments confirm the presence and crucial importance of drug-specific T cells in nonimmediate reactions to RCM.

Another argument against an immunologic reaction in nonimmediate hypersensitivity reactions has been the lack of a hapten. Nonionic RCM are chemically nonreactive and unable to bind covalently to proteins;[30] however, it has been shown that drugs without haptenic properties are able to stimulate T cells noncovalently in an HLA-restricted pattern.[73,74] This concept has been termed the *p-i concept* (pharmacologic interaction of drugs with immune receptors) and does not require drug metabolism or protein processing. Pichler and colleagues provided evidence for this concept reminiscent of other drug-receptor cross-talks. This model can be applied for RCM reactions and would explain the cross-reactivity observed between different compounds.

DIAGNOSIS

Because different mechanisms are involved in RCM hypersensitivity, the allergologic work-up of immediate and nonimmediate reactions must be regarded separately.

Immediate Hypersensitivity Reactions

Immediately after the reaction, elevated plasma histamine and serum or plasma levels of histamine and tryptase have been found, especially in patients with severe or fatal immediate reactions.[48,53,54] In cases in question for anaphylaxis, blood samples for histamine analysis should be drawn as soon as possible after the reaction and for tryptase 1 to 2 hours after the onset of symptoms.[48] Tryptase values should be compared with baseline levels.

Further allergologic work-up is recommended between 2 and 6 months after the reaction (**Table 3**) because positive skin tests are more seldom found afterward.[3] Patients are only rarely skin prick test (SPT) positive with undiluted RCM. Afterward, IDTs with readings after 20 minutes are recommended with the RCM (300–320 mg I/mL) diluted 10-fold in sterile saline, because this concentration has been shown to give a low frequency of false-positive reactions in controls (0% to 4%).[3] Because cross-reactivity is frequent, a panel of several different RCMs should be tested in an attempt to find a skin test–negative product, which might be tolerated in future RCM examinations.

No commercial assay is available for routine measurement of serum levels of RCM-specific IgE antibodies. The reliability of other in vitro tests, such as the basophil activation test, has not yet been established. Results from individual patients and the author's unpublished study indicate that the basophil activation test may be helpful;[62] however, currently, it may only be used on an experimental scientific basis. Provocation is generally not recommended because intravenous applications of as low as 0.5 to 1 mL of RCM have led to severe anaphylaxis.[75]

Nonimmediate Hypersensitivity Reactions

In patients with RCM-induced nonimmediate skin reactions, systemic involvement has been described;[64] therefore, hematology and clinical chemistry should be determined in more severe exanthemas. A skin biopsy is sometimes needed for differential diagnosis.

Based on available data, further allergologic work-up should be performed within 6 months after the reaction.[3] Both delayed IDTs (**Fig. 2**) and patch tests are frequently positive when read after 48 and 72 hours (and optionally at other time points, such as at 24 hours or 96 hours in cases of local pruritus or erythematous plaques). Because some patients test positive with only one of these tests, it is recommended to use both tests in parallel to enhance test sensitivity (see **Table 3**). Patch tests should be conducted with undiluted contrast media, whereas 10-fold diluted products in physiologic saline are recommended when performing delayed IDTs. In cases of non-severe reactions, an IDT and late readings with undiluted RCM may be discussed to increase sensitivity; however, this approach has not yet been evaluated in a sufficient number of controls. A panel of several different RCM should be tested to identify skin test–negative substances.

A response involving RCM-related T-cell activity may be assessed in vitro by the lymphocyte transformation test.[9,14] In addition, CD69 up-regulation (lymphocyte

Table 3			
Presently recommended skin test concentrations for radiocontrast media			
		Readings	
Test	Concentration[a]	Immediate Reaction	Nonimmediate Reaction
Skin prick test	Undiluted	20 min	20 min, 48 h, 72 h[b]
Intradermal test	1/10 diluted	20 min	20 min, 48 h, 72 h[b]
Patch test	Undiluted	—	20 min, 48 h, 72 h[b]

[a] Undiluted RCM with an iodine concentration of 300–320 mg/mL.
[b] If the patient notices a positive reaction (pruritus, erythema) at the skin test site at other time points, additional readings may be performed (eg, after 24 or 96 hours).

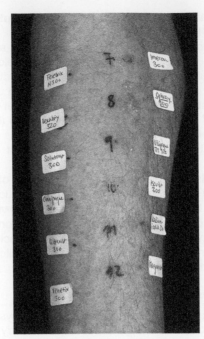

Fig. 2. Positive skin test reactions after 72 hours in the IDT in a patient with nonimmediate RCM hypersensitivity. The patient developed a disseminated maculopapular exanthema 1 day after contrasted CT with ioversol (Optiray). Ioversol tested positive in a 1/10 dilution with vesicle formation. Several other positive skin test reactions indicate cross-reactivity between RCM.

activation test) has been observed in patients with a positive lymphocyte transformation test.[14,72] These tests appear to be promising tools to identify drug-reactive T cells in the peripheral blood of patients with RCM-induced drug hypersensitivity reactions; however, because the sensitivity and specificity remain unknown, the tests cannot be recommended for routine use at present. Further research on the specificity and sensitivity is indicated.

Provocation tests with progressive increases of the injected RCM dose over several days are useful to confirm a negative skin test result before the patient is exposed to the full dose of contrast media.[7,76] Safe readministration of a skin test–negative contrast media has only been published for individual case reports and in a series of 15 patients with nonimmediate skin eruptions.[7] In that study, nonserious skin symptoms after exposition of the dimeric agents iodixanol (n = 4) or ioxaglate (n = 1) were described despite negative skin tests for these agents in five patients. It remains unknown whether false-negative skin tests are a phenomenon specific for dimeric contrast media. Skin test results are currently being validated in a European multicenter follow-up study by provocation tests and data on re-exposure. Until these results are available, a positive skin test to a given RCM dictates that this RCM should not be chosen for a future exposure, but a negative test does not necessarily guarantee tolerance. In this situation, graded provocation tests are helpful depending on the time course of the primary reaction (eg, one-tenth of the full dose on day 1, one half of this issue on day 2, and the full dose on day 3 at the radiology department).[7] This procedure has also been performed in the author's department without problems. Although a previous nonimmediate exanthematous reaction does not pose a higher risk for a subsequent immediate anaphylactic reaction, due to the potential risk involved, provocation tests should generally be performed only in centers with experience in performing monitoring and emergency treatment.

PREVENTION OF IMMEDIATE REACTIONS

In patients with risk factors, such as bronchial asthma or a previous contrast media–induced immediate adverse reaction, radiologists routinely administer nonionic RCM because of their lower incidence of total reactions.[77] If a patient with a previous immediate hypersensitivity reaction to a RCM needs a new contrasted examination, the culprit preparation should not be readministered. In patients with a history of previous anaphylaxis, skin tests (SPT and IDT) with RCM and a reading after 20 minutes are recommended.[16] In a patient with a positive reaction, a panel of several different contrast media should be tested in an attempt to find a skin test–negative product;[3] however, only a few case reports have described the successful use of skin tests or in vitro tests for selection of a safe, alternative contrast media in patients with a previous immediate reaction.[54,57,58] The results from multicenter studies with re-exposure of RCM are needed to clarify the negative predictive value of these tests. In the majority of cases with immediate reactions, skin tests will remain negative and the pathomechanism will not be identified; therefore, on theoretical grounds, a structurally unrelated RCM should be chosen for the next examination.

The prophylactic use of premedication in patients at high risk of immediate RCM reaction is becoming more controversial.[78–80] Corticosteroids and H1- and H2-antihistamines are the most frequently used agents.[81,82,83] Despite different protocols and administration routes, severe reactions may still develop in patients who receive corticosteroid premedication.[82,83] The estimated recurrence rate of RCM reaction after corticosteroid administration has been estimated to be almost 10%.[82] In a recent systematic review, it was concluded that, in unselected patients, the usefulness of premedication is doubtful because a large number of patients would need to receive premedication to prevent one potentially serious reaction.[79] In addition, sufficient data supporting the use of premedication in patients with a history of allergic reactions are lacking. Physicians treating these patients should not rely on the efficacy of premedication.[79]

PREVENTION OF NONIMMEDIATE REACTIONS

Patients with previous nonimmediate skin exanthemas to RCM are at risk for developing new eruptions on re-exposure to the same RCM.[37,38,66–70] Consequently, another product should be chosen if re-exposure is required. Due to frequent cross-reactivity between different RCM, a change of product is no guarantee against a repeat reaction.

Patch tests and delayed IDTs are recommended to confirm an allergic reaction to the culprit RCM.[3] Although it has not yet been proven whether skin testing is a suitable tool for the selection of an alternative CM that can be safely used, in the case of positive skin tests, the substances that are able to elicit test reactions should be avoided. Currently, the administration of skin test–negative contrast media in previous reactors should be done with caution because reactions have been observed after administration of skin test–negative dimeric contrast media in five patients.[7] A fractionated provocation test, which is performed in the author's department before the final procedure, may be indicated.

In current practice, steroid prophylaxis is often given to patients with previous serious nonimmediate adverse reactions if new contrast media exposure is required.

An even stronger pretreatment protocol that has been used involved intramuscular 6-methyl-prednisolone (40 mg daily) and oral cyclosporine (100 mg twice daily) 1 week before and 2 weeks after each of four angiograms in a patient with two previous episodes of maculopapular reactions after RCM administration, the last despite steroid premedication.[6] No studies have been conducted to establish the optimum pretreatment regimen. Repeated nonimmediate reactions, including a case of toxic epidermal necrolysis, have been reported despite corticosteroid premedication.[6,38,41,68] There are not enough data to support the efficacy of pharmacologic prevention in patients with nonimmediate reactions to RCM.

ACKNOWLEDGMENTS

The author thanks Cathrine Christiansen, Werner Pichler, MD, PhD, and Johannes Ring, MD, PhD, for many stimulating discussions and the great input they provided in clarifying the underlying mechanism of RCM hypersensitivity.

REFERENCES

1. Christiansen C. X-ray contrast media: an overview. Toxicology 2005;209:185–7.
2. Brockow K, Christiansen C, Kanny G, et al. Management of hypersensitivity reactions to iodinated contrast media. Allergy 2005;60:150–8.
3. Brockow K, Romano A, Aberer W, et al. Skin testing in patients with hypersensitivity reactions to iodinated contrast media: a European multicenter study. Allergy 2009;64:234–41.
4. Christiansen C, Dreborg S, Pichler WJ, et al. Macular exanthema appearing 5 days after x-ray contrast medium administration. Eur Radiol 2002;3(Suppl 12):S94–7.
5. Kvedariene V, Martins P, Rouanet L, et al. Diagnosis of iodinated contrast media hypersensitivity: results of a 6-year period. Clin Exp Allergy 2006;36:1072–7.
6. Romano A, Artesani M, Andriolo M, et al. Effective prophylactic protocol in delayed hypersensitivity to contrast media: report of a case involving lymphocyte transformation studies with different compounds. Radiology 2002;225:466–70.
7. Vernassiere C, Trechot P, Commun N, et al. Low negative predictive value of skin tests in investigating delayed reactions to radiocontrast media. Contact Derm 2004;50:359–66.
8. Brockow K, Becker EW, Worret WI, et al. Late skin test reactions to radiocontrast medium. J Allergy Clin Immunol 1999;104:1107–8.
9. Kanny G, Pichler W, Morisset M, et al. T cell–mediated reactions to iodinated contrast media: evaluation by skin and lymphocyte activation tests. J Allergy Clin Immunol 2005;115:179–85.
10. Arnold AW, Hausermann P, Bach S, et al. Recurrent flexural exanthema (SDRIFE or baboon syndrome) after administration of two different iodinated radiocontrast media. Dermatology 2007;214:89–93.
11. Laroche D. Immediate reactions to contrast media: mediator release and value of diagnostic testing. Toxicology 2005;209:193–4.
12. Brockow K, Kiehn M, Kleinheinz A, et al. Positive skin tests in late reactions to radiographic contrast media. Allerg Immunol (Paris) 1999;31:49–51.
13. Lerch M, Keller M, Britschgi M, et al. Cross-reactivity patterns of T cells specific for iodinated contrast media. J Allergy Clin Immunol 2007;119:1529–36.
14. Torres MJ, Mayorga C, Cornejo-Garcia JA, et al. Monitoring non-immediate allergic reactions to iodine contrast media. Clin Exp Immunol 2008;152:233–8.

15. Mita H, Tadokoro K, Akiyama K. Detection of IgE antibody to a radiocontrast medium. Allergy 1998;53:1133–40.
16. Brockow K. Contrast media hypersensitivity: scope of the problem. Toxicology 2005;209:189–92.
17. Gueant-Rodriguez RM, Romano A, Barbaud A, et al. Hypersensitivity reactions to iodinated contrast media. Curr Pharm Des 2006;12:3359–72.
18. Katayama H, Yamaguchi K, Kozuka T, et al. Adverse reactions to ionic and nonionic contrast media: a report from the Japanese committee on the safety of contrast media. Radiology 1990;175:621–8.
19. Wolf GL, Arenson RL, Cross AP. A prospective trial of ionic versus nonionic contrast agents in routine clinical practice: comparison of adverse effects. AJR Am J Roentgenol 1989;152:939–44.
20. Palmer FJ. The RACR survey of intravenous contrast media reactions: final report. Australas Radiol 1988;32:426–8.
21. Caro JJ, Trindade E, McGregor M. The risks of death and of severe nonfatal reactions with high- vs low-osmolality contrast media: a meta-analysis. AJR Am J Roentgenol 1991;156:825–32.
22. Webb JA, Stacul F, Thomsen HS, et al. Late adverse reactions to intravascular iodinated contrast media. Eur Radiol 2003;13:181–4.
23. Munechika H, Yasuda R, Michihiro K. Delayed adverse reaction of monomeric contrast media: comparison of plain CT and enhanced CT. Acad Radiol 1998; 1(Suppl 5):S157–8.
24. Yasuda R, Munechika H. Delayed adverse reactions to nonionic monomeric contrast-enhanced media. Invest Radiol 1998;33:1–5.
25. Hosoya T, Yamaguchi K, Akutsu T, et al. Delayed adverse reactions to iodinated contrast media and their risk factors. Radiat Med 2000;18:39–45.
26. Sutton AG, Finn P, Grech ED, et al. Early and late reactions after the use of iopamidol 340, ioxaglate 320, and iodixanol 320 in cardiac catheterization. Am Heart J 2001;141:677–83.
27. Kalimo K, Jansen CT, Kormano M. Allergological risk factors as predictors of radiographic contrast media hypersensitivity. Ann Allergy 1980;45:253–5.
28. Choyke PL, Miller DL, Lotze MT, et al. Delayed reactions to contrast media after interleukin-2 immunotherapy. Radiology 1992;183:111–4.
29. Witten J, Hirsch F, Hartman G. Acute reactions to urographic contrast medium. Am J Roentgenol 1973;119:832–40.
30. Idee JM, Pines E, Prigent P, et al. Allergy-like reactions to iodinated contrast agents: a critical analysis. Fundam Clin Pharmacol 2005;19:263–81.
31. Ring J, Messmer K. Incidence and severity of anaphylactoid reactions to colloid volume substitutes. Lancet 1977;1:466–9.
32. Vavricka SR, Halter J, Furrer K, et al. Contrast media triggering cutaneous graft-vs-host disease. Bone Marrow Transplant 2002;29:899–901.
33. Belhadjali H, Bouzgarrou L, Youssef M, et al. DRESS syndrome induced by sodium meglumine ioxitalamate. Allergy 2008;63:786–7.
34. Laffitte E, Nenadov Beck M, Hofer M, et al. Severe Stevens-Johnson syndrome induced by contrast medium iopentol (Imagopaque). Br J Dermatol 2004;150: 376–8.
35. Goodfellow T, Holdstock GE, Brunton FJ, et al. Fatal acute vasculitis after high-dose urography with iohexol. Br J Radiol 1986;59:620–1.
36. Savill JS, Barrie R, Ghosh S, et al. Fatal Stevens-Johnson syndrome following urography with iopamidol in systemic lupus erythematosus. Postgrad Med J 1988;64:392–4.

37. Schmidt BJ, Foley WD, Bohorfoush AG. Toxic epidermal necrolysis related to oral administration of diluted diatrizoate meglumine and diatrizoate sodium. AJR Am J Roentgenol 1998;171:1215–6.
38. Rosado A, Canto G, Veleiro B, et al. Toxic epidermal necrolysis after repeated injections of iohexol. AJR Am J Roentgenol 2001;176:262–3.
39. Miranda-Romero A, Sanchez-Sambucety P, Esquivias Gomez JI, et al. Vegetating iododerma with fatal outcome. Dermatology 1999;198:295–7.
40. Vaillant L, Pengloan J, Blanchier D, et al. Iododerma and acute respiratory distress with leucocytoclastic vasculitis following the intravenous injection of contrast medium. Clin Exp Dermatol 1990;15:232–3.
41. Savader S, Brodkin J, Osterman F. Delayed life-threatening reaction to non-ionic contrast media. Invest Radiol 1995;10:115–6.
42. Miamoto Y, Tatei T, Ichijima S, et al. [Delayed eruption caused with non-ionic contrast material injection]. Nippon Igaku Hoshasen Gakkai Zaschi 1990;50(3): 295–7 [in Japanese].
43. Ring J, Arroyave CM, Frizler MJ, et al. In vitro histamine and serotonin release by radiographic contrast media (RCM): complement-dependent and -independent release reaction and changes in ultrastructure of human blood cells. Clin Exp Immunol 1978;32:105–18.
44. Lasser EC, Lyon SG. Inhibition of angiotensin-converting enzyme by contrast media. I. In vitro findings. Invest Radiol 1990;25(6):698–702.
45. Krause W, Niehues D. Biochemical characterization of x-ray contrast media. Invest Radiol 1996;31:30–42.
46. Amon EU, Ennis M, Schnabel M, et al. Radiographic contrast media–induced histamine release: a comparative study with mast cells from different species. Agents Actions 1989;27:104–6.
47. Stellato C, de Crescenzo G, Patella V, et al. Human basophil/mast cell releasability. XI. Heterogeneity of the effects of contrast media on mediator release. J Allergy Clin Immunol 1996;97:838–50.
48. Laroche D, Aimone-Gastin I, Dubois F, et al. Mechanisms of severe, immediate reactions to iodinated contrast material. Radiology 1998;209:183–90.
49. Westaby S, Dawson P, Turner MW, et al. Angiography and complement activation. Evidence for generation of C3a anaphylaxtoxin by intravascular contrast agents. Cardiovasc Res 1985;19:85–8.
50. Ring J, Endrich B, Intaglietta M. Histamine release, complement consumption, and microvascular changes after radiographic contrast media infusion in rabbits. J Lab Clin Med 1978;92:584–94.
51. Ring J, Simon RA, Arroyave CM. Increased in vitro histamine release by radiographic contrast media in patients with history of incompatibility. Clin Exp Immunol 1978;34:302–9.
52. Brockow K, Vieluf D, Puschel K, et al. Increased postmortem serum mast cell tryptase in a fatal anaphylactoid reaction to nonionic radiocontrast medium. J Allergy Clin Immunol 1999;104:237–8.
53. Dewachter P, Mouton-Faivre C, Felden F. Allergy and contrast media. Allergy 2001;56:250–1.
54. Yamaguchi K, Katayama H, Takashima T, et al. Prediction of severe adverse reactions to ionic and nonionic contrast media in Japan: evaluation of pretesting. A report from the Japanese committee on the safety of contrast media. Radiology 1991;178:363–7.
55. Fischer HW, Doust VL. An evaluation of pretesting in the problem of serious and fatal reactions to excretory urography. Radiology 1972;103:497–501.

56. Wakkers-Garritsen BG, Houwerziji J, Nater JP, et al. IgE-mediated adverse reactivity to a radiographic contrast medium. Ann Allergy 1976;36:122–6.
57. Kanny G, Maria Y, Mentre B, et al. Case report: recurrent anaphylactic shock to radiographic contrast media. Evidence supporting an exceptional IgE-mediated reaction. Allerg Immunol (Paris) 1993;25:425–30.
58. Alvarez-Fernandez JA, Valero AM, Pulido Z, et al. Hypersensitivity reaction to ioversol. Allergy 2000;55:581–2.
59. Laroche D, Dewachter P, Mouton-Faivre C, et al. Immediate reactions to iodinated contrast media: the CIRTACI study [abstract]. Allergologie 2004;27:165.
60. Blanca M, Torres MJ, Garcia JJ, et al. Natural evolution of skin test sensitivity in patients allergic to beta-lactam antibiotics. J Allergy Clin Immunol 1999;103:918–24.
61. Trcka J, Schmidt C, Seitz CS, et al. Anaphylaxis to iodinated contrast material: nonallergic hypersensitivity or IgE-mediated allergy? AJR Am J Roentgenol 2008;190:666–70.
62. Mertes PM, Laxenaire MC, Lienhart A, et al. Reducing the risk of anaphylaxis during anaesthesia: guidelines for clinical practice. J Investig Allergol Clin Immunol 2005;15:91–101.
63. Hari Y, Frutig-Schnyder K, Hurni M, et al. T cell involvement in cutaneous drug eruptions. Clin Exp Allergy 2001;31:1398–408.
64. Kanny G, Marie B, Hoen B, et al. Delayed adverse reaction to sodium ioxaglic acid-meglumine. Eur J Dermatol 2001;11:134–7.
65. Watanabe H, Sueki H, Nakada T, et al. Multiple fixed drug eruption caused by iomeprol (Iomeron), a nonionic contrast medium. Dermatology 1999;198:291–4.
66. Good AE, Novak E, Sonda LP III. Fixed eruption and fever after urography. South Med J 1980;73:948–9.
67. Courvoisier S, Bircher AJ. Delayed-type hypersensitivity to a nonionic, radiopaque contrast medium. Allergy 1998;53:1221–4.
68. Kanzaki T, Sakagami H. Late phase allergic reaction to a CT contrast medium (Iotrolan). J Dermatol 1991;18:528–31.
69. Gall H, Pillekamp H, Peter RU. Late-type allergy to the x-ray contrast medium Solutrast (Iopamidol). Contact Derm 1999;40:248–50.
70. Akiyama M, Nakada T, Sueki H, et al. Drug eruption caused by nonionic iodinated x-ray contrast media. Acad Radiol 1998;1(Suppl 5):S159–61.
71. Beeler A, Zaccaria L, Kawabata T, et al. CD69 upregulation on T cells as an in vitro marker for delayed-type drug hypersensitivity. Allergy 2008;63:181–8.
72. Pichler WJ. Immune mechanism of drug hypersensitivity. Immunol Allergy Clin North Am 2004;24:373–97.
73. Pichler WJ. Delayed drug hypersensitivity reactions. Ann Intern Med 2003;139:683–93.
74. Kwak R. [A case of shock by pretesting of contrast media]. Rinsho Hoshasen 1985;30:407–9 [in Japanese].
75. Gonzalo-Garijo MA, de Argila D, Pimentel JJ, et al. Skin reaction to contrast medium. Allergy 1997;52:875–6.
76. Morcos SK, Thomsen HS, Webb JA. Prevention of generalized reactions to contrast media: a consensus report and guidelines. Eur Radiol 2001;11:1720–8.
77. Dewachter P, Mouton-Faivre C. [Severe reactions to iodinated contrast agents: is anaphylaxis responsible?]. J Radiol 2001;82:973–7 [in French].
78. Tramer MR, von Elm E, Loubeyre P, et al. Pharmacological prevention of serious anaphylactic reactions due to iodinated contrast media: systematic review. BMJ 2006;333:675–81.

79. Kopp AF, Mortele KJ, Cho YD, et al. Prevalence of acute reactions to iopromide: postmarketing surveillance study of 74,717 patients. Acta Radiol 2008;49: 902–11.

80. Greenberger PA, Patterson R. The prevention of immediate generalized reactions to radiocontrast media in high-risk patients. J Allergy Clin Immunol 1991;87: 867–72.

81. Ring J, Rothenberger KH, Clauss W. Prevention of anaphylactoid reactions after radiographic contrast media infusion by combined histamine H1- and H2-receptor antagonists: results of a prospective controlled trial. Int Arch Allergy Appl Immunol 1985;78:9–14.

82. Freed KS, Leder RA, Alexander C, et al. Breakthrough adverse reactions to low-osmolar contrast media after steroid premedication. AJR Am J Roentgenol 2001; 176:1389–92.

83. Roberts M, Fisher M. Anaphylactoid reaction to iopamiro (after pretreatment). Australas Radiol 1992;36:144–6.

Heparin Allergy: Delayed-Type Non–IgE-Mediated Allergic Hypersensitivity to Subcutaneous Heparin Injection

Axel Trautmann, MD[a],*, Cornelia S. Seitz, MD[b]

KEYWORDS

- Adverse drug reaction • Delayed-type hypersensitivity
- Heparin • Heparinoid • Intravenous challenge

Pathologic immune reactions during ongoing anticoagulation with heparins may present as heparin-induced thrombocytopenia (HIT), erythematous or eczematous lesions around injection sites, or, in extremely rare cases, IgE-mediated urticaria or anaphylaxis.[1–3] From an allergologist's perspective, however, delayed-type non–IgE-mediated allergic hypersensitivity (DTH) to subcutaneously injected heparin is the most common and clinically relevant issue.[4–6] Frequently, changing the subcutaneous therapy from unfractionated heparin (UFH) to low molecular weight heparin (LMWH) or treatment with heparinoids does not provide improvement because of extensive cross-reactivity of these anionic polysaccharides. DTH may be verified by skin testing (intradermal and patch tests) or, in cases of false-negative skin test results, by subcutaneous challenge tests.[7]

For the treating physician and patient, diagnosis of allergy to subcutaneously applied heparins usually implies discontinuation of subcutaneously and intravenously applied heparins because, at least theoretically, intravenously applied heparin in sensitized individuals (ie, patients with DTH to subcutaneously injected heparins) may reach the skin by way of blood circulation and may trigger a hematogenous generalized eczematous or exanthematic eruption. Data in the literature[8,9] and in

---

[a] Allergy Unit, Department of Dermatology, Venereology, and Allergology, University of Würzburg, Josef Schneider Strasse 2, 97080 Würzburg, Germany
[b] Department of Dermatology, Venereology, and Allergology, University of Göttingen, Von Siebold Strasse 3, 37075 Göttingen, Germany
* Corresponding author.
E-mail address: trautmann_a@klinik.uni-wuerzburg.de (A. Trautmann).

Immunol Allergy Clin N Am 29 (2009) 469–480
doi:10.1016/j.iac.2009.04.006
0889-8561/09/$ – see front matter © 2009 Elsevier Inc. All rights reserved.

the authors' studies[10–13] show that patients with DTH to heparins tolerate intravenous heparin application, however.

PHARMACOLOGY

Heparins are anionic polysaccharides extracted from porcine intestinal mucosa; during the processing process, they are fractionated and depolymerized.[14] Therefore, heparin preparations are not pure substances but a composite of heterogeneous molecules varying in size and chemical structure. For this reason, heparin dose is not recorded in milligrams but in international units (IU). Depending on the average molecular weight, unfractionated high molecular weight heparins (UFH; 12–15 kDa) and LMWHs (4–6 kDa) are distinguished.[15–17] Anticoagulation capacity depends on anionic charge of carboxy and sulfate groups of the heparin molecule (**Fig.** 1A). UFH binding to antithrombin leads to inactivation of thrombin and factor Xa, whereas LMWH inhibits factor Xa activity. Like other anionic polysaccharides, UFH unspecifically binds to plasma and tissue macromolecules, resulting in bioavailability of 15% to 30% after subcutaneous application. In contrast, LMWH, such as enoxaparin, reviparin, dalteparin, nadroparin, tinzaparin, and certoparin, has a significantly decreased unspecific binding capacity, resulting in almost 100% bioavailability. Heparins are

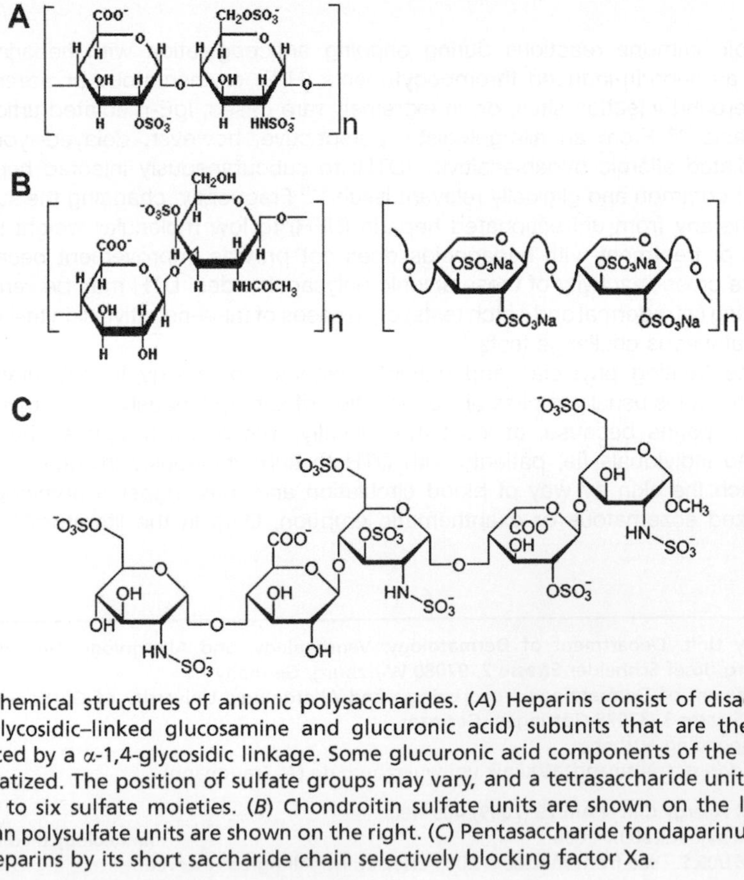

Fig. 1. Chemical structures of anionic polysaccharides. (*A*) Heparins consist of disaccharide (α-1,4-glycosidic–linked glucosamine and glucuronic acid) subunits that are themselves connected by a α-1,4-glycosidic linkage. Some glucuronic acid components of the polymer are sulfatized. The position of sulfate groups may vary, and a tetrasaccharide unit consists of four to six sulfate moieties. (*B*) Chondroitin sulfate units are shown on the left, and pentosan polysulfate units are shown on the right. (*C*) Pentasaccharide fondaparinux differs from heparins by its short saccharide chain selectively blocking factor Xa.

indicated for prophylaxis of thrombosis and for treatment of thromboembolic complications.

Heparinoids are sulfated polysaccharides with antithrombotic effects similar to heparins. Danaparoid (average molecular weight of 6 kDa) is a mixture of heparan sulfate, dermatan sulfate, and chondroitin sulfate (see **Fig. 1**B). Pentosan polysulfate (average molecular weight of 6 kDa) is a semisynthetically produced polysaccharide, derived from pentosan extracted from the bark of the beech tree (see **Fig. 1**B). Although pentosan polysulfate is approved for thrombosis prophylaxis, it is not mentioned in international treatment guidelines.[17]

Fondaparinux (average molecular weight of 1.7 kDa) is a chemically synthesized sulfatized pentasaccharide specifically inhibiting factor Xa after binding to antithrombin (see **Fig. 1**C).[18] In contrast to heparins and heparinoids, fondaparinux is a chemically defined molecule without unspecific binding characteristics and with fast and complete resorption after subcutaneous injection (100% bioavailability).

Hirudins are polypeptides originally extracted from the leech *Hirudo medicinalis* that function as direct thrombin inhibitors without affecting antithrombin.[19] There are multiple hirudin variants (average molecular weight of 7 kDa). Recently, recombinant hirudins and hirudin variants, such as lepirudin, desirudin, and bivalirudin, were approved as antithrombotic substances.

SYMPTOMS

In case of DTH to subcutaneously applied heparins, itchy erythematous or eczematous plaques develop around injection sites (**Fig. 2**A).[4–6,20,21] The usual latency for development of characteristic lesions during ongoing therapy is 7 to 10 days; in case of prior sensitization and re-exposure, skin lesions appear within 1 to 3 days.

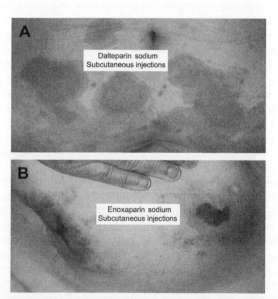

Fig. 2. DTH to subcutaneously applied heparins and heparin-induced skin necrosis. (*A*) Itchy erythematous and eczematous plaques 12 days after initiation of subcutaneously applied dalteparin. (*B*) Painful heparin-induced skin necrosis at injection sites 10 days after initiation of subcutaneous enoxaparin injections. (*From* Gaigl Z, Klein CE, Großmann R, et al. [Managing allergy to heparins]. Dtsch Arztebl 2006;103:2878; with permission.)

The spectrum of skin lesions ranges from mild erythema with little infiltration to typical eczematous plaques with papulovesicles located on an infiltrated erythematous ground. Less frequently, in cases with continuation of subcutaneous injections despite local reactions, a generalized eczema or exanthema with accentuation around injection sites may be observed.[12,22–25] In early erythematous lesions, histopathologic examination reveals a dense mononuclear infiltrate of predominantly CD4+ lymphocytes with scattered eosinophils. Eczematous lesions additionally show epidermal spongiosis.[5,6,12,26] These findings are consistent with a DTH reaction of the skin. Potential antigenic determinants of the heparin molecule have not yet been determined, however.

DTH reactions to subcutaneously injected heparin are mostly described in obese women, which is in agreement with findings in the authors' patients.[11,27] Therefore, gender and obesity seem to be risk factors for the development of DTH to heparin. It is tempting to speculate that hormonal and metabolic influences may play a role in the pathogenesis.[28]

DIFFERENTIAL DIAGNOSIS

The differential diagnosis of erythematous and eczematous plaques after subcutaneous heparin administration includes hematomas, local infections, and eczema attributable to skin disinfectants.[7,29] The most important differential diagnosis is heparin-induced skin necrosis, however.

HIT is the most common serious side effect of heparin treatment.[30] Patients undergoing hip arthroplasty, thoracic surgery, or coronary artery bypass surgery have a risk of 1% to 5% for developing HIT. Interestingly, UFH has a 10-fold risk for HIT compared with LMWH.[31] Immune complexes composed of heparin, platelet factor 4, and specific antibodies activate thrombocytes and induce the characteristic decline of thrombocytes of more than 50% or a decrease to a total less than 100,000 thrombocytes/μL. In case of HIT, thromboembolic complications occur despite thrombocytopenia (deep vein thrombosis or pulmonary embolism) and arterial thrombosis, leading to ischemia of extremities, cerebrovascular insult, or myocardial infarction (the so-called "white-clot syndrome"). Arterial embolisms are often the result of the false diagnosis of "thrombosis despite anticoagulation," with a subsequent increase in heparin dosage. The usual latency for development of characteristic lesions during ongoing therapy is 5 to 14 days; in case of prior sensitization (exposure to heparins within the past 100 days) and re-exposure, skin lesions appear within 3 to 5 days. Functional assays (serotonin-release test or platelet activation test) and antigen assays (ELISA) may confirm the clinical diagnosis of HIT.[32]

Heparin-induced skin necrosis is the cutaneous manifestation of HIT.[33–36] Typically, painful and mildly infiltrated erythema is followed by a central bullous and necrotic area surrounded by a hemorrhagic rim (see **Fig. 2**B). Skin necrosis as a symptom of HIT is not always restricted to heparin application sites but may also occur at distant sites, with a predilection for locations with increased subcutaneous fat tissue, such as mammae, abdomen, buttocks, and thighs. Skin biopsy of typical lesions shows thrombosis of skin vessels without signs of vasculitis. In case of suspected HIT, immediate discontinuation of heparin treatment is required and alternative compounds, such as danaparoid or hirudins, are indicated for treatment of thromboembolic complications.[37,38] Re-exposure to heparins has to be strictly avoided in the future. Similar clinical and histologic features may be observed for coumarin-induced skin necrosis.[39–41]

In the beginning of 2008, the Centers for Disease Control and Prevention (CDC) registered a cluster of heparin-associated allergy-like reactions. Among patients receiving UFH during hemodialysis, reactions included dyspnea, facial edema, urticaria, nausea or vomiting, tachycardia and hypotension, and life-threatening shock. In addition to dermatan sulfate, a known contaminant of heparin, spectroscopy identified oversulfated chondroitin sulfate (OSCS) in tested samples of one heparin manufacturer.[42] Although chondroitin sulfate is a natural substance derived from animal cartilage, its oversulfated form (ie, OSCS) does not occur naturally. OSCS exerts its effects by activation of the kinin-kallikrein system, leading to generation of bradykinin, and by activation of C3a and C5a, which are potent anaphylatoxins.[43,44] The contaminated heparin could be traced back to China, where heparins are regularly processed by small and often unregistered plants. Until now, however, it has not been clearly elucidated where the contamination had occurred.

ALLERGOLOGIC WORKUP

Patients referred to the authors' department with suspected DTH to heparins are consecutively subjected to an allergologic workup, including skin tests and subcutaneous challenge tests. In cases in which DTH to heparins is verified, intravenous challenge tests are performed (**Fig. 3**). As part of the standard practice in the authors' allergy clinic, all patients are informed of any risks involved with the testing and written informed consent for allergologic workup (skin tests and challenge tests) is obtained.

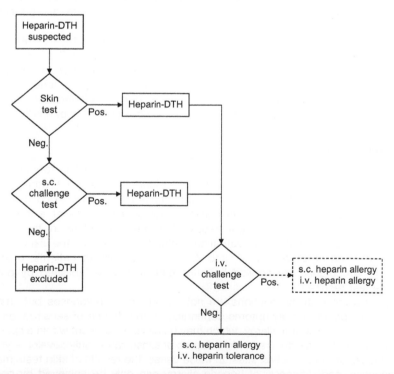

Fig. 3. Recommended steps of the allergologic workup in patients with a history of DTH to subcutaneously injected heparins. The diagnosis in case of a positive intravenous challenge test result is depicted in dotted lines because this has not occurred in our studies, in which all patients tolerated intravenous challenge tests. i.v., intravenous; Pos., positive; Neg., negative; s.c., subcutaneous.

Skin Tests

The authors perform intradermal tests on the volar forearm and patch tests on the back with a panel of heparin and heparinoid preparations, including UFH and the LMWHs nadroparin, dalteparin, and enoxaparin; the heparinoids danaparoid and pentosan polysulfate; and fondaparinux (**Table 1**). For intradermal tests, heparin preparations are used in a 1:10 dilution (using sodium chloride 0.9% solution). Patch tests are performed after tape stripping for better antigen penetration with pure heparin solutions.[45] Allergologic testing of patients with a panel of different heparin preparations can reveal cross-reactivity among heparins and exclude a causal role of preservatives sometimes added to heparin multidose products, such as sodium metabisulfite, benzyl alcohol, or chlorocresol. Most single-dose heparin products contain salts, acids, or bases for pH adjustment but no preservatives (see **Table 1**). Skin tests are read on days 2, 3, and 4 according to the 1+ to 3+ scoring system recommended by the International Contact Dermatitis Research Group. The 2+ to 3+ reactions can be considered unequivocally positive. In approximately 60% of all cases, crescendo reactions to skin tests develop only after 3 to 4 days. Therefore, skin tests should be read for at least 4 days. In 70% to 80% of all patients, allergy to heparins may be diagnosed by skin tests alone. Frequently, several positive test reactions throughout the panel of UFH and LMWH may be observed. Single negative skin test reactions are usually false-negative, and subsequent subcutaneous challenge usually proves cross-reactivity. Overall, correctly performed skin tests with heparins are safe, and generalized reactions usually do not occur.

Immediate-type reactions may be observed in approximately 10% of intradermal tests despite the 1:10 dilution of testing solutions; in most cases, they are attributable to histamine liberation of heparin, and therefore should not be interpreted naively as proof of an IgE-mediated allergy. Anaphylactic reactions or immediate-type skin test reactions may also be caused by accidental or deliberate contaminants (eg, histamine, OSCS) during the processing of heparins.[42,43,46]

Subcutaneous Challenge

All challenge tests should be performed and interpreted according to international standards by experienced allergologists.[47,48] Mandatory is strict adherence to contraindications, side effects, and drug interactions of heparins. In case of negative skin test results, subcutaneous challenge tests of heparins at a therapeutic dosage are indicated. The subcutaneous challenge procedure in the authors' department is performed in an outpatient setting. Reading of the skin injection site is performed on days 2, 3, 4, and 7. In 20% to 30% of patients, diagnosis of DTH to subcutaneously applied heparins can only be established by positive challenge test results.

Allergic hypersensitivity reactions are not "all or none" responses but, instead, present as a spectrum of symptoms depending on the degree of sensitization. This is also the case for heparin allergy, which may be clinically present within a spectrum of symptoms. Patients with a rather low degree of sensitization only develop erythematous plaques around injection sites. In these cases, the results of skin tests may be false-negative, and diagnosis of heparin allergy can only be achieved by positive subcutaneous challenge test results. Strong sensitization presents clinically as a pronounced local eczematous reaction, and continuation of heparin injections in such cases may lead to development of a generalized eczema. Skin tests in these cases usually show at least 2+, and sometimes 3+, reactions.

Table 1
Panel of heparins and heparinoids tested in the authors' allergy clinic

Heparins/Heparinoids	Product	Preservatives, Additives for pH Adjustment
Heparin sodium (UFH)	Heparin-natrium-5000 ratiopharm (ratiopharm, Ulm, Germany)	None
Nadroparin calcium	Fraxiparin-0.3 (GlaxoSmithKline, München, Germany)	Calcium hydroxide, hydrochloric acid
Dalteparin sodium	Fragmin/D (Pharmacia, Karlsruhe, Germany)	Sodium chloride
Enoxaparin sodium	Clexane-40 mg (Sanofi-Aventis, Frankfurt, Germany)	None
Danaparoid sodium	Orgaran (Organon, Oberschleissheim, Germany)	Sodium metabisulfite, sodium chloride, hydrochloric acid
Pentosan polysulfate sodium	Fibrezym (bene Arzneimittel, München, Germany)	Levulinic acid, sodium chloride
Fondaparinux sodium	Arixtra-2.5 mg (GlaxoSmithKline, München, Germany)	Sodium chloride, hydrochloric acid, sodium hydroxide

Intravenous Challenge

In the authors' department, intravenous challenge is a standardized procedure using UFH (5000 IU heparin-natrium/0.5 mL). On day 1, patients receive an intravenously administered bolus of 2500 IU. On day 2, another bolus of 2500 IU is administered, followed by intravenous administration of 7500 IU over a period of 6 hours. A time interval of at least 6 weeks between positive skin test results or positive subcutaneous challenge test results and intravenous challenge tests should be strictly adhered to.

HEPARIN ALLERGY: SUBCUTANEOUS ALLERGY AND INTRAVENOUS TOLERANCE

In case of DTH to subcutaneously injected heparin, intravenous application of this drug theoretically implies the risk for a generalized eczematous reaction. Evidence that intravenous administration of heparin is tolerated despite DTH was previously observed in single patients, however.[8,10,49,50] In two prospective studies, the authors demonstrated that intravenous administration of heparin was well tolerated without side effects in 64 patients who developed eczema-like infiltrated plaques after subcutaneous injection of heparin.[11,13] Therefore, intravenous application of heparin is a safe alternative for anticoagulation in these patients. Furthermore, in case of therapeutic necessity, the shift from subcutaneous to intravenous heparin administration without prior tests may be justified even in cases with generalized eczema.[12]

Currently it is unknown, why some patients initialize an immune reaction after subcutaneous application of UFH and LMWH, whereas intravenous administration of heparin is well tolerated. Eczematous plaques after subcutaneously injected heparins are likely real DTH caused by heparin-specific T lymphocytes. Subtle differences in the absorption of heparin from the skin and differential processing or presentation of antigens depending on the route of application may be the responsible factors. In addition to its traditional anticoagulant activity, anti-inflammatory effects of heparin have been described.[51] It has been shown that UFH and, to a lesser extent, LMWH down-regulate L-selectin.[52] Because L-selectin has a crucial role in lymphocyte homing, this effect may therefore inhibit the migration of activated T cells, preventing clinically obvious inflammation.

In case of premature intravenous challenge tests performed less than 4 to 6 weeks after positive skin testing results, flare-up reactions at previously positive skin testing sites may develop. A single reported case of generalized eczema after intravenous heparin challenge tests may have been attributable to a too short interval between a positive skin test or positive subcutaneous challenge test result and intravenous challenge.[53] This observation supports the hypothesis that depot effects may play an important pathogenic role. Alternatively, intravenous heparin administration may activate residual specific T lymphocytes in skin test areas, similar to mechanisms discussed for fixed drug eruptions.

CROSS-REACTIVITY AND ALTERNATIVE ANTICOAGULATION

Typical for DTH against subcutaneously administered heparins is the extensive cross-reactivity between all UFH and LMWH. Potential alternative antithrombotic compounds are the heparinoids danaparoid and pentosan polysulfate.[54] Heparinoids were initially developed as alternatives in case of antibody-mediated HIT. Although danaparoid indeed shows low cross-reactivity with heparin in terms of heparin-induced antibody binding, it may cross-react with heparin in case of DTH. Heparinoids sometimes have negative skin test results. Most of these test results are false-negative, however, and in subcutaneous challenge tests, skin lesions also develop after heparinoid application because of cross-reactivity. Tolerance of a single challenge test should also not be overinterpreted. Several of the authors' patients also developed eczematous plaques around injection sites despite an initial negative subcutaneous challenge test result to heparinoids after a longer anticoagulation period and increasing number of heparinoid injections. As already suggested by the chemical structure, cross-reactivity between heparinoids and heparins is quite common.[26]

Previously, fondaparinux was considered another potential alternative anticoagulant compound.[55,56] In one of the authors' studies,[11] however, positive skin test results with fondaparinux were observed in 6 of 16 patients with DTH to subcutaneously applied heparins. Meanwhile, several studies confirmed that only up to 50% of patients with DTH to subcutaneous heparins tolerate fondaparinux.[57–60] This is not surprising because fondaparinux is an anionic polysaccharide like heparin; therefore, cross-reactivity develops after continued anticoagulation for a longer period despite initial tolerance of the compound in skin and subcutaneous challenge tests.

Because of their completely different chemical structure, hirudins are the only safe alternative for subcutaneously applied anticoagulation. Available for clinical use are recombinant hirudins, including lepirudin, desirudin, bivalirudin, and other direct thrombin inhibitors, such as argatroban. Because of the lack of antidotes for neutralization, application of these compounds is always associated with increased risk for bleeding complications. Lepirudin is indicated for treatment of thromboembolic complications and HIT.[61] In Germany, desirudin, bivalirudin, and argatroban are only approved for limited indications: desirudin is approved for prophylaxis of deep vein thrombosis after hip and knee replacement surgery, whereas bivalirudin is indicated as an anticoagulant in patients undergoing percutaneous coronary intervention. Argatroban is approved for anticoagulation in patients who have HIT. Despite approval of these new anticoagulants (direct thrombin inhibitors, Xa-inhibitors), heparin remains the medication of first choice, especially for intravenous anticoagulation.[16]

CONCLUDING REMARKS

- DTH reactions to subcutaneously injected heparins are relatively common and clinically present as erythematous or eczematous plaques restricted to the injection site. In case of continuation of heparin injections, there is a risk for generalized eczema or exanthema.
- The most important differential diagnosis of DTH to subcutaneous heparins is heparin-induced skin necrosis, the leading cutaneous symptom of HIT.
- For diagnosis of DTH to subcutaneous heparins, a step-by-step allergologic workup, including skin and subcutaneous challenge tests, is a safe procedure with a high predictive value when performed and interpreted by experienced allergologists.
- Extensive cross-reactivity among different heparins is the rule, including all UFH and LMWH preparations of all manufacturers.
- Heparinoids (eg, danaparoid, pentosan polysulfate) or fondaparinux, as anionic polysaccharides, are not suitable alternative substances in most cases. Because of their similar chemical structure, cross-reactivity is likely, especially if prolonged treatment periods are necessary.
- The only safe alternative compounds are thrombin inhibitors (eg, lepirudin, desirudin, bivalirudin). In case of DTH reactions to subcutaneously injected heparin, diagnostic testing of these compounds before application is not necessary.

- In patients with hypersensitivity reactions to subcutaneously injected heparin, intravenous challenge tests usually demonstrate intravenous tolerance. The risk for a generalized reaction after intravenous application appears to be minimal. However, substantial uncertainty still exists as to whether intravenous administration is really safe in all these patients.
- In clinical practice, there is frequently no time for the recommended complex and time-consuming allergologic workup. In case of therapeutic necessity, the shift from subcutaneous to intravenous heparin administration without prior allergologic tests may be justified according to current data.

REFERENCES

1. Harenberg J, Hoffmann U, Huhle G, et al. Cutaneous reactions to anticoagulants. Recognition and management. Am J Clin Dermatol 2001;2:69–75.
2. Harr T, Scherer K, Tsakiris DA, et al. Immediate type hypersensitivity to low molecular weight heparins and tolerance of unfractioned heparin and fondaparinux. Allergy 2006;61:787–8.
3. Rajka G, Skog E. On the question of heparin hypersensitivity. Acta Derm Venereol 1962;42:27–34.
4. Trautmann A, Hamm K, Bröcker EB, et al. [Delayed hypersensitivity to heparins. Clinical signs, diagnosis, therapeutic alternatives]. Z Hautkr 1997;72:447–50 [in German].
5. Bircher AJ, Flückiger R, Buchner SA. Eczematous infiltrated plaques to subcutaneous heparin: a type IV allergic reaction. Br J Dermatol 1990;123:507–14.
6. Klein GF, Kofler H, Wolf H, et al. Eczema-like, erythematous, infiltrated plaques: a common side effect of subcutaneous heparin therapy. J Am Acad Dermatol 1989;21:703–7.
7. Bircher AJ, Harr T, Hohenstein L, et al. Hypersensitivity reactions to anticoagulant drugs: diagnosis and management options. Allergy 2006;61:1432–40.
8. Boehncke WH, Weber L, Gall H. Tolerance to intravenous administration of heparin and heparinoid in a patient with delayed-type hypersensitivity to heparins and heparinoids. Contact Dermatitis 1996;35:73–5.
9. Irion R, Gall H, Peter RU. Delayed-type hypersensitivity to heparin with tolerance of its intravenous administration. Contact Dermatitis 2000;43:249–50.
10. Trautmann A, Bröcker EB, Klein CE. Intravenous challenge with heparins in patients with delayed-type skin reactions after subcutaneous administration of the drug. Contact Dermatitis 1998;39:43–4.
11. Gaigl Z, Klein CE, Großmann R, et al. [Managing allergy to heparins]. Dtsch Arztebl 2006;103:2877–81 [in German].
12. Seitz CS, Bröcker EB, Trautmann A. Management of allergy to heparins in postoperative care: subcutaneous allergy and intravenous tolerance. Dermatol Online J 2008;14(9):4.
13. Gaigl Z, Pfeuffer P, Raith P, et al. Tolerance to intravenous heparin in patients with delayed-type hypersensitivity to heparins: a prospective study. Br J Haematol 2005;128:389–92.
14. Hirsh J, Warkentin TE, Shaughnessy SG, et al. Heparin and low-molecular-weight heparin: mechanisms of action, pharmacokinetics, dosing, monitoring, efficacy, and safety. Chest 2001;119:64–94.
15. Blann AD, Landray MJ, Lip GY. ABC of antithrombotic therapy: an overview of antithrombotic therapy. BMJ 2002;325:762–5.
16. Hyers TM. Management of venous thromboembolism: past, present, and future. Arch Intern Med 2003;163:759–68.

17. Geerts WH, Bergqvist D, Pineo GF, et al. Prevention of venous thromboembolism: American College of Chest Physicians evidence-based clinical practice guidelines (8th edition). Chest 2008;133:381–453.
18. Keam SJ, Goa KL. Fondaparinux sodium. Drugs 2002;62:1673–85.
19. Weitz JI, Crowther M. Direct thrombin inhibitors. Thromb Res 2002;106:275–84.
20. Guillet G, Delaire P, Plantin P, et al. Eczema as a complication of heparin therapy. J Am Acad Dermatol 1989;20:1130–2.
21. Korstanje MJ, Bessems PJ, Hardy E, et al. Delayed-type hypersensitivity reaction to heparin. Contact Dermatitis 1989;20:383–4.
22. Kim KH, Lynfield Y. Enoxaparin-induced generalized exanthem. Cutis 2003;72: 57–60.
23. Patrizi A, DiLernia V, Patrone P. Generalized reaction to subcutaneous heparin. Contact Dermatitis 1989;20:309–10.
24. Greiner D, Schöfer H. [Allergic drug exanthema to heparin. Cutaneous reactions to high molecular and fractionated heparin]. Hautarzt 1994;45:569–72 [in German].
25. Estrada Rodriguez JL, Gozalo RF, Ortiz U, et al. Generalized eczema induced by nadroparin. J Investig Allergol Clin Immunol 2003;13:69–70.
26. Grassegger A, Fritsch P, Reider N. Delayed-type hypersensitivity and cross-reactivity to heparins and danaparoid: a prospective study. Dermatol Surg 2001;27: 47–52.
27. Mendez J, Sanchis ME, de la Fuente R, et al. Delayed-type hypersensitivity to subcutaneous enoxaparin. Allergy 1998;53:999–1003.
28. Kroon C, de Boer A, Kroon JM, et al. Influence of skinfold thickness on heparin absorption. Lancet 1991;337:945–6.
29. James RF. Rectus sheath haematoma. Lancet 2005;365:1824.
30. Greinacher A, Warkentin TE. Recognition, treatment, and prevention of heparin-induced thrombocytopenia: review and update. Thromb Res 2006;118:165–79.
31. Warkentin TE, Greinacher A. Heparin-induced thrombocytopenia: recognition, treatment, and prevention: the Seventh ACCP Conference on Antithrombotic and Thrombolytic Therapy. Chest 2004;126:311–37.
32. Eichler P, Raschke R, Lubenow N, et al. The new ID-heparin/PF4 antibody test for rapid detection of heparin-induced antibodies in comparison with functional and antigenic assays. Br J Haematol 2002;116:887–91.
33. Warkentin TE, Roberts RS, Hirsh J, et al. Heparin-induced skin lesions and other unusual sequelae of the heparin-induced thrombocytopenia syndrome: a nested cohort study. Chest 2005;127:1857–61.
34. Yates P, Jones S. Heparin skin necrosis—an important indicator of potentially fatal heparin hypersensitivity. Clin Exp Dermatol 1993;18:138–41.
35. Shelley WB, Sayen JJ. Heparin necrosis: an anticoagulant-induced cutaneous infarct. J Am Acad Dermatol 1982;7:674–7.
36. Balestra B. [Skin necrosis: a paradoxical complication of anticoagulation]. Schweiz Med Wochenschr 1995;125:361–4 [in German].
37. Hirsh J, Heddle N, Kelton JG. Treatment of heparin-induced thrombocytopenia: a critical review. Arch Intern Med 2004;164:361–9.
38. Alving BM. How I treat heparin-induced thrombocytopenia and thrombosis. Blood 2003;101:31–7.
39. Argaud L, Guerin C, Thomas L, et al. Extensive coumarin-induced skin necrosis in a patient with acquired protein C deficiency. Intensive Care Med 2001;27:1555.
40. Wattiaux MJ, Herve R, Robert A, et al. Coumarin-induced skin necrosis associated with acquired protein S deficiency and antiphospholipid antibody syndrome. Arthritis Rheum 1994;37:1096–100.

41. Bauer KA. Coumarin-induced skin necrosis. Arch Dermatol 1993;129:766–8.
42. Guerrini M, Beccati D, Shriver Z, et al. Oversulfated chondroitin sulfate is a contaminant in heparin associated with adverse clinical events. Nat Biotechnol 2008;26:669–75.
43. Kishimoto TK, Viswanathan K, Ganguly T, et al. Contaminated heparin associated with adverse clinical events and activation of the contact system. N Engl J Med 2008;358:2457–67.
44. Blossom DB, Kallen AJ, Patel PR, et al. Outbreak of adverse reactions associated with contaminated heparin. N Engl J Med 2008;359:2674–84.
45. Oldhoff JM, Bihari IC, Knol EF, et al. Atopy patch test in patients with atopic eczema/dermatitis syndrome: comparison of petrolatum and aqueous solution as a vehicle. Allergy 2004;59:451–6.
46. Hermann K, Frank G, Ring J. Contamination of heparin by histamine: measurement and characterization by high-performance liquid chromatography and radioimmunoassay. Allergy 1994;49:569–72.
47. Demoly P, Bousquet J. Drug allergy diagnosis work up. Allergy 2002;57:37–40.
48. Aberer W, Bircher A, Romano A, et al. Drug provocation testing in the diagnosis of drug hypersensitivity reactions: general considerations. Allergy 2003;58:854–63.
49. Liew G, Campbell C, Thursby P. Delayed-type hypersensitivity to subcutaneous heparin with tolerance of i.v. administration. ANZ J Surg 2004;74:1020–1.
50. Jappe U, Reinhold D, Bonnekoh B. Arthus reaction to lepirudin, a new recombinant hirudin, and delayed-type hypersensitivity to several heparins and heparinoids, with tolerance to its intravenous administration. Contact Dermatitis 2002;46:29–32.
51. Tyrrell DJ, Horne AP, Holme KR, et al. Heparin in inflammation: potential therapeutic applications beyond anticoagulation. Adv Pharmacol 1999;46:151–208.
52. Derhaschnig U, Pernerstorfer T, Knechtelsdorfer M, et al. Evaluation of antiinflammatory and antiadhesive effects of heparins in human endotoxemia. Crit Care Med 2003;31:1108–12.
53. Schiffner R, Glassl A, Landthaler M, et al. Tolerance of desirudin in a patient with generalized eczema after intravenous challenge with heparin and a delayed-type skin reaction to high and low molecular weight heparins and heparinoids. Contact Dermatitis 2000;42:49.
54. Lindhoff-Last E, Kreutzenbeck HJ, Magnani HN. Treatment of 51 pregnancies with danaparoid because of heparin intolerance. Thromb Haemost 2005;93:63–9.
55. Ludwig RJ, Beier C, Lindhoff-Last E, et al. Tolerance of fondaparinux in a patient allergic to heparins and other glycosaminoglycans. Contact Dermatitis 2003;49: 158–9.
56. Ludwig RJ, Schindewolf M, Alban S, et al. Molecular weight determines the frequency of delayed type hypersensitivity reactions to heparin and synthetic oligosaccharides. Thromb Haemost 2005;94:1265–9.
57. Utikal J, Peitsch WK, Booken D, et al. Hypersensitivity to the pentasaccharide fondaparinux in patients with delayed-type heparin allergy. Thromb Haemost 2005;94:895–6.
58. Hirsch K, Ludwig RJ, Lindhoff-Last E, et al. Intolerance of fondaparinux in a patient allergic to heparins. Contact Dermatitis 2004;50:383–4.
59. Hohenstein E, Tsakiris D, Bircher AJ. Delayed-type hypersensitivity to the ultra-low-molecular-weight heparin fondaparinux. Contact Dermatitis 2004;51:149–51.
60. Maetzke J, Hinrichs R, Staib G, et al. Fondaparinux as a novel therapeutic alternative in a patient with heparin allergy. Allergy 2004;59:237–8.
61. Kam PC, Kaur N, Thong CL. Direct thrombin inhibitors: pharmacology and clinical relevance. Anaesthesia 2005;60:565–74.

The Variable Clinical Picture of Drug-Induced Hypersensitivity Syndrome / Drug Rash with Eosinophilia and Systemic Symptoms in Relation to the Eliciting Drug

Yoko Kano, MD, PhD*, Tetsuo Shiohara, MD, PhD

KEYWORDS

- Anticonvulsant hypersensitivity syndrome
- Drug-induced hypersensitivity syndrome
- Drug rash with eosinophilia and systemic symptoms
- Eosinophilia • Human herpesvirus 6
- Liver dysfunction • Skin rash

Drug-hypersensitivity syndrome is a life-threatening adverse reaction characterized by skin rashes, fever, leukocytosis with eosinophilia or atypical lymphocytosis, lymph node enlargement, and liver or renal dysfunctions.[1] The syndrome develops 2 to 6 weeks or longer after initiation of administration of a specific drug. It has been estimated to occur in between 1 in 1000 and 1 in 10,000 exposures with antiepileptic drugs.[2] Mortality is approximately 10% and is primarily associated with systemic organ involvement, such as liver dysfunction, renal impairment, and interstitial pneumonitis.[3] Previously, there had been no consistent term for this syndrome; various

This work was supported in part by grants from the Ministry of Education, Sports, Science, and Culture of Japan (to Y.K. and T.S.) and Health and Labo Sciences Research grants from the Ministry of Health, Labor, and Welfare of Japan (to T.S.).

Department of Dermatology, Kyorin University School of Medicine, 6-20-2 Shinkawa Mitaka, Tokyo, 181-8611, Japan

* Corresponding author.

E-mail address: kano@ks.kyorin-u.ac.jp (Y. Kano).

Immunol Allergy Clin N Am 29 (2009) 481–501

doi:10.1016/j.iac.2009.04.007

0889-8561/09/$ – see front matter © 2009 Elsevier Inc. All rights reserved.

immunology.theclinics.com

terms had been used to refer to this syndrome after generic names of the culprit drugs or the pathophysiologic consequence, such as *phenytoin syndrome*, *allopurinol hypersensitivity syndrome*, *dapsone syndrome*, *eosinophilic pneumonia*, and *exfoliative dermatitis*. All these entities may represent different clinicopathologic expressions of a single pathologic process. Bocquet and colleagues[4] proposed the term *drug rash with eosinophilia and systemic symptoms* (DRESS) to simplify the nomenclature of drug-hypersensitivity syndromes. Then, Descamps and colleagues,[5] the authors' group,[6] and Hashimoto's group[7] demonstrated a relation between this drug reaction and human herpesvirus (HHV)-6 reactivation. Subsequently, the authors' group and Hashimoto's group coined the term *drug-induced hypersensitivity syndrome* (DIHS) to reflect the association with HHV-6.[8,9] There have been no significant differences in the clinical findings of cases reported under the name of DRESS or DIHS, although it seems that patients fulfilling the criteria of DIHS may represent those with more severe DRESS. Although the reaction is caused by a limited number of drugs, there are some differences in the clinical and laboratory findings depending on the drug given, underlying physiologic state, and genetic background. It is useful to know these differences in clinical appearance depending on the causative drugs for the early diagnosis of this life-threatening adverse drug reaction. In this review, the authors have focused on the clinical picture of DIHS/DRESS in relation to different eliciting drugs.

DIAGNOSIS OF DRUG-INDUCED HYPERSENSITIVITY SYNDROME/DRUG RASH WITH EOSINOPHILIA AND SYSTEMIC SYMPTOMS

The criteria for the diagnosis of DRESS proposed by Bocquet and colleagues[4] are as follows: (1) cutaneous drug eruption; (2) hematologic abnormalities, including eosinophilia greater than 1.5×10^9 eosinophils/L or the presence of atypical lymphocytes; and (3) systemic involvement, including adenopathies greater than 2 cm in diameter, hepatitis (liver transaminases values >2 N), interstitial nephritis, interstitial pneumonia, or carditis. The criteria emphasize two important characteristics: multiple organ involvement and eosinophilia.[10]

The criteria for the diagnosis of DIHS established by the Japanese groups are as follows: (1) maculopapular rash developing longer than 3 weeks after starting a limited number of drugs; (2) prolonged clinical symptoms 2 weeks after discontinuation of the causative drug; (3) fever higher than 38°C; (4) liver abnormalities (alanine aminotransferase [ALT] >100 U/L); (5) leukocyte abnormalities, including leukocytosis (>11 × 10^9 leukocytes/L), atypical lymphocytosis (>5%), or eosinophilia (>1.5×10^9 eosinophils/L); (6) lymphadenopathies; and (7) HHV-6 reactivation. Diagnosis of definite or typical DIHS requires the presence of the seven criteria. Probable or atypical DIHS is diagnosed in patients with typical clinical presentations (criteria 1–5) in whom HHV-6 reactivation cannot be detected, probably because of inappropriate timing of sampling. Renal dysfunction can serve as a substitute for liver abnormalities. Considering that HHV-6 reactivation is rarely detected in patients who develop a milder form of the disease, the detection of this viral reactivation is a useful marker for the diagnosis of DIHS.[9] The authors have recently demonstrated that various herpesvirus reactivations, in addition to HHV-6, contribute to internal organ involvement and the relapse of symptoms observed long after discontinuation of the causative drugs.[11] The criteria proposed by Bocquet and colleagues[4] are fundamentally similar to those of the authors with regard to the clinical and laboratory findings, except for HHV-6 reactivation. Using the authors' criteria, other types of drug reactions, such as the maculopapular-type drug eruption, Stevens-Johnson syndrome (SJS), and toxic epidermal necrolysis (TEN), can be differentiated from DIHS/DRESS. Differential diagnoses attributable to the most likely infectious diseases, such as measles and infectious mononucleosis, need to be excluded, however. Other differential diagnoses include Kawasaki syndrome, serum sickness-like reaction, hypereosinophilic syndrome, and drug-induced pseudolymphoma (**Box 1**).[4,12] Pseudolymphomas have also been reported to develop in association with phenytoin and carbamazepine (CBZ).[13,14] A diagnosis of drug-induced pseudolymphoma can be based on the histologic findings or the clinical presentation, ranging from solitary nodules to multiple infiltrative papules or plaques, without evidence of extracutaneous lymphoma, or resolution of the eruption with cessation of the drug.[15] The delay between the start of the drug and the eruption was up to 110 days, which is longer than that in DIHS/DRESS. No fever or multiple organ involvement is observed. Thus, the drug-induced pseudolymphomas represent a distinct entity from DIHS/DRESS, with different clinical and histologic features and outcomes.

The clinical features of this syndrome include the stepwise development of multiorgan failure and frequent deterioration of clinical signs, such as fever, skin rashes, and liver or renal dysfunction, occurring even after discontinuation of the causative drug.[12] Internal organ involvement, which can be asymptomatic, may occur even several months after the onset. It includes hepatitis, renal insufficiency, pneumonitis, myocarditis, and thyroiditis.[8–12] Recently, encephalitis[16] and type 1 diabetes mellitus[17] have been reported to develop during the course of DIHS/DRESS (**Box 2**). The highly variable waxing and waning nature of the clinical manifestations occurring in different organs is the most prominent feature of DIHS/DRESS. There is great variability in the target organs involved and in severity. Such variability allows for a delay in diagnosis, which can lead to significant morbidity. A recent survey of cases from the French Pharmacovigilance database and the literature revealed particular clinical patterns in DIHS/DRESS caused by certain drugs (eg, renal dysfunction was associated with allopurinol-induced DRESS/DIHS, peripheral lymphadenopathy and eosinophilic pneumopathy in cases with minocycline, and, only rarely, eosinophilia with lamotrigine).[18]

In this article, the authors have included cases that were reported using various denominations, most of which fulfill their criteria for DIHS or the criteria of Bocquet and colleagues[4] for DRESS.

CHARACTERISTICS OF THE CAUSATIVE DRUGS

DIHS/DRESS is caused by a limited number of specific drugs, such as anticonvulsants, allopurinol, and sulfonamides. **Box 3** lists drugs that reportedly cause DIHS/DRESS. It remains unknown, however, why a limited number of drugs can cause

---

Box 1
Differential diagnosis in DIHS/DRESS

Drug-induced lupus erythematosus

Hypereosinophilic syndrome

Infectious mononucleosis

Kawasaki disease

Measles

Pseudolymphoma/immunoblastic lymphadenopathy

Serum sickness-like reaction

Staphylococcal toxic shock syndrome

> **Box 2**
> **Internal organ involvement in DIHS/DRESS**
>
> Colitis/Intestinal bleeding
> Diabetes mellitus
> Encephalitis/aseptic meningitis
> Hepatitis
> Interstitial nephritis
> Interstitial pneumonitis/respiratory distress syndrome
> Myocarditis
> Serositis
> Syndrome of inappropriate secretion of antidiuretic hormone
> Thyroiditis

the development of DIHS/DRESS because they do not have any pharmacologic actions or structural similarities in common.

Various factors may contribute to the development of DIHS/DRESS. The authors have demonstrated that there is a decrease in serum immunoglobulin levels, including IgG and IgA, and of circulating B cells at onset in patients who have anticonvulsant[19] and allopurinol[20] hypersensitivity syndromes. Several reports have also demonstrated a transient hypogammaglobulinemia at the onset of DIHS/DRESS.[21] More importantly, these drugs have been shown to inhibit B-cell differentiation to immunoglobulin-producing cells in vitro when purified B-cell populations were used.[22,23] Taken together, the causative drugs of DIHS/DRESS may have a pharmacologically mediated immunomodulatory effect on B cells and possibly other cells of the immune system, and thus contribute to the development of DIHS/DRESS. The long latency period before the onset of DIHS/DRESS after starting therapy with causative drugs would represent the time required for immunoglobulin levels to decrease to lower than a threshold level. During the course of DIHS/DRESS, a variety of antiviral T cells

> **Box 3**
> **Causative drugs of DIHS/DRESS**
>
> Anticonvulsant
> CBZ
> Phenytoin
> Phenobarbital
> Zonisamide
> Lamotrigine
> Allopurinol
> Minocycline
> Dapsone
> Sulfasalazine
> Mexiletine

are generated that may cross-react with the culprit drug; human leukocyte antigen (HLA) molecules are thereby reactivated, and thus play a key role in mediating DIHS/DRESS, similar to graft-versus-host disease.[24] These immunologic alterations occur initially subclinically, induced by the protracted administration of the causative drug, and may then lead to the development of DIHS/DRESS by means of sequential reactivations of herpesviruses.

CLINICAL PICTURE OF DRUG-INDUCED HYPERSENSITIVITY SYNDROME/DRUG RASH WITH EOSINOPHILIA AND SYSTEMIC SYMPTOMS INDUCED BY DIFFERENT ELICITING DRUGS
Aromatic Anticonvulsants

Anticonvulsant hypersensitivity syndrome is a life-threatening syndrome that occurs after exposure to aromatic anticonvulsants, including CBZ, phenytoin, and phenobarbital. The incidence of this syndrome induced by these anticonvulsants is thought to be in the range of 1 per 1000 to 10,000 exposures.[2] Cross-reactivity between CBZ, phenytoin, and phenobarbital may be as high as 70% to 80%;[25] this may explain why symptoms persist or recur after switching to another aromatic anticonvulsant. In addition, there is a familial tendency to hypersensitivity to anticonvulsants; this is not related to the dosage or serum concentration of these drugs. The frequency of this reaction is higher with CBZ and phenytoin than with phenobarbital, which may reflect a greater use of the two former agents.

Although SJS and TEN are often regarded in the literature as the most severe form of drug eruptions induced by these anticonvulsants, these two drug eruptions are not extensively reviewed in this article.

Carbamazepine
CBZ is an iminostilbene derivative chemically related to the tricyclic antidepressants. CBZ is currently the primary drug used for the treatment of partial and tonic-clonic seizures.[26] The drug is also effective in treating pain of neurologic origin and psychiatric disorders, such as bipolar affective disorders and schizophrenia. These numerous uses of CBZ explain the widespread utilization of the drug. Cutaneous adverse effects, such as erythematous rashes, urticaria, pruritus, or alopecia, are not unusual with the use of CBZ.[27] More serious adverse reactions, such as SJS, TEN, and DIHS/DRESS, may occur. Of these three aromatic anticonvulsants, CBZ is the most commonly implicated drug for DIHS/DRESS because of the frequency of use. Therefore, the clinical and laboratory findings of CBZ-induced DIHS/DRESS (CBZ-DIHS/DRESS) are the major prototype of this syndrome.

CBZ-DIHS/DRESS is a severe reaction characterized by skin rash, fever, leukocytosis with eosinophilia or atypical lymphocytosis, lymph node enlargement, and liver or renal dysfunction, as described in the previous section. According to the authors' analyses, the mean interval between drug intake and onset is 36.8 days (**Table 1**). In some cases, the interval was longer than 6 months. It is likely that the time interval between drug intake and onset is longer for phenobarbital.[25] The initial symptoms of CBZ-DIHS/DRESS include general fatigue, low-grade fever, and sore throat, any of which can precede cutaneous manifestations by 1 to 4 days. This stage is usually interpreted as an upper respiratory infection by most patients. Maculopapular rashes, which are frequently accompanied by facial and neck edema, tend to appear first over the trunk and face and spread to the proximal upper extremities. Marked periorbital edema is frequently observed, which is a characteristic cutaneous manifestation of DIHS/DRESS (**Fig. 1**). Small crusts and scales along the nasolabial sulci are often observed at the initial stage. The maculopapular rashes coalesce to form larger plaques and often progress to diffuse erythema over the trunk with a high-grade fever

Table 1
Clinical characteristics in relation to causative drugs

	Carbamazepine	Phenytoin	Phenobarbital	Allopurinol	Minocycline	Dapsone	Mexiletine
	36.8 (n = 8)	40.5 (n = 2)	31.7 (n = 4)	32.2 (n = 4)	(n = 0)	19.0 (n = 1)	32.6 (n = 3)
Duration[a]							
Skin eruption Facial edema	++	++	++	++	++	+	++
Others	Maculopapular EM-like Purpuric Exfoliative	Maculopapular EM-like Purpuric	Maculopapular EM-like Purpuric Pustular Exfoliative	Maculopapular EM-like Pustular Exfoliative	Maculopapular EM-like Pustular Exfoliative	Maculopapular Exfoliative	Maculopapular EM-like Pustular Exfoliative
Leukocytosis	++	++	++	++	++	++	++
Eosinophilia	++	++	++	++	+++	+	++
Atypical lymphocytosis	++	++	+++	++	++	+++	+
Lymphadenopathy	++	++	+++	+	+++	+++	+
Liver dysfunction	++	+++	++	+	+++	+++	+
Renal dysfunction	+	+	+	+++	+	+	+
Pulmonary insufficiency	+	+	+	+	+++	+	+

Frequencies were described using scales ranging from + to +++.

Abbreviation: EM, erythema multiforme.

[a] Duration between initial drug intake and onset in the authors' analyses.

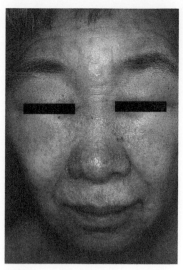

Fig. 1. Marked facial edema (CBZ).

(**Fig. 2**). Purpuric lesions are noted on the lower extremities (**Fig. 3**). This process can take several days after withdrawal of CBZ. Marked edema in the upper dermis over the upper extremities often gives rise to blisters, which may mimic those of TEN (**Fig. 4**). Mucosal involvement in buccal and genital regions is not frequently observed. Most mucosal lesions are hyperemic with petechia but resolve rapidly on withdrawal of the drug; this finding is in sharp contrast to those of SJS or TEN.

Histopathologic findings of a skin biopsy specimen obtained from maculopapular rashes at an early stage include exocytosis of lymphocytes in the epidermis and focal hydropic degeneration of the basal cell layer. A lymphocytic infiltrate containing eosinophils is often observed in the edematous papillary dermis. The cellular infiltration in the dermis is generally denser in DIHS/DRESS than in other types of drug reaction. Blister may be formed beneath the epidermis because of the prominent edema in the upper dermis. Histochemical staining of the skin lesion reveals that CD8+ cells are more frequently observed than CD4+ cells.

Bilateral cervical, axillary, and inguinal lymphadenopathies with tenderness are commonly present. Because of the severe lymphadenopathy and

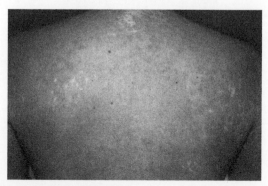

Fig. 2. Diffuse erythema on the back (CBZ).

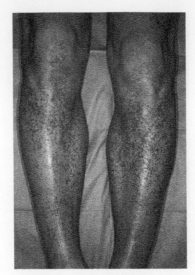

Fig. 3. Erythema with purpuric lesions on the legs (CBZ).

hepatosplenomegaly associated with the skin eruption, immunoblastic lymphadenopathy or pseudolymphoma is often suspected. The clinical and laboratory findings, showing skin rashes with facial edema, atypical lymphocytosis with severe lymphadenopathies, and hepatosplenomegaly, may mimic those of infectious mononucleosis. A lymph node biopsy may show paracortical hyperplasia and eosinophilia suggestive of dermatopathic lymphadenopathy or lymphadenitis.

Hematologic abnormalities, especially eosinophilia and mononucleosis-like atypical lymphocytosis, are common. Marked leukocytosis with eosinophilia or atypical lymphocytosis is observed at the acute stage, a finding different from that observed

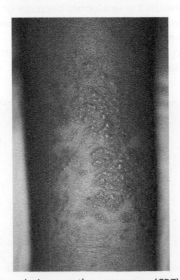

Fig. 4. Blisters on erythematous lesions on the upper arm (CBZ).

in SJS or TEN. Internal organ involvement is usually observed from 2 weeks to several months after discontinuation of CBZ and includes hepatitis, interstitial nephritis, interstitial lung disease, or myocardial involvement with or without any clinical symptoms.[10,25] The liver is the organ most frequently involved, ranging from mild elevation in transaminase levels to fulminant hepatic necrosis.[28] ALT levels are commonly increased more than three times the reference range. In most patients, aspartate aminotransferase (AST) and ALT levels increase more than those of γ-glutamyl transpeptidase (γ-GTP) and alkaline phosphatase (ALP); however, isolated elevation of γ-GTP may occur in the absence of actual liver disease. The renal failure in CBZ-DIHS/DRESS is considered to be attributable to acute interstitial nephritis. Acute interstitial nephritis is typically reversible after withdrawal of the causative agent.

Empiric treatment with antibiotics often exacerbates the clinical condition attributable to unexplained cross-reactivity to multiple drugs, which is a unique characteristic of this syndrome. CBZ-DIHS/DRESS requires immediate discontinuation of the drug. Valproic acid can usually be substituted with minimal concern for cross-reactivity but should be cautiously used for seizure control in the face of liver dysfunction. Recovery is usually slow, and it takes 3 to 8 weeks for skin rashes and all laboratory abnormalities to return to normal.

Phenytoin

Phenytoin (diphenylhydantoin) belongs to the hydantoin family, which includes mephenytoin, phenylethylhydantoin, and fosphenytoin. Phenytoin has been demonstrated to be a highly effective anticonvulsant in the treatment of generalized and focal epilepsy. A broad spectrum of cutaneous and immunologic reactions to phenytoin has been reported. These reactions include tissue proliferative syndromes, such as gingival hyperplasia and coarse facies, DIHS/DRESS, and a possible association with lymphoma. Although cutaneous eruptions occur in up to 19% of patients receiving phenytoin, only a small percentage of these patients experience phenytoin-induced DIHS/DRESS (phenytoin-DIHS/DRESS).[29]

Phenytoin-DIHS/DRESS usually occurs within 3 weeks to 3 months after initiation of therapy. The major manifestations of this syndrome include fever, dermatitis, hepatitis, and lymphadenopathy. Often, the initial symptoms are fever with malaise and pharyngitis, sometimes with strawberry tongue, followed by eruptions similar to those of CBZ-DIHS/DRESS.[29] The eruption usually begins as patchy erythema; it evolves into a typical pruritic maculopapular eruption (**Fig. 5**) and may later progress to become erythroderma. The eruption can manifest various types of skin rashes; they include infectious mononucleosis-like eruption, staphylococcal toxic shock syndrome-like exanthema, and a generalized pustular eruption. Prominent facial edema occurs periorbitally.[30] Anemia and diarrhea may also be present.[31]

Systemic involvement is common in phenytoin-DIHS/DRESS; the liver, kidney, lung, or central nervous system can be involved. According to Shear and Spielberg,[28] kidney involvement is more frequently observed in phenytoin-DIHS/DRESS compared with CBZ-DIHS/DRESS and phenobarbital-induced (PB) DIHS/DRESS. Although most patients who have phenytoin-DIHS/DRESS are initially anicteric, severe cholestatic hepatitis with jaundice and peripheral eosinophilia is sometimes observed (see **Table 1**). Severe hepatitis portends a prolonged course characterized by multiple exacerbations and remissions of the rash and liver disease. Most deaths occur from hepatic necrosis in the setting of coagulopathy, and sepsis and 30% to 40% mortality have been reported in such patients.[32] Other manifestations include hypothyroidism, which may occur within 2 months after onset of the syndrome.[29]

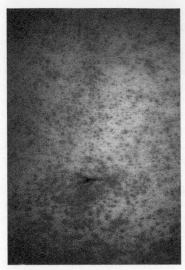

Fig. 5. Violaceous lesions on the trunk (phenytoin).

Phenobarbital

The clinical picture of PB-DIHS/DRESS is similar to CBZ-DHIS/DRESS or phenytoin-DIHS/DRESS. Skin eruptions vary, ranging from erythema multiforme-like (**Fig. 6**), pustular, and purpuric eruptions to exfoliative dermatitis. With pustular eruptions, pinhead-sized pustules are often superimposed on diffuse erythema of the face and trunk (**Fig. 7**). According to a report by Shear and Spielberg,[28] atypical lymphocytosis is detected more frequently in PB-DIHS/DRESS compared with CBZ-DHIS/DRESS or phenytoin-DIHS/DRESS (see **Table 1**). A case of PB-DIHS/DRESS was misdiagnosed as cutaneous T-cell lymphoma because prominent T-lymphocytosis (ie, lymphoid leukemoid reaction) was observed.[33]

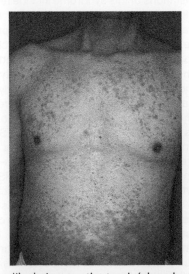

Fig. 6. Erythema multiforme-like lesions on the trunk (phenobarbital).

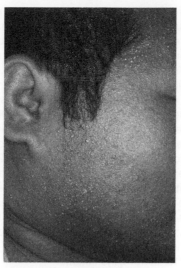

Fig. 7. Pustular eruption on the face (phenobarbital).

In some cases, systemic organ involvement is present in PB-DIHS/DRESS. For example, Descamps and colleagues[5] described a patient who had severe PB-DIHS/DRESS in whom a fulminant heamophagocytic syndrome associated with HHV-6 reactivation was noted. The authors also reported a case of syndrome of inappropriate secretion of antidiuretic hormone and limbic encephalitis associated with PB-DIHS/DRESS.[34] They also experienced a case of PB-DIHS/DRESS with an erythema multiforme-like eruption and severe prolonged liver dysfunction, in which various herpesvirus reactivations, including HHV-6, were observed. It has also been demonstrated that PB-DIHS/DRESS can share many clinical and laboratory findings with drug-induced lupus erythematosus, such as systemic involvement and serum immunologic abnormalities.[35]

Zonisamide

Zonisamide is an anticonvulsant that contains a sulfa moiety with potential to trigger hypersensitivity reactions. It displays similarity to sulfamethoxazole. The drug is generally regarded as a safe antiepileptic with minimal side effects. In the English literature, zonisamide-induced DIHS/DRESS has rarely been reported. According to the manufacturer, skin rash occurs in 1% to 2% of Japanese patients. Maculopapular and purpuric eruptions have been noted in addition to mild oral mucosal involvement. Teraki and colleagues[36] have recently reported a patient with clinical features of TEN attributable to zonisamide. In this case, however, significant increases in HHV-6 IgG titers and detection of HHV-6 DNA in leukocytes were observed during the course of the illness, indicating that HHV-6 reactivation occurred.

Lamotrigine

Lamotrigine is an antiepileptic drug that is structurally unrelated to aromatic anticonvulsants. It acts on voltage-sensitive sodium channels, stabilizes neuronal membranes, and inhibits the release of excitatory neurotransmitter glutamate or aspartate. The drug is considered effective for multiple types of seizures.[37] Despite a structural difference from the aromatic anticonvulsants, lamotrigine has been recently reported to cause a potentially life-threatening adverse drug reaction resembling DIHS/DRESS induced by these anticonvulsants.[38] It has been estimated that the incidence of potentially life-threatening skin reactions, such as DIHS/DRESS, occurs in 1 in 1000 adults treated with lamotrigine and in 1 in 50 to 100 children, which is higher than that associated with the aromatic anticonvulsants.[37] In addition to age, the risk for exanthema is strongly associated with high initial serum levels and with a rapid increase in doses of lamotrigine.[39] Conversely, slow introduction of the drug has been reported to reduce the incidence of rash. The risk for lamotrigine-induced DIHS/DRESS (lamotrigine-DIHS/DRESS) has also been attributed to valproic acid comedication.[37]

According to the analyses of 26 cases by Schlienger and colleagues,[40] eosinophilia was noted in 19%, lymphadenopathy was reported in only 12% of the cases, and multiorgan involvement was reported in 46%; these rates are markedly lower than in other anticonvulsant hypersensitivity syndromes. Clinically, in the severe form of lamotrigine-DIHS/DRESS, severe maculopapular exanthema, fever, lymphadenopathy, and internal organ involvement are observed; however, many of the reported cases represent an abortive form. Cutaneous eruption, usually severe, occurs typically within the first 4 weeks of treatment in approximately 10% of patients but has been reported to develop up to 6 months after lamotrigine initiation.[40]

Cutaneous findings include a polymorphous eruption consisting of blanchable, erythematous, urticarial papules predominantly on the trunk, which spread to the face but spare the palms. The face becomes severely edematous and erythematous. Mucous membranes are rarely involved. Tender, firm, enlarged lymph nodes are found in the cervical, axillary, and inguinal regions. Lymphadenopathy and hepatomegaly are commonly present. Early rechallenge with this drug may cause a quick reappearance of the symptoms in patients who have lamotrigine-DIHS/DRESS.[37] As far as the authors were able to determine, HHV-6 reactivation was not detected during the course of lamotrigine-DIHS/DRESS. It has been reported that an adult patient developed transient diffuse alopecia and transverse onychodystrophy of all nails after resolution of lamotrigine-DIHS/DRESS.[39]

Allopurinol

Allopurinol is an inhibitor of xanthine oxidase in clinical use. It is an effective urate-lowering drug that has been the mainstay treatment for hyperuremia and gout. The most serious side effects, which occur in less than 1 in 1000 cases, are exfoliative dermatitis, fever, liver dysfunction, eosinophilia, and acute interstitial nephritis (see **Table 1**). Numerous cases of allopurinol hypersensitivity syndrome have been reported. Up to 20% of patients with this type of reaction become extremely ill. According to Elasy and colleagues,[41] mortality is approximately 20% to 25%. Death is more likely to occur in patients who have preexisting renal disease or in those receiving diuretic therapy.[42] In more than 80% of cases of allopurinol-induced DIHS/DRESS (allopurinol-DIHS/DRESS), patients had evidence of renal impairment before commencing allopurinol.[43] Because renal function declines steadily with age, the elderly are most vulnerable to developing the reaction.[43] Other risk factors for the development of allopurinol DIHS/DRESS include chronic alcoholism and severe liver disease. Hung and colleagues[44] have recently reported a strong association between HLA-B*5801 allele and allopurinol-related severe cutaneous reactions, including DIHS/DRESS, SJS, and TEN. Although HLA-B* 5801 has been linked to the allopurinol-DIHS/DRESS in a series of Japanese patients, a strong association between HLA-B*5801 and Japanese patients who have allopurinol-DIHS/DRESS has not been detected in the authors' series.[45]

The average interval between onset of the syndrome and initiation of allopurinol treatment is 2 to 6 weeks, but it can be up to 728 days.[41,43] The rash may take the form of erythema multiforme, diffuse maculopapular rash (**Fig. 8**), or exfoliative dermatitis. A fine papular rash or erythema multiforme usually evolves to a diffuse maculopapular rash in association with facial edema and erythema (**Fig. 9**). Edema is often observed on the extremities. In severe cases, blisters on the hands and feet are observed with superficial ulceration, mimicking TEN; however, the lesions originate from the severe edema in the upper dermis and not from the epidermal necrosis. Erythematous skin lesions later desquamate. Occasionally, superficial oral ulcers are observed.

With respect to the hematologic findings, leukocytosis is often characterized by eosinophilia and by the presence of band forms without clear evidence of infection.[41,43]

Regarding visceral involvement, renal involvement is particularly observed in allopurinol-DIHS/DRESS. In many cases, laboratory studies demonstrate worsening renal insufficiency, ranging from mild elevation in serum creatinine levels to severe interstitial nephritis. Severe renal insufficiency increases the risk for mortality. In addition to renal involvement, there has been a reported case of HHV-6 encephalitis after reduction of systemic corticosteroids in a patient who had allopurinol-DIHS/DRESS.[13] Another case presented with a diffuse erythematous rash and erosive lesions, and the clinical course was complicated by cytomegalovirus and HHV-6 reactivation in addition to sepsis during the course of DIHS/DRESS.[46] Sommers and Schoene[47] reported that fulminant type 1 diabetes mellitus developed 1 month after the onset of allopurinol-DIHS/DRESS. The authors have experienced a case of allopurinol-DIHS/DRESS with intestinal bleeding accompanied by the appearance of urticarial eruptions and scratch dermatitis during cytomegalovirus reactivation in the course of DIHS/DRESS.

Minocycline

Minocycline is a semisynthetic tetracycline derivative commonly used to treat acne vulgaris that has antibiotic and anti-inflammatory activities. Serious adverse reactions

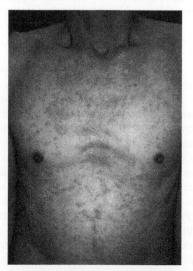

Fig. 8. Maculopapular eruption and erythema multiforme-like lesions on the trunk (allopurinol).

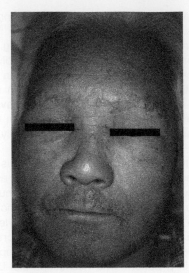

Fig. 9. Prominent facial edema (allopurinol).

include a serum sickness-like reaction, drug-induced systemic lupus erythematosus, and DIHS/DRESS. Minocycline-induced DIHS/DRESS (minocycline-DIHS/DRESS) occurs most frequently in young patients. Minocycline-DIHS/DRESS presents with fever, skin eruption, lymphadenopathy, and internal organ involvement developing within 8 weeks after initiation of therapy. Minocycline-DIHS/DRESS commonly begins with a fever 2 to 4 weeks after initiation of therapy, followed by atypical lymphocytosis, eosinophilia, lymphadenopathy, skin rash, and visceral organ involvement. Eosinophilia often persists during the entire course of this reaction. Patients complain of symptoms of headache and a nonproductive cough at the onset. The skin rashes may take the form of a morbilliform eruption, erythema multiforme-like lesions, exfoliative dermatitis, or pustular eruptions.[48,49] Macular eruptions progress to become purpuric, spreading to involve most of the body. Prominent facial edema or swelling of the scrotum secondary to lymphadenopathy is also observed. Arthralgia or arthritis is infrequently observed, which differentiates minocycline-DIHS/DRESS from serum sickness-like reaction.[49]

Lymphadenopathy is frequently observed in minocycline-DIHS/DRESS (see **Table 1**). Cervical posterior occipital, axillary, and inguinal lymph nodes are enlarged, soft, mobile, and tender to palpitation. With the prominent lymphadenopathy and atypical lymphocytosis seen in the peripheral blood, lymphoma and pseudolymphoma are also considered in the differential diagnosis. These differential diagnoses are excluded by skin and lymph node biopsy results.[49]

Cases of minocycline-DIHS/DRESS have been reported in terms of the most prominent single organ involvement, such as hepatitis, pneumonitis, and nephritis. Closer inspection of these cases often reveals the presence of a rash and fever, however, suggesting a diagnosis of DIHS/DRESS. Internal organ involvement usually manifests as hepatic injury. Although pulmonary involvement is rarely reported in DIHS/DRESS, interstitial pneumonia with eosinophilia is often observed in patients who have minocycline-DIHS/DRESS. Most patients who have this pneumonia survive with no permanent sequelae, but it may be life-threatening in some patients and show characteristic findings of adult respiratory distress syndrome.[50] Other systemic involvement includes myocarditis, interstitial nephritis, and rhabdomyolysis.[50,51]

Dapsone

Dapsone (4, 4′-diaminodiphenylsulfone), a potent antiparasitic and anti-inflammatory compound, is mainly used in the treatment of leprosy. It has also been the drug of choice for the management for bullous dermatoses and inflammatory skin diseases, such as leukocytoclastic vasculitis and erythema elevatum diutinum. Common side effects include headache, methemoglobulinemia, agranulocytosis, and hemolytic anemia. Dapsone-induced DIHS/DRESS (dapsone-DIHS/DRESS) occurs in less than 1% of patients treated with dapsone, however.[52,53] Dapsone-induced agranulocytosis and dapsone-DIHS/DRESS are two different adverse reactions; therefore, these two adverse reactions are not simultaneously observed. Dapsone-DIHS/DRESS has been reported in cases other than those associated with leprosy, such as *Pneumocystis carinii* pneumonia in patients who have AIDS.

The constellation of symptoms in this reaction includes fever, malaise, exfoliative dermatitis, lymphadenopathy, atypical lymphocytosis, and hepatitis. Cyanosis on the lips, fingers, and toes, is observed, followed by hemolytic anemia and methemoglobinemia. Dapsone-DIHS/DRESS usually begins 4 weeks or more after starting the drug.[52,54] The rash, which is often a morbilliform eruption (**Fig. 10**), may develop into diffuse erythematous dermatitis, which disappears with desquamation. Icterus and lymphadenopathy are observed in 80.7% of patients who have leprosy with dapsone-DIHS/DRESS, and hepatomegaly is seen in 73.0% of patients who have leprosy with this reaction (see **Table 1**).[55]

Rather common in dapsone-DIHS/DRESS is the absence of eosinophilia. Liver involvement displays a mixed hepatocellular and cholestatic pattern. ALT, AST, and total bilirubin levels are elevated. Hyperbilirubinemia is present in 85% of patients who have leprosy with dapsone-DIHS/DRESS,[55] which may be partly attributable to hemolysis in addition to hepatotoxicity. A liver biopsy reveals hepatitis, cholestasis, or granuloma formation.[54] Hepatitis may progress to liver failure and death; a cholestatic pattern may have a less severe clinical course and is characterized by high ALP and moderate transaminase levels. Cholangitis has also been reported in a patient who had dapsone-DIHS/DRESS.[54] Hypoalbuminemia is also a feature of dapsone-DIHS/DRESS, which is probably attributable to binding of dapsone to the circulating

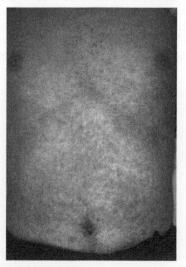

Fig. 10. Maculopapular eruption (dapsone).

serum albumin.[54] A case with visceral involvement, including myocarditis, thyroiditis, serositis, and hepatitis, has been reported.[56] DIHS/DRESS has been reported to develop during treatment with dapsone for pemphigus foliaceus. In this case, anti-desmoglein 1 IgG antibodies decreased during the course of the illness, and not only HHV-6 reactivation but cytomegalovirus and Epstein-Barr virus reactivations were detected.[57]

Sulfasalazine

Sulfasalazine is a drug used to treat inflammatory bowel diseases, rheumatoid arthritis, and some forms of spondyloarthropathy. Serious side effects with systemic involvement are less frequent. Nevertheless, a severe adverse reaction to sulfasalazine has been identified as a type of hypersensitivity reaction. Sulfasalazine-induced DIHS/DRESS is referred to as the "3-week sulfasalazine syndrome" that occurs 3 weeks after first administration of the drug. According to an analysis of 23 patients who had sulfasalazine-induced DIHS/DRESS, the period between drug administration and onset ranges from 1 week to 4 months.[58] The clinical features of sulfasalazine-induced DIHS/DRESS are similar to those of infectious mononucleosis. A high-grade fever, skin eruptions, lymphadenopathy, and hepatomegaly are usually seen. Skin eruptions manifest as erythematous papules and macules that become confluent (**Fig. 11**); this rash progresses over the whole body with the appearance of purpuric lesions. There is notable facial edema, especially on the eyelids.

Visceral complications are characterized by fulminant hepatitis, interstitial nephropathy, eosinophilic interstitial pneumonitis pericarditis, myocarditis, or pancreatitis. Pleural effusion is also observed. Symptoms often persist for several weeks after discontinuation of the drug. Laboratory tests reveal increases in serum transaminases and total bilirubin levels, reflecting hepatic cytolysis and cholestasis.[59] Some of these cases present with life-threatening fulminant hepatitis with symptoms of jaundice and persistent high-grade fever.

Mexiletine Hydrochloride

Mexiletine hydrochloride is an antiarrhythmic drug. A variety of drug eruptions attributable to mexiletine hydrochloride have been reported, including maculopapular eruption (**Fig. 12**), erythema multiforme, erythroderma, urticaria, and pustular eruptions. Several cases of mexiletine-induced DIHS/DRESS (mexiletine-DIHS/DRESS) have been reported in Japan.[60–62] In affected patients, prominent edema is usually observed on the periorbital lesions. There is an erythematous periorbital edema at

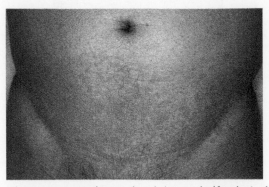

Fig. 11. Confluent erythematous macules on the abdomen (sulfasalazine).

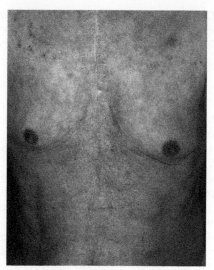

Fig. 12. Diffuse erythema on the trunk (mexiletine).

the onset, which changes to a violaceous color. Edema on the lower legs is also observed; however, this may be related to preexisting cardiovascular disease. Erythema multiforme-like eruptions are observed on the trunk and extremities. Less frequently, tiny pustules are disseminated on the surface of large confluent erythematous plaques on the face and chest. This finding may resemble acute generalized exanthematous pustulosis (AGEP);[63] however, the pustules are not localized on the skin folds, such as the neck, axilla, and groin. The pustules gradually regress soon after discontinuation of mexiletine hydrochloride. It takes several weeks for the erythematous eruptions to disappear.

In regard to laboratory findings, eosinophilia is more frequently detected than atypical lymphocytosis (see **Table 1**). The neutrophil count is not prominently elevated as observed in AGEP. Liver dysfunction is usually mild.

Regarding herpesvirus reactivations, it has been reported that DIHS/DRESS developed 33 months after the onset of herpes zoster,[60] in which mexiletine hydrochloride was administered for 1 month. Sekiguchi and colleagues[61] have reported a patient who had mexiletine-DIHS/DRESS with evidence of HHV-6 reactivation and cytomegalovirus reactivation. In a separate case, HHV-7 reactivation, in addition to HHV-6, was detected during the course of DIHS/DRESS using polymerase chain reaction analysis and a serologic assay.[62] A patient who had fulminant type 1 diabetes mellitus after mexiletine-DIHS/DRESS has been reported.[64]

Other Culprit Drugs

Other causative drugs, such as cyanamide,[65] tribenoside,[66] methimazole,[67] and clomipramine,[68] have also been reported to induce DIHS/DRESS.

SUMMARY

DIHS/DRESS exhibits a broad range of clinical manifestations and laboratory abnormalities that are a result of the interplay of host immune status, the extent of sensitization to the drug, immunologic and pharmacokinetic properties of the drug, and the sites and types of viral reactions associated with this syndrome. They could also induce reactions with a different time sequence. Despite a variable clinical appearance, however, DIHS/DRESS is a distinct clinical entity with highly reproducible clinical and immunopathologic features. A better understanding of the interplay in the development of DIHS/DRESS has implications for safer and more efficient treatment of this syndrome.

REFERENCES

1. Sullivan JR, Shear NH. The drug hypersensitivity syndrome: what is the pathogenesis? Arch Dermatol 2001;137(3):357–64.
2. Gennis MA, Vemuri R, Burns EA, et al. Familial occurrence of hypersensitivity to phenytoin. Am J Med 1991;91(6):631–4.
3. Ghislain PD, Roujeau JC. Treatment of severe drug reactions: Stevens-Johnson syndrome, toxic epidermal necrolysis and hypersensitivity syndrome. Dermatol Online J 2002;8(1):5. Available at: http://dermatology.cdlib.org/DOJvol8num1/reviews/drugrxn/ghislain.html.
4. Bocquet H, Martine B, Roujeau JC. Drug-induced pseudolymphoma and drug hypersensitivity syndrome (drug rash with eosinophilia and systemic symptoms: DRESS). Semin Cutan Med Surg 1996;15(4):250–7.
5. Descamps V, Bouscarat F, Laglenne S, et al. Human herpesvirus 6 infection associated with anticonvulsant hypersensitivity syndrome and reactive haemophagocytic syndrome. Br J Dermatol 1997;137(4):605–8.
6. Suzuki Y, Inagi R, Aono T, et al. Human herpesvirus 6 infection as a risk factor of the development of severe drug-induced hypersensitivity. Arch Dermatol 1998;134(9):1108–12.
7. Tohyama M, Yahata Y, Yasukawa M, et al. Severe hypersensitivity syndrome due to sulfasalazine associated with reactivation of human herpesvirus 6. Arch Dermatol 1998;134(9):1113–7.
8. Hashimoto K, Yasukawa M, Tohyama M. Human herpesvirus 6 and drug allergy. Curr Opin Allergy Clin Immunol 2003;3(4):255–60.
9. Shiohara T, Iijima M, Ikezawa Z, et al. The diagnosis of a DRESS syndrome has been sufficiently established on the basis of typical clinical features and viral reactivations. Br J Dermatol 2007;156(5):1083–4.
10. Roujeau JC. Clinical heterogeneity of drug hypersensitivity. Toxicology 2005;209(2):123–9.
11. Kano Y, Hirahara K, Sakuma K, et al. Several herpesviruses can reactivate in a severe drug-induced multiorgan reaction in the same sequential order as in graft-versus-host disease. Br J Dermatol 2006;155(2):301–6.
12. Shiohara T, Takahashi R, Kano Y. Drug-induced hypersensitivity syndrome and viral reactivation. In: Pichler WJ, editor. Drug hypersensitivity. Basel (Switzerland): Karger; 2007. p. 251–66.
13. Rijlaarsdam U, Scheffer E, Meijer CJ, et al. Mycosis fungoides-like lesions associated with phenytoin and carbamazepine therapy. J Am Acad Dermatol 1991;24(2 Pt 1):216–20.
14. Callot V, Roujeau JC, Bagot M, et al. Drug-induced pseudolymphoma and hypersensitivity syndrome; two different clinical entities. Arch Dermatol 1996;132(11):1315–21.
15. Rijlaarsdam JU, Scheffer E, Meijer CJ, et al. Cutaneous pseudo-T cell lymphomas; a clinicopathologic study of 20 patients. Cancer 1992;69(3):717–24.
16. Masaki T, Fukunaga A, Tohyama M, et al. Human herpes virus 6 encephalitis in allopurinol-induced hypersensitivity syndrome. Acta Derm Venereol 2003;83(2):28–31.

17. Sekine N, Motokura T, Oki T, et al. Rapid loss of insulin secretion in a patient with fulminant type 1 diabetes mellitus and carbamazepine hypersensitivity syndrome. JAMA 2001;285(9):1153–4.
18. Peyrière H, Dereure O, Breton P, et al. Variability in the clinical pattern of cutaneous side-effects of drugs with systemic symptoms: does a DRESS syndrome really exist? Br J Dermatol 2006;155(2):422–8.
19. Kano Y, Inaoka M, Shiohara T. Association between anticonvulsant hypersensitivity syndrome and human herpesvirus 6 reactivation and hypogammaglobulinemia. Arch Dermatol 2004;140(2):183–8.
20. Kano Y, Seishima M, Shiohara T. Hypogammaglobulinemia as an early sign of drug-induced hypersensitivity syndrome. J Am Acad Dermatol 2006;55(4):727–8.
21. Boccara O, Valeyrie-Allanore L, Crickx B, et al. Association of hypogammaglobulinemia with DRESS (drug rash with eosinophilia and systemic symptoms). Eur J Dermatol 2006;16(6):666–8.
22. Wangel AG, Arvilommi H, Jokinen I. The effect of phenytoin in vitro on normal human mononuclear cells and on human lymphoblastoid B cell lines of different Ig isotype specificities. Immunobiology 1985;170(3):232–8.
23. Go T. Carbamazepine-induced IgG1 and IgG2 deficiency associated with B cell maturation defect. Seizure 2004;13(3):187–90.
24. Shiohara T, Kano Y. A complex interaction between drug allergy and viral infection. Clin Rev Allergy Immunol 2007;33(1–2):124–33.
25. Knowles SR, Shapiro LE, Shear NH. Anticonvulsant hypersensitivity syndrome: incidence, prevention and management. Drug Saf 1999;21(6):489–501.
26. Ganeva M, Gancheva T, Lazarova R, et al. Carbamazepine-induced drug reaction with eosinophilia and systemic symptoms (DRESS) syndrome: report of four cases and brief review. Int J Dermatol 2008;47(8):853–60.
27. Kansky A, Vodnik A, Stanovnik L. Serious drug reactions to carbamazepine in oncologic patients after x-ray treatment: report of four cases. Acta Dermatovenerol Alp Panonica Adriat 2002;11(3):105–10.
28. Shear NH, Spielberg SP. Anticonvulsant hypersensitivity syndrome. In vitro assessment of risk. J Clin Invest 1988;82(6):1826–32.
29. Scheinfeld N. Impact of phenytoin therapy on the skin and skin disease. Expert Opin Drug Saf 2004;3(6):655–65.
30. Potter T, DiGregorio F, Stiff M, et al. Dilantin hypersensitivity syndrome imitating staphylococcal toxic shock. Arch Dermatol 1994;130(7):856–8.
31. Conger LA Jr, Grabski WJ. Dilantin hypersensitivity reaction. Cutis 1996;57(4):223–6.
32. Ting S, Maj MC, Dunsky EH. Diphenylhydantoin-induced hepatitis. Ann Allergy 1982;48(6):331–2.
33. Sakai C, Takagi T, Oguro M, et al. Erythroderma and marked atypical lymphocytosis mimicking cutaneous T-cell lymphoma probably caused by phenobarbital. Intern Med 1993;32(2):182–4.
34. Sakuma K, Kano Y, Fukuhara M, et al. Syndrome of inappropriate secretion of antidiuretic hormone associated with limbic encephalitis in a patient with drug-induced hypersensitivity syndrome. Clin Exp Dermatol 2007;33(3):287–90.
35. Giordano N, Amendola A, Papakostas P, et al. A clinical case of drug hypersensitivity syndrome with phenobarbital administration: drug-induced rash with eosinophilia and systemic symptoms or lupus-like syndrome? [letter]. Clin Exp Rheumatol 2007;25(2):339.
36. Teraki Y, Murota H, Izaki S. Toxic epidermal necrolysis due to zonisamide associated with reactivation of human herpesvirus 6. Arch Dermatol 2008;144(2):232–5.

37. Iannetti P, Raucci U, Zuccaro P, et al. Lamotrigine hypersensitivity in child hood epilepsy. Epilepsia 1998;39(5):502–7.
38. Parri N, Bernardini R, Pucci N, et al. Drug rash with eosinophilia and systemic symptoms induced by lamotrigine therapy. Int J Immunopathol Pharmacol 2007;20(3):643–5.
39. Schaub N, Bircher AJ. Severe hypersensitivity syndrome to lamotrigine confirmed by lymphocyte stimulation in vitro. Allergy 2000;55(2):191–3.
40. Schlienger RG, Knowles SR, Shear NH. Lamotrigine-associated anticonvulsant hypersensitivity syndrome. Neurology 1998;51(4):1172–5.
41. Elasy T, Kaminsky D, Tracy M, et al. Allopurinol hypersensitivity syndrome revisited. West J Med 1995;162(4):360–1.
42. Emmerson BT. The management of gout. N Engl J Med 1996;334(7):445–51.
43. Kumar A, Edward N, White MI, et al. Allopurinol, erythema multiforme, and renal insufficiency. BMJ 1996;312(7024):173–4.
44. Hung SI, Chung WH, Liou LB, et al. HLA-B*5801 allele as a genetic marker for severe cutaneous adverse reactions caused by allopurinol. Proc Natl Acad Sci U S A 2005;102(11):4134–9.
45. Kano Y, Hirahara K, Asano Y, et al. HLA-B allele association with certain drugs are not confirmed in Japanese patients with severe cutaneous drug reactions. Acta Derm Venereol 2008;88(6):616–8.
46. Arakawa M, Kakuto Y, Ichikawa K, et al. Allopurinol hypersensitivity syndrome associated with systemic cytomegalovirus infection and systemic bacteremia. Intern Med 2001;40(4):331–5.
47. Sommers LM, Schoene RB. Allopurinol hypersensitivity syndrome associated with pancreatic exocrine abnormalities and new-onset diabetes mellitus. Arch Intern Med 2002;162(10):1190–2.
48. Colvin JH, Sheth AP. Minocycline hypersensitivity syndrome with hypotension mimicking septic shock. Pediatr Dermatol 2001;18(4):295–8.
49. Knowles SR, Shapiro L, Shear NH. Serious adverse reactions induced by minocycline. Report of 13 patients and review of the literature. Arch Dermatol 1996; 132(8):934–9.
50. Roca B, Calvo B, Ferrer D. Minocycline hypersensitivity reaction with acute respiratory distress syndrome. Intensive Care Med 2003;29(2):338.
51. Gough A, Chapman S, Wagstaff K, et al. Minocycline-induced autoimmune hepatitis and systemic lupus erythematosus-like syndrome. BMJ 1996;312(7024):169–72.
52. Leslie KS, Gaffney K, Ross CN, et al. A near fatal case of the dapsone hypersensitivity syndrome in a patient with urticarial vasculitis. Clin Exp Dermatol 2003; 28(5):496–8.
53. Sener O, Doganci L, Safali M, et al. Severe dapsone hypersensitivity syndrome. J Investig Allergol Clin Immunol 2006;16(4):268–70.
54. Itha S, Kumar A, Dhingra S, et al. Dapsone induced cholangitis as a part of dapsone syndrome: a case report. BMC Gastroenterol 2003;3:21. Available at: http://www.biomedcentral.com/1471-230X/3/21.
55. Agrawal S, Agarwalla A. Dapsone hypersensitivity syndrome: a clinico-epidemiological review. J Dermatol 2005;32(11):883–9.
56. Teo RY, Tay YK, Tan CH, et al. Presumed dapsone-induced drug hypersensitivity syndrome causing reversible hypersensitivity myocarditis and thyrotoxicosis. Ann Acad Med Singap 2006;35(11):833–6.
57. Takahashi H, Tanaka M, Tanikawa A, et al. A case of drug-induced hypersensitivity syndrome showing transient immunosuppression before viral reactivation during treatment for pemphigus foliaceus. Clin Exp Dermatol 2006;31(1):33–5.

58. Kunisaki Y, Goto H, Kitagawa K, et al. Salazosulfapyridine induced hypersensitivity syndrome associated with reactivation of human herpesvirus 6. Intern Med 2003;42(2):203–7.

59. Descloux E, Argaud L, Dumortier J, et al. Favourable issue of a fulminant hepatitis associated with sulfasalazine DRESS syndrome without liver transplantation. Intensive Care Med 2005;31(12):1727–8.

60. Higa K, Hirata K, Dan K. Mexiletine-induced severe skin eruption, fever, eosinophilia, lymphocytosis, and liver dysfunction. Pain 1997;73(1):97–9.

61. Sekiguchi A, Kashiwagi T, Ishida-Yamamoto A, et al. Drug-induced hypersensitivity syndrome due to mexiletine associated with human herpesvirus 6 and cytomegalovirus reactivation. J Dermatol 2005;32(4):278–81.

62. Yagami A, Yoshikawa T, Asano Y, et al. Drug-induced hypersensitivity syndrome due to mexiletine hydrochloride associated with reactivation of human herpesvirus 7. Dermatology 2006;213(4):341–4.

63. Sasaki K, Yamamoto T, Kishi M, et al. Acute exanthematous pustular drug eruption induced by mexiletine. Eur J Dermatol 2001;11(5):469–71.

64. Seino Y, Yamauchi M, Hirai C, et al. A case of fulminant Type 1 diabetes associated with mexiletine hypersensitivity syndrome. Diabet Med 2004;21(10):1156–7.

65. Mitani N, Aihara M, Yamakawa Y, et al. Drug-induced hypersensitivity syndrome due to cyanamide associated with multiple reactivation of human herpesviruses. J Med Virol 2005;75(3):430–4.

66. Hashizume H, Takigawa M. Drug-induced hypersensitivity syndrome associated with cytomegalovirus reactivation: immunological characterization of pathogenic T cells. Acta Derm Venereol 2005;85(1):47–50.

67. Ozaki N, Miura Y, Sakakibara A, et al. A case of hypersensitivity syndrome induced by methimazole for Graves' disease. Thyroid 2005;15(12):1333–6.

68. Nishimura Y, Kitoh A, Yoshida Y, et al. Clomipramine-induced hypersensitivity syndrome with unusual clinical features. J Am Acad Dermatol 2005;53(Suppl 1): S231–3.

Skin Testing for IgE-Mediated Drug Allergy

Birger Kränke, MD*, Werner Aberer, MD

KEYWORDS

- Drug hypersensitivity • Drug allergy • Adverse drug reaction
- Immediate reaction • Prick test • Intradermal test

Adverse drug reactions (ADRs) are a frequent problem of the daily clinical praxis. Although patients who have experienced ADRs often refer to them as drug allergies, true allergic reactions—hypersensitivities with the involvement of one or more immunologic mechanisms—represent approximately 15% of all ADRs. As a consequence, this often results in avoidance of one or more drug classes, which may lead to the prescription of less effective or more expensive alternative drugs. Therefore, an adequate diagnostic work-up is recommended and widely done in Europe, less so in the United States.[1–13]

Every work-up has to start with a detailed case history and accurate determination of the reaction type, followed by skin tests or, if available, in vitro tests. If this procedure remains inconclusive, drug provocation tests with the suspicious or an alternative drug could be performed by a physician experienced in the field of drug allergy.

In general, drug hypersensitivities can be classified as immediate, accelerated, or delayed, according to the time interval between intake of the drug and occurrence of the reaction. This classification was set up by Levine on the basis of his experience with penicillin allergy.[14] From a clinical standpoint, immediate and nonimmediate reactions differ in the time interval between drug intake and beginning of clinical manifestations. In immediate reactions, symptoms appear within 1 hour and sometimes within just a few minutes of drug intake. Main clinical manifestations are urticaria or angioedema and anaphylaxis, often due to drug-specific IgE. These ADRs are the principal indications for skin prick tests (SPTs) and intradermal tests (IDTs) in drug allergy work-up (**Box 1**).

INDICATION FOR SKIN TESTS

A detailed history is the prerequisite for an accurate diagnosis of a drug-induced (skin) reaction. It must comprise any details of the drug administration (all active ingredients, formulation, dose, route, previous exposure to and tolerance of the drug incriminated,

Department of Dermatology and Venereology, Medical University of Graz, Auenbruggerplatz 8, 8036 Graz, Austria
* Corresponding author.
E-mail address: birger.kraenke@medunigraz.at (B. Kränke).

Immunol Allergy Clin N Am 29 (2009) 503–516
doi:10.1016/j.iac.2009.04.003   immunology.theclinics.com
0889-8561/09/$ – see front matter © 2009 Published by Elsevier Inc.

> **Box 1**
> **Indications for skin prick test and intradermal test in drug allergy work-up**
>
> Erythematous eruption/flushing
> Urticaria
> Angioedema
> Anaphylaxis
> Conjunctivitis
> Rhinitis
> Bronchospasm/asthma

review of an anesthetic chart, and so forth) and the definite nature of the adverse reaction. Use of the European Network for Drug Allergy questionnaire may be helpful.[1] If an immediate allergic reaction can be stated based on the presence of a sensitization period, reaction to low drug doses, and the typical symptomatology and course of type I allergic reactions, SPTs and IDTs may be recommended depending on the drug class involved. SPTs and IDTs are read at 15 to 20 minutes and then are indicative only for an IgE-mediated drug allergic reaction.[3] Later readings of IDTs are used for delayed, non–IgE-mediated allergies. A list of ADRs that represent no indications or even contraindications for IDTs with immediate readings or where IDT may cause exacerbations of an allergy is given in **Box 2**.

Drugs with well-standardized test procedures are β-lactams (penicillins and cephalosporins), neuromuscular blocking agents, local anesthetics, iodinated contrast media, and chemotherapeutics (platinum salts).

> **Box 2**
> **No indications for skin prick test and intradermal tests in drug allergy work-up (sample)**
>
> Drug-induced autoimmune diseases
>
>   Bullous pemphigoid
>   Pemphigus vulgaris
>   Systemic lupus erythematosus
>
> Severe exfoliative skin reactions
>
>   Acute generalized exanthematic pustulosis
>   Drug reaction with eosinophilia and systemic symptoms or drug hypersensitivity syndrome
>   Exfoliative dermatitis
>   Multilocalized bullous fixed drug eruption
>   Stevens-Johnson syndrome
>   Toxic epidermal necrolysis
>
> Severe vasculitis syndromes
>
> Late reading of intradermal tests is useful in delayed reactions but bears risk for flare-up reactions to the intradermally applied drug.

In addition, SPTs can be performed with other drugs and IDTs, if sterilized solutions used for parenteral applications are available (subject to investigator experience).[5] Some indications for nonirritative concentrations can be obtained from published case reports. These experimental tests have to be interpreted cautiously, however, as many drugs may cause wheal and flare reactions spontaneously; the sensitivity for such reactions may differ individually and positive controls often are missing.

Additionally, (immediate) skin tests are of educational value, because they provide a visual illustration that may reinforce the verbal advice given to patients.[4]

TIMING FOR SKIN TEST PERFORMANCE

A few guidelines have been published for performing SPTs and IDTs with drugs in the investigation of ADRs.[2–4] Generally, it is advised to perform the tests 6 weeks to 6 months after the hypersensitivity reaction because it is not known whether or not positive results will persist and whether or not some drug reactivities last longer.[2,5,6] Ideally, immediate skin testing should be performed after an interval that allows resolution of clinical symptoms and clearance of a suspected drug.

It is important to avoid antihistamines (up to 7 days) before testing. Higher doses of systemic corticosteroids and other immunosuppressive therapy and antidepressants with antihistamine side effects also may interfere and hamper the interpretation of a negative result; hence, these drugs should be stopped for 3 days to 1 month before testing (**Table 1**).[2,3,7]

WORKFLOW AND PERFORMANCE

Patients preferably should be in good condition and give informed verbal or (preferably) written consent.[8]

Finding a suitable test reagent may be a problem as most drugs have low molecular weight and are not immunogenic, and, furthermore, drug metabolites may have caused the adverse reaction. Moreover, investigators must be aware of appropriate starting dilutions and the concentrations likely to induce irritant, nonallergic skin responses. Unfortunately, for the vast majority of drugs, commercial test preparations are not available, and if adequate test concentrations for a suspected drug are not known, it is recommended to test the drug at concentrations comparable to that of a related drug for which data already are published.

Table 1
Drug-free intervals demanded for immediate skin testing

Medication	Route	Free Interval
H1-antihistamines, phenothiazines	Oral, intravenous	5 days
β-Adrenergic drugs	Oral, intravenous	5 days
Glucocorticosteroids		
Long-term	Oral, intravenous	3 weeks
Short-term, high-dose	Oral, intravenous	1 week
Short-term, <50 mg prednisolone	Oral, intravenous	3 days
Topical corticosteroids	Topical (at the test site)	>2 weeks

Data from Barbaud A, Goncalo M, Bruynzeel D, et al. Guidelines for performing skin tests with drugs in the investigation of cutaneous adverse drug reactions. Contact Derm 2001;45:321–8 and Brockow K, Romano A, Blanca M, et al. General considerations for skin test procedures in the diagnosis of drug hypersensitivity. Allergy 2002;57:45–51.

Because it is a safe and easy way to perform test, prick testing should be done initially. It is performed by pricking the skin percutaneously with a prick test needle (lancet) through the test (drug) solution. The drug is, if necessary, appropriately diluted (eg, 1:10 or sometimes 1:1000) with normal saline (0.9% NaCl). Whenever possible, the pure drug and excipients should be tested as is, but in patients who have developed anaphylaxis, sequential solutions (10^{-3} to 10^{-1}) should be tested.[2] An additional application of a positive control (histamine) and negative control (normal saline, diluent) is essential for correct interpretation of the test results. Reading is done after 15 minutes,[3,4,7] but some investigators propose 20 minutes[2,3,5,6] or even 30 minutes[9] after application of the test solution to skin. The SPT is considered positive in cases of a wheal with a diameter larger than that of the negative control and larger than 3 mm, typically surrounded by a red flare.[3] For the purpose of comparison, a morphologic description or, even better, a morphologic score also should be applied.

If SPT is negative, IDTs are done with serial dilutions of the suspected drug, usually starting with 1/100 of the concentration used for SPT. The skin of the volar forearm is injected intradermally with 0.02 to 0.05 mL of the lowest concentration (1:10,000 to 1:100, depending on the drug and patient history), resulting in a wheal of 4 to 6 mm in diameter. If no reaction can be elicited, the test solution is injected again in a concentration increased in logarithmic steps ($\times 10$). In the literature it is recommended to prepare dilutions (in an optimal way under laminar flow) no more than 2 hours before administration.[2,5] As with SPT, negative (0.9% NaCl) and positive (histamine, 1 mg/mL) control testing are strongly recommended. IDT readings are recommended at 15,[3,7] 20,[3,10] or 30[2] minutes in cases of evaluating immediate-type ADR and at 24 hours if a delayed-type reaction is evaluated (IDT then is performed in addition to or instead of patch testing). IDT is considered positive when the diameter of the reaction is enlarged by a minimum 3-mm diameter, is found twice the diameter of the injection papula, or is a wheal larger than 8 mm (summarized by Barbaud[5]). The painfulness of IDT may limit its use in (young) children. IDTs in patients who have severe reactions, such as drug reaction with eosinophilia and systemic symptoms, and possibly also in patients who have Stevens-Johnson syndrome/toxic epidermal necrolysis (see **Box 2**), may cause a (mostly mild) flare up of the reaction (**Table 2**).

REASONS FOR FALSE-POSITIVE RESULTS

False-positive results are those in which the skin test response to the tested drug is interpreted as positive, but a patient does not develop adequate symptoms if re-exposed to the drug. Common causes include the following:

1. Patient is sensitized and may have (low-affinity) drug/hapten–specific IgE antibodies but does not react clinically

Table 2	
Maximum concentrations recommended for prick and intradermal testing with β-lactams	
Allergen/Hapten	**Dose/Units**
BPO	5×10^{-5} mmol/L
MDM	2×10^{-2} mmol/L
Amoxicillin	20–25 mg/mL
Ampicillin	20–25 mg/mL

Data from Torres MJ, Blanca M, Fernandez J, et al. Diagnosis of immediate allergic reactions to beta-lactam antibiotics. Allergy 2003;58:961–72.

2. Drug may cause spontaneous mast cell degranulation (eg, opiates or quinolones)
3. Test dilution is too highly concentrated, thus producing an immediate reaction on the basis of nonspecific irritation of mast cells
4. Physical trauma of skin testing in patients who have dermographism or urticaria (factitia)
5. Reaction to the diluent, preservative (phenol, glycerol, and so forth), or contaminants[15]
6. Improper interpretation of results, reading erythema rather than wheals
7. Lack of negative and positive skin test controls; because individuals react differently to drugs, at least 20 controls also should be analyzed

Even when correct technique and proper drug dilution are used, a positive skin test result does not necessarily validate the diagnosis. The diagnostic value of skin test positivity depends on the demonstration, by drug re-exposure, that clinical symptoms of the ADR are elicited by exposure to the drug allergen that induced the skin test reaction.

REASONS FOR FALSE-NEGATIVE RESULTS

Skin tests may be interpreted incorrectly as "negative" in individuals for various, mainly technical, reasons:

1. Application of too little antigen because of inappropriate dilution, loss of potency during storage, and so forth
2. Insufficient penetration of the antigen to the dermal mast cells, improper introduction of antigen (eg, poor technique), or exclusive use of a relatively insensitive method (eg, scratch test)
3. Blocking effect by medications, such as antihistamines, and, less often, tricyclic antidepressants or theophylline
4. Improper reading of reactions or inadequate scoring systems

In addition, there are some important, nontechnical reasons that may cause a lack of skin test reactivity:[9]

1. Cofactors of critical importance at the time of ADR manifestation, such as viral infections or drug-drug interactions, may be absent when performing SPT and IDT
2. Reaction requires metabolism, which cannot occur within 20 minutes to the intradermally applied drug or it happens only in the liver
3. The presentation of the relevant antigen or hapten to the immune system may be different after epicutaneous, oral, or otherwise parenteral challenge
4. SPT or IDT is performed in a time period when the mast cells have degranulated and are not yet restored

ADVERSE REACTIONS INDUCED BY SKIN PRICK TESTS OR INTRADERMAL TESTS

SPT is a safe diagnostic approach. IDTs, however, also are safe, but several fatal or near-fatal reactions have been reported.[16–19] Urticaria and, rarely, anaphylaxis are described after intradermal testings, in particular with β-lactams.[17–19] In general, patients who have previous anaphylaxis or complicating conditions, such as systemic mastocytosis, may be considered at higher risk (ie, they may react more readily to the minute amounts applied).

As a consequence, it is prudent and recommended to perform SPT first, followed by IDT, in severe immediate reactions. For practical purposes, most tests are done simultaneously (**Fig. 1**). In addition, adequate equipment and a specialist environment to treat anaphylaxis must be available.[16]

VALUE OF IMMEDIATE SKIN TESTS ACCORDING TO SELECTED DRUGS

Unfortunately, the usefulness of SPT and IDT in determining the cause of cutaneous ADRs has not been evaluated as much as that of drug patch tests, except for the β-lactams.[9] Even at the beginning of the current millennium, it had to be stated that the sensitivity and predictive value of immediate skin tests vary from excellent (penicillins, neuromuscular blocking agents, heterologous sera, and enzymes) to satisfactory (vaccines, hormones, opiates, and thiopental) and poor or unknown (local anesthetics, nonsteroidal anti-inflammatory drugs, iodine radiocontrast media, quinolones, and other anti-infectious drugs).[6] In recent years, however, some projects in Europe (mainly under the auspices of European Network for Drug Allergy) and some United States investigators have improved this situation considerably for selected drug groups.

β-LACTAMS AND OTHER ANTIBIOTICS

Allergic reactions to β-lactams (eg, penicillins, cephalosporins, imipenem, and monobactam) are the most common cause of ADRs mediated by immunologic mechanisms.[20–26] The β-lactams all possess a characteristic β-lactam ring structure. When the ring is fused to a 5-membered thiazolidine ring (penam), the drug is classified as a penicillin; when fused to a 6-membered dihydrothiazine ring (cephem), it is classified as a cephalosporin. Penicillins and cephalosporins may incorporate different salt forms at the ester-binding site, but penicillins have only one side chain (6 position)

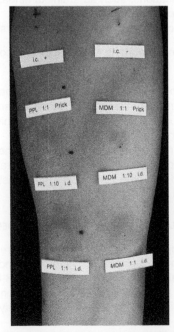

Fig. 1. Positive reactions in the SPT and IDT with the major and minor determinats of penicillin.

whereas cephalosporins have two side chains (3 and 7 positions). These chains differentiate the activity and metabolic parameters of each drug within each class, and this is recognized as the major source of cross reactivity (called structural activity relationship), replacing the concept of a class effect.[23]

Unlike many diagnostic tests for drug allergies, the positive and negative predictive values of skin tests using penicillin reagents have been well studied.[24] For immediate skin testing purpose, the antigenic determinant benzylpenicilloyl (BPO) has been conjugated to a carrier molecule, polylysine (PPL), which results in BPO-PPL. This compound is well suited to cross-link neighboring IgE molecules bound to high-affinity crystallizable fragment-IgE receptors. Other β-lactam antigens, such as the minor determinant mixture (MDM; composed of benzylpenicillin, sodium benzylpenicilloat, and benzylpenicilloic acid), amoxicillin, or some cephalosporins are applied in uncoupled form[22,27] and nevertheless are able to cause mast cell degranulation, if specific IgE is present. How IgE is cross-linked by these small haptens is unknown. Perhaps rapid in vivo haptenization of proteins occurs during the skin testing, allowing cross-linking of IgEs by the larger, hapten-modified molecule.

Most studies performed in recent decades, mainly in the United States, have shown that PPL in combination with MDM is adequate (sensitivity up to 70% and high specificity reaching 97% to 100%) to evaluate patients by SPT and IDT with immediate-type allergies to β-lactams (see **Fig. 1**).[20,21] Unfortunately, in 2004, Hollister-Stier removed BPO-PPL (Pre-Pen) from the United States market, and Allergopharma in 2005 ceased production of PPL and MDM in Europe, so that the diagnostic evaluation had been hampered.[25,28] PPL and MDM now are on the market again, commercialized (with a substantially higher price) by Diater Laboratories (Madrid, Spain), and recent studies in Europe and Australia indicate that they are equivalent to those from Allergopharma.[22,29] Moreover, a new United States company (AllerQuest, Plainville, Connecticut) has the patent rights to produce Pre-Pen, so that this diagnostic gap should be closed in the near future.[26] If PPL and MDM are not available, SPT and IDT with benzylpenicillin (10,000 to 25,000 IU/mL) can be considered as a compensating test procedure.[25]

Data from the United States suggest that in the presence of a positive history for β-lactam hypersensitivity and negative immediate skin tests for PPL and MDM, patients have only a 0% to 6% risk for reacting with an oral challenge and an approximately 6% risk for reacting on re-exposure.[4] Working groups from Europe, particularly from Spain, however, challenged this conclusion, as they showed that the sensitivity is far lower, approximately 70%.[30] Therefore, controlled drug provocation tests are recommended in cases of skin test negativity and a positive history.[4]

Cephalosporins are the second most prescribed group of β-lactams, and their chemical structures are more heterogenous than those of the penicillins. Immediate skin testing with cephalosporins raises several questions and problems: the tests are not widely standardized, and different test concentrations, from 2 mg/mL up to 30 mg/mL, are reported by different groups. The degradation process of the β-lactam ring is more rapid for cephalosporins than penicillins. Therefore (as discussed previously) the immune response in cephalosporin allergy may be directed to the side chain and individual degradation components but not the β-lactam ring. As a consequence, the shared β-lactam ring of penicillins and cephalosporins is not predictive of cross-reactivity, and penicillin testing does not reliably predict sensitization to cephalosporins unless the side chain of the penicillin or aminopenicillin reagent is similar to the individual side chain of the cephalosporin under evaluation. Thus, skin testing with penicillin determinants shows some cross-reactivity between penicillins and first-generation cephalosporins, such as cephalothin or cephaloridine, and between amoxicillin and first-generation cephalosporins, such as cephalexin and cefadroxil, but not between penicillin/amoxicillin and later-generation cephalosporins (**Box 3**).[31–34]

Moreover, most oral cephalosporins are only poorly soluble.[27,29,32,35] In patients who have negative skin test results, drug provocation tests with the suspect cephalosporin may be performed.[29] SPT and IDT with cephalosporins also may help find safe alternatives. In a study enrolling 128 patients who had IgE-mediated allergy to penicillins, all 101 patients who had negative skin tests for cefuroxime, ceftazidime, ceftriaxone, and cefotaxime tolerated cefuroxime axetil and ceftriaxone in drug provocation testing.[36] In patients allergic to cephalosporins but who have negative immediate skin testing to penicillin determinants, penicillins may be administered safely.[35]

Recent data on cross-reactivity of penicillin and carbapenems indicate a low degree of cross-reactivity in IgE-mediated reactions: of 112 patients who had immediate reactions to penicillins (mainly amoxicillin, ampicillin, piperacillin, and bacampicillin) and who had positive skin test to penicillins, only 1 of 112 reacted in skin test to imipenem. The remaining 111 were provoked with imipenem and tolerated this carbapenem.[37] The Romano group[37] also evaluated the cross-reactivity to another carbapenem (meropenem): only 1 of 104 (all who had immediate penicillin allergy and positive skin tests to penicillins) had a positive skin test to meropenem, and the 103 remaining penicillin-allergic individuals tolerated a provocation test with meropenem.[38] Thus, IgE-mediated cross-reactivity between penicillins and carbapenem

---

Box 3
Cross-reactivity between penicillins and cephalosporins based on 6- and 7-position (R1) side chain similarity, respectively

Penicillin G

    Cephaloridine (first generation)

    Cephalothin (first generation)

Ampicillin

    Amoxicillin

    Cefaclor (second generation)

    Cefadroxil (first generation)

    Cephalexin (first generation)

    Cephradine (first generation)

Ceftizoxime (third generation):

    Cefepime (fourth generation)

    Cefotaxime (third generation)

    Cefpirome (fourth generation)

    Cefpodoxime (third generation)

    Ceftriaxone (third generation)

Data from Yates AB. Management of patients with a history of allergy to beta-lactam antibiotics. Am J Med 2008;121:572–6 Pichichero ME. Use of selected cephalosporins in penicillin-allergic patients: a paradigm shift. Diagn Microbiol Infect Dis 2007;57:13s–18s.

seems rare and skin testing with the carbapenem may exclude the few double reactors. For other non–β-lactam antibiotics, immediate skin testing is only marginally validated. Ciprofloxacin, for example, shows a wide variance in skin test responsiveness, as quinolones cause some direct mast cell degranulation. This degranulating potency may differ among quinolones and individuals, which explains why irritating skin test concentrations differ by up to 1000-fold in several subjects on testing.[39] Test concentrations for cephalosporines, macrolides, aminoglycosides, and other antibiotics are given in **Table 3**.

MYORELAXANTS AND ANESTETHICS

Perioperative anaphylaxis may be induced by a variety of agents, including local anesthetics, myorelaxants, inhaled anesthetics, induction drugs, opioids, antibiotics, and so forth.[40–42] Determination of the causative agent is complicated by simultaneous exposure to multimedications and other products, such as latex. Hence, a thorough work-up to identify the allergic trigger must be completed. The majority of anaphylactic reactions are induced by neuromuscular blocking agents, followed by antibiotics and latex, hypnotics, plasma substitutes, chlorhexidine, and, occasionally, opioids and colorants, such as patent blue.[43] Allergy to local anesthetic agents ("caines") is believed rare (0.7%).[43–45]

SPT and IDT are essential diagnostic measures, because more than 50% of adverse reactions to myorelaxants seem to be IgE mediated.[40–42] Skin tests are performed after obtaining information on the chronology of the event documented by an anesthetist, accompanied by a (readable) copy of the anesthesia record. SPT and IDT are performed by using the commercial solutions. Usually, IDT is started with a 1/1000 dilution of the reagent, except with muscle relaxants and morphine, for

Table 3
Nonirritating test concentrations for commonly used antibiotic agents

Antimicrobial Drug	Full-Strength Concentration	Nonirritating Concentration for Intradermal Tests (as dilution from Full-Strength Concentration)
Cefotaxime	100 mg/mL	10 mg/mL
Cefuroxime	100 mg/mL	10 mg/mL
Cefazolin	330 mg/mL	33 mg/mL
Ceftazidime	100 mg/mL	10 mg/mL
Tobramycin	40 mg/mL	4 mg/mL
Ticarcillin	200 mg/mL	20 mg/mL
Clindamycin	150 mg/mL	15 mg/mL
Gentamicin	40 mg/mL	4 mg/mL
Cotrimoxazole	80 mg/mL	0.8 mg/mL
Levofloxacin	25 mg/mL	0.025 mg/mL
Erythromycin	50 mg/mL	0.05 mg/mL
Azithromycin	100 mg/mL	0.01 mg/mL
Nafcillin	250 mg/mL	0.025 mg/mL
Vancomycin	50 mg/mL	0.005 mg/mL

Data from Empedrad R, Darter AM, Earl HS, et al. Nonirritating intradermal skin test concentrations for commonly prescribed antibiotics. J Allergy Clin Immunol 2003;112:629–30.

which a 1/10.000 dilution is suggested (see Mertes and colleagues[43]). Diagnostic work-up regarding local anesthetics comprises, in addition to SPT and IDT with products free of preservatives, subcutaneous challenge tests.[44–46] In the majority, tests are uneventful, so that the test procedure in most cases have an educative nature.

CHEMOTHERAPEUTICS (PLATINUM SALTS)

Platinum salts are cytotoxic agents and currently components of many chemotherapy regimens. Hypersensitivity reactions to platinum components are well described among refinery workers, who inhaled complex salts of platinum. The extensive chemotherapeutical use of carboplatin, cisplatin, and oxaliplatin has led to an increase in cases of platinum salt hypersensitivity reactions.[47–50] Hypersensitivity to carboplatin (12% to 30%) seems more frequent than that to cisplatin (5% to 20%) or oxaliplatin (mild reaction 10% to 12%, severe reactions <1%).[49] Early-onset symptoms are believed IgE mediated (rather than induced by direct histamine release). The allergy hypothesis is supported by the usually long (and uneventful) therapy intervals before onset of hypersensitivity symptoms (this may be interpreted as the sensitization phase).[47,48] SPTs should be performed with pure injectable drugs; for IDTs, sequentially diluted solutions (1:1000 to 1:10) are recommended with a maximum concentration of 0.1 mg/mL for oxaliplatin.[49,50] In total, skin testing seems safe because no serious systemic reaction has been reported, and, moreover, negative test results are helpful in identifying suitable platinum salts for the continuation of chemotherapy.[49] For details on desensitization see the article by Castells and colleagues elsewhere in this issue.

CONTRAST MEDIA

Iodinated contrast media are regarded as safe but are capable of inducing immediate and nonimmediate hypersensitivity reactions in susceptible patients. Contrast media–induced reactions traditionally have been classified as nonallergic, and skin tests have been regarded as inappropriate tools.[51,52] In a recent prospective multicenter study, 32 of 122 patients who had immediate reactions positive skin tests were observed with the highest frequency of positive reactions in the first 6 months after the adverse event: 4 of 122 patients had positive SPT (undiluted contrast media) and 30 of 121 patients had positive IDT (10-fold diluted contrast media, reading after 20 minutes).[52] As the reactions were occurring mostly to the eliciting contrast medium, whereas other contrast media failed to cause a reaction, the hypersensitivity often was specific for one contrast medium, supporting the hypothesis that at least 50% of the hypersensitivity reactions to contrast media are caused by immunologic mechanism and that skin testing was rated as a useful tool.[52] Positive reactions by immediate skin testing were found for iobitridol, iohexol, iomeprol, iopamidol, iopentol, iopromide, ioversol, iodixanol, ioxithalamate, and ioxaglate. For details, see the article by Brockow and coworkers elsewhere in this issue.

CORTICOSTEROIDS

Although delayed-type, T-cell–mediated allergic reactions to corticosteroids are well documented, the existence of IgE-mediated allergic reactions due to systemically applied corticosteroid therapy is controversial. Immediate reactions with positive skin tests are mainly due to the content of stabilizing or suspending agents, such as carboxymethylcellulose in injectable preparations. Such reactions are well

Table 4
Corticosteroid concentrations used in immediate skin tests

Corticosteroid	Skin Prick Test (mg/mL)	Intradermal Test (mg/mL)
Bethamethasone	4	
Dexamethasone	4	0.04–0.4
Hydrocortisone	1.00	0.04–0.4
Methylprednisolone	40	1–10
Budesonide	0.25	0.4–4
Triamcinolone	40	0.0025–0.025
Prednisone	30	0.4–4
Prednisolone	13	

Data from Venturini M, Lobera T, del Pozo, MD, et al. Immediate hypersensitivity to corticosteroids. J Investig Allergol Clin Immunol 2006;16:51–6.

documented by positive SPT and IDT[15,53] and positive basophil activation tests (see article by Hausmann and Ebo elsewhere in this issue).

In rare cases, however, a true type I allergy to steroids has been postulated with SPT and IDT as useful diagnostic tools;[53,54] in one study, seven patients who had immediate allergic symptoms to corticosteroids was described: the reaction was caused by the steroid molecule (triamcinolone or methylprednisolone succinate) in four patients and by the suspending agent carboxymethylcellulose in two, and the sensitized molecule was not identified in one patient.[55] For test concentrations see **Table 4**.

SUMMARY

In the diagnostic work-up of immediate-type ADRs, skin testing is an important component of identifying the relevant drug. SPTs and IDTs can be regarded as bioassays that rapidly detect a biologic response to mediators released from stimulated mast cells. The mediators lead to local reactions with formation of a wheal and flare, which suggest but do not prove an IgE-mediated reaction. There is a great variability, however, of skin reactivity in individual patients, which may be related to factors, such as age, skin color, time of day, timing in relation to exposure, and placement on the body.

The diagnostic validity of SPT and intracutaneous testing has been confirmed by additional in vitro or provocation testing. Thus, skin tests provide useful confirmatory evidence for a diagnosis of specific allergy that has been made on clinical grounds. Their characteristics—simplicity, rapidity of performance, low cost, and high sensitivity (at least for some reactions)—explain their key position in allergy diagnosis.[56]

The main limitation of skin tests is that a positive test is more relevant than a negative test, as the sensitivity is limited. A negative test cannot absolutely exclude a drug allergy. In addition, a positive reaction does not mean that a patient is allergic, as it reflects solely a sensitization, not allergy. Although in the past, reliable skin test procedures have been defined for some drug classes (β-lactams, neuromuscular blocking agents, and iodinated contrast media), potency and stability of the test reagents and test concentrations have been insufficiently validated for the majority of other drugs, mostly because such events are not frequent and a sufficient number of patients to serve as positive controls in a single center is lacking. Thus, progress in this field depends on (supranational) collaboration.

REFERENCES

1. Demoly P, Kropf R, Bircher A, et al. Drug hypersensitivity: questionnaire. Allergy 1999;54:999–1003.
2. Barbaud A, Goncalo M, Bruynzeel D, et al. Guidelines for performing skin tests with drugs in the investigation of cutaneous adverse drug reactions. Contact Derm 2001;45:321–8.
3. Brockow K, Romano A, Blanca M, et al. General considerations for skin test procedures in the diagnosis of drug hypersensitivity. Allergy 2002;57:45–51.
4. Mirakian R, Ewan PW, Durham SR, et al. BSACI guidelines for the management of drug allergy. Clin Exp Allergy 2009;39:43–61.
5. Barbaud A. Place of drug skin tests in investigating systemic cutaneous drug reactions. In: Pichler WJ, editor. Drug hypersensitivity. Basel, Switzerland: Karger; 2007. p. 366–79.
6. Demoly P, Bousquet J. Drug allergy diagnosis work up. Allergy 2002;57(s72): 37–40.
7. Li TJ. Allergy testing. Am Fam Physician 2002;66:621–4.
8. Benahmed S, Picot MC, Dumas F, et al. Accuracy of a pharmacovigilance algorithm in diagnosing drug hypersensitivity reactions. Arch Intern Med 2005;165: 1500–5.
9. Choquet-Kastylevsky G, Vial T, Descotes J. Drug allergy diagnosis in humans: possibilities and pitfalls. Toxicology 2001;158:1–10.
10. Wöhrl S, Vigl K, Stingl G. Patients with drug reactions—is it worth testing? Allergy 2006;61:928–34.
11. Aberer W, Kränke B. Clinical manifestations and mechanisms of skin reactions after systemic drug administration. Drug Discov Today Dis Mech 2008;5: e237–47.
12. Lammintausta K, Kortekangas-Savolainen O. The usefulness of skin tests to prove drug hypersensitivity. Br J Dermatol 2005;152:968–74.
13. Gomes ER, Fonseca J, Araujo L, et al. Drug allergy claims in children: from self-reporting to confirmed diagnosis. Clin Exp Allergy 2007;38:191–8.
14. Levine BB. Immunologic mechanisms of penicillin allergy. A haptenic model system for the study of allergic diseases. N Engl J Med 1994;331:1272–85.
15. Grims RH, Kränke B, Aberer W. Pitfalls in drug allergy skin testing: false-positive reactions due to (hidden) additives. Contact Derm 2006;54:290–4.
16. Liccardi G, D'Amato G, Canonica GW, et al. Systemic reactions from skin testing: literature review. J Investig Allergol Clin Immunol 2006;16:75–8.
17. Koshak EA. Could a routine skin test to penicillin lead to fatal anaphylaxis? East Mediterr Health J 2000;6:526–31.
18. Gaig Jane P, Casas Ramisa R, Nevot Falco S, et al. Anaphylactic reaction during performance of skin tests in a patient allergic to amoxicillin. Med Clin (Barc) 1997; 13:319.
19. Weber-Mani U, Pichler WJ. Anaphylactic shock after intradermal testing with betalactam antibiotics. Allergy 2008;63:785.
20. Torres MJ, Blanca M, Fernandez J, et al. Diagnosis of immediate allergic reactions to beta-lactam antibiotics. Allergy 2003;58:961–72.
21. Torres MJ, Romano A, Mayorga C, et al. Diagnostic evaluation of a large group of patients with immediate allergy to penicillins: the role of skin testing. Allergy 2001; 56:850–6.
22. Blanca M, Romano A, Torres MJ, et al. Update on the evaluation of hypersensitivity reactions to betalactams. Allergy 2009;64:183–93.

23. DePestel DD, Benninger MS, Danzinger L, et al. Cephalosporin use in treatment of patients with penicillin allergies. J Am Pharm Assoc 2008;48:530–40.
24. Weiss ME, Adkinson NF. Diagnostic testing for drug hypersensitivity. Immunol Allergy Clin North Am 1998;18:731–44.
25. Romano A, Bousquet-Rouanet L, Viola M, et al. Benzylpenicillin skin testing is still important in diagnosing immediate hypersensitivity reactions to penicillins. Allergy 2009;64:249–53.
26. Yates AB. Management of patients with a history of allergy to beta-lactam antibiotics. Am J Med 2008;121:572–6.
27. Blanca M, Romano A, Torres MJ, et al. Continued need of appropriate betalactam-derived skin test reagents for the management of allergy to betalactams. Clin Exp Allergy 2007;37:166–73.
28. Rodriguez-Bada JL, Montanez MI, Torres MJ, et al. Skin testing for immediate hypersensitivity to betalactams: comparison between two commercial kits. Allergy 2006;61:947–51.
29. Romano A, Gaeta F, Valluzzi RL, et al. Diagnosing hypersensitivity reactions to cephalosporins in children. Pediatrics 2008;122:521–7.
30. Bousquet PJ, Kvedariene V, Co-Minh HB, et al. Clinical presentation and time course in hypersensitivity reactions to ß-lactams. Allergy 2007; 62:872–6.
31. Pichichero ME. Use of selected cephalosporins in penicillin-allergic patients: a paradigm shift. Diagn Microbiol Infect Dis 2007;57:13s–8s.
32. Pichichero ME. A review of evidence supporting the American Academy of Pediatrics recommendation for prescribing cephalosporin antibiotics for penicillin-allergic patients. Pediatrics 2005;115:1048–57.
33. Romano A, Quaratino D, Venuti A, et al. Selective type-1 hypersensitivity to ceftriaxone. J Allergy Clin Immunol 1998;101:564–5.
34. Romano A, Mayorga C, Torres MJ, et al. Immediate allergic reactions to cephalosporins: cross-reactivity and selective responses. J Allergy Clin Immunol 2000;106:1177–83.
35. Antunez C, Blanca-Lopez N, Torres MJ, et al. Immediate allergic reactions to cephalosporins: evaluation of cross-reactivity with a panel of penicillins and cephalosporins. J Allergy Clin Immunol 2006;117:404–10.
36. Romano A, Gueant-Rodriguez RM, Viola M, et al. Cross-reactivity and toleralibility of cephalosporins in patients with immediate hypersensitivity to penicillins. Ann Intern Med 2004;141:16–22.
37. Romano A, Viola M, Guéant-Rodriguez RM, et al. Imipenem in patients with immediate hypersensitivity to penicillins. N Engl J Med 2006;354:2835–7.
38. Romano A, Viola M, Guéant-Rodriguez RM, et al. Brief communication: tolerability of meropenem in patients with IgE-mediated hypersensitivity to penicillins. Ann Intern Med 2007;146:266–9.
39. Empedrad R, Darter AM, Earl HS, et al. Nonirritating intradermal skin test concentrations for commonly prescribed antibiotics. J Allergy Clin Immunol 2003;112: 629–30.
40. Mertes PM, Laxenaire MC, Alla F. Anaphylactic and anaphylactoid reactions occurring during anesthesia in France in 1999–2000. Anesthesiology 2003;99: 536–45.
41. Lobera T, Audicana MT, Pozo MD, et al. Study of hypersensitivity reactions and anaphylaxis during anaesthesia in Spain. J Investig Allergol Clin Immunol 2008; 18:350–6.

42. Harboe T, Johansson SGO, Florvaag E, et al. Pholcodine exposure raises serum IgE in patients with previous anaphylaxis to neuromuscular blocking agents. Allergy 2007;62:1445–50.

43. Mertes PM, Laxenaire MC, Lienhart A, et al. Reducing the risk of anaphylaxis during anaesthesia: Guidelines for clinic practice. J Investig Allergol Clin Immunol 2005;15:91–101.

44. Thyssen JP, Menne T, Elberling J, et al. Hypersensitivity to local anaesthetics—update and proposal of evaluation algorithm. Contact Derm 2008;59:69–78.

45. Gall H, Kaufmann R, Kalveram CM. Adverse reactions to local anesthetics: analysis of 197 cases. J Allergy Clin Immunol 1996;97:933–7.

46. Jacobsen RB, Borch JE, Bindslev-Jensen C. Hypersensitivity to local anaesthetics. Allergy 2005;60:262–4.

47. Zanotti KM, Rybicki LA, Kennedy AW, et al. Carboplatin skin testing: a skin-testing protocol for predicting hypersensitivity to carboplatin chemotherapy. J Clin Oncol 2001;19:3126–9.

48. Markman M, Zanotti K, Peterson G, et al. Expanded experience with an intradermal skin test to predict for the presence or absence of carboplatin hypersensitivity. J Clin Oncol 2003;21:4611–4.

49. Leguy-Seguin V, Jolimoy G, Coudert B, et al. Diagnostic and predictive value of skin testing in platinum salt hypersensitivity. J Allergy Clin Immunol 2007;119: 726–30.

50. Pagani M, Bonadona P, Senna GE, et al. Standardization of skin tests for diagnosis and prevention of hypersensitivity reactions to oxaliplatin. Int Arch Allergy Immunol 2008;145:54–7.

51. Johansson SG, Hourihane JO, Bousquet J, et al. A revised nomenclature for allergy. An EAACI position statement from the EAACI nomenclature task force. Allergy 2001;56:813–24.

52. Brockow K, Romano A, Aberer W, et al. Skin testing in patients with hypersensitivity reactions to iodinated contrast media—a European multicenter study. Allergy 2009;64:234–41.

53. Caduff C, Reinhart WH, Hartmann K, et al. Immediate hypersensitivity reactions to parenteral glucocorticoids? Analysis of 14 cases. Schweiz Med Wochenschr 2000;130:977–83.

54. Nettis E, Muratore L, Calogiuri G, et al. Urticaria to hydrocortisone. Allergy 2001; 56:802–3.

55. Venturini M, Lobera T, del Pozo MD, et al. Immediate hypersensitivity to corticosteroids. J Investig Allergol Clin Immunol 2006;16:51–6.

56. Wallace DV, Bahna SL, Goldstein S, et al. American Academy of Allergy, Asthma & Immunology Work Group Report: allergy diagnosis in clinical practice. J Allergy Clin Immunol 2007;120:967–9.

Skin Testing in Delayed Reactions to Drugs

Annick Barbaud, MD, PhD

KEYWORDS

- Maculopapular rash
- Acute generalized exanthematous pustulosis
- Drug reaction with eosinophilia and systemic symptoms
- Toxic epidermal necrolysis (TEN) • Drug patch tests
- Intradermal tests • Antibiotics • Corticosteroids

During recent years, numerous reports have emphasized the usefulness of drug skin tests (patch tests, prick tests, intradermal tests [IDT]) for the investigation of cutaneous adverse drug reactions (CADR) caused by delayed hypersensitivity to drugs.[1–6] The following CADR are supposed to be caused totally or partially by a delayed cell-mediated hypersensitivity: maculopapular rash (MPR), photosensitivities to drugs, heparin-induced cell-mediated reactions, acute generalized exanthematous pustulosis (AGEP), drug reactions with eosinophilia and systemic symptoms (DRESS), fixed drug eruption (FDE), Stevens Johnson syndrome (SJS) or toxic epidermal necrolysis (TEN).[7] Drug patch testing (or prick/IDT with delayed reading) are the logical first step in defining the relevant drug in these reactions.[1,6–12] They can also help to better understand the pathomechanism of these reactions.[1,8,13,14] However, although some drugs have been used widely and are standardized (eg, amoxicillin), many compounds are still not standardized for skin-testing and their use remains experimental. Because frequently no other possibility exists to pinpoint the relevant drug, these tests are nevertheless widely used, but they should be interpreted cautiously.

Different guidelines for performing drug skin tests (patch tests, prick tests, and IDT) with drugs in the investigation CADR have been published.[3,15] It is advised to perform drug skin tests during the 6 months following the CADR[4] because the persistence of drug allergies seem to vary substantially and cannot be predicted in the individual case. Patch tests and prick tests can be done with any commercialized form of a drug. Intradermal tests can be done only if an injectable form of the drug is commercialized. If one uses IDR in patients with severe CADR, one should be aware that skin testing may reactivate the disease.

Department of Dermatology, Fournier Hospital, University Hospital of Nancy, Nancy, France
E-mail address: a.barbaud@chu-nancy.fr

Immunol Allergy Clin N Am 29 (2009) 517–535
doi:10.1016/j.iac.2009.04.010
0889-8561/09/$ – see front matter © 2009 Elsevier Inc. All rights reserved.

immunology.theclinics.com

DRUG PATCH TESTS
Drug Concentration in Drug Patch Tests

The threshold of sensitivity for many pure substances has not been determined in drug patch tests. Therefore, a practical approach would be to use a 10% concentration in petrolatum and, if necessary, in other vehicles, although for some drugs, smaller concentrations may be sufficient.[1,3,4] Recently, standardized material to do patch test with pure molecules diluted in petrolatum has been commercialized for some drugs (Chemotechnique laboratory, Malmö, Sweden) (**Table 1**).

Using a pulverized tablet, 30% is the highest concentration possible to get a homogeneous dilution in petrolatum, in water or in alcohol.[3] When the commercialized form of the drug is used, it is advised to use a 30% concentration of the final product. It is also possible to use a concentration that leads to a final 10% concentration of the active drug, when the weight of the active drug and excipients are known in the commercialized form. With commercialized forms of the drugs, each preparation is done for only one patient. As the stability of these freshly made substances may vary, they cannot be kept more than a few hours.[1,3] Whenever possible, preservatives, coloring agents and excipients should also be tested, undiluted or diluted at 10% in petrolatum, or in the vehicles and concentrations usually proposed for testing allergic contact dermatitis. Testing with acyclovir, carbamazepine or pseudoephedrin have been reported to reinduce the CADR symptoms during patch testing (see **Table 1**).[1,2,4] Therefore, it is recommended that patch tests are performed, first diluted at 1% and, when negative, up to 10% (either with the commercialized form of the drug or the pure substance). Moreover, to avoid false positive results, some drugs have to be tested at higher dilutions. The content of capsules of celecoxib (Celebrex) should be tested at 5% or at 10% in petrolatum and not with any higher concentration.[16] Desloratadine has to be tested at 1% in petrolatum (see **Table 1**).[17] Colchicin at 10% in petrolatum induces false positive results, the threshold of specificity is unknown.[18] Captopril in commercialized forms diluted at 1% and chloroquine in commercialized forms diluted at 30% in petrolatum sometimes induce false positive results.[18] Misoprostol in commercialized forms has to be diluted at 1% in petrolatum.[18]

In investigating a photosensitivity reaction induced by a drug, both drug patch tests and drug photopatch tests with the responsible drug have to be performed. The irradiation for drug photopatch tests is performed on day 1, or for practical reasons, can be performed on day 2 with a 5 Joules/cm2 UVA irradiation.[3] Photoscratch patch tests are more irritating, do not have a better value than photopatch tests, and should consequently be avoided.[19]

The results of patch testing are reported according to the International Contact Dermatitis Research Group (ICDRG) criteria for patch test reading[20] with negative, doubtful or positive (+, ++, +++) results on days 2 and 4.

The best vehicle to prepare drug patch test has not yet been determined. Petrolatum seemed to be convenient in most of the cases.[1,3] Steroid hormones have to be tested diluted in alcohol because false negative results have been observed in testing estrogens diluted in water or petrolatum.[3]

Under chambers, patch tests are performed on the upper back, but it could also be of value to test on the most affected site of the initial CADR. Testing in the affected area is recommended in FDE[9] but could also be of value in other forms of CADR, as reported in TEN with co-trimoxazole[21] or with tetrazepam in a patient with MPR.[22]

Drug Patch Tests and Topical Application in Fixed Drug Eruption

In FDE, it is well known that patch tests[9] or open application tests[23–25] with the suspected drug are more positive when performed on the residual pigmented skin site of the CADR but not when applied on the previously nonaffected skin of the back. In 312/523 topical provocation tests, which were done with the suspected drug diluted at 5% in petrolatum, Mahboob and colleagues[25] had positive results in FDE, mainly caused by sulfamethoxazole. They performed the application test on the normal skin of the forearm. Seghal and Srivastava[26] proposed to perform at first patch tests on the nonaffected skin area, followed—if negative—by a topical provocation test. Finally, if the cutaneous tests are negative, it can be suggested to do an oral provocation test,[27] while starting with amounts lower than those used for the therapeutic use of the offending drug.

PRICK TESTS

Prick tests are performed to identify immediate reactions or in unclear cases. They are done on the volar forearm with the commercialized form of the drug. In delayed CADR, they have to be read at 20 min and also at 24 hours after the tests, because delayed positive results can occur also in prick tests[2,3,13] in patients with drug-induced MPR.

INTRADERMAL TESTS

Intradermal tests are performed only when prick tests show negative results 20 min after testing with the suspected drug. Because they could re-induce the adverse drug reactions, IDTs in SJS, TEN, leucocytoclastic vasculitis or DRESS are normally not recommended.[3,4] Patients with DRESS are particularly sensitive to IDT that have been reported to induce immediate or delayed[3,28] relapses of the CADR.

Because the techniques used in performing IDT are not standardized, thresholds for specificity are impossible to compare from one study to another.[18,29,30] Considering the two papers written on guidelines in doing drug skin tests,[3,15] it should be advised to determine the volume (0.03 mL to 0.05 mL), wherever the site of injection, which leads to a diameter of the injection wheal of 3 mm. Read at 20 min, IDT would be considered as having positive results when the diameter of the reaction is equal or greater than 6 mms. In delayed reactions, IDT have to be read after 24 hours or later. Delayed reactions are considered positive when there is an infiltrated erythematous reaction.[3,4,15,29,30]

THE VALUE OF DRUG SKIN TESTS (SENSITIVITY AND SPECIFICITY)

In populations with various or unknown imputabilities for the tested drug, drug patch tests were positive in 89/826 patients (10.8%).[31] In patients with a high probability that a given drug would cause a CADR, drug (photopatch) patch tests had positive results in 50% of 108 patients.[4] Lammintausta and Kortekangas-Savolainen[31] with an unknown imputability of the tested drugs obtained 10 (1.1%) positive reactions on 935 prick tests.

Photopatch tests may be useful in studying drug photosensitivity, but patch tests have a low sensitivity in investigating SJS or TEN,[32] pruritus or vasculitis.[1–4]

Except for betalactam antibiotics, the usefulness of prick tests and IDT in determining the cause of delayed CADR has not been evaluated as widely as that of drug patch tests. With a high imputability for a drug having induced a CADR, positive results were obtained in 24% of 46 cases with prick tests and in 64% of the 30 patients undergoing IDT.[3]

IDT is generally more sensitive than patch testing: Among 60 patients with CADR and negative patch tests with the suspected drug, 35 (58%) had positive results on IDT.[3] Among 94 patients with a suspected delayed sensitization to betalactam

Table 1
Drugs with reported positive patch tests, in investigating systemic cutaneous adverse drug reactions or commercialized material for drug patch test available

Drug or Drug Class	References	Concentrations Used and Controls (when available)	Relapse of the CADR Caused by Drug Patch Tests
Acetylsalicylic acid	—	C*: 10% in petrolatum	—
Acyclovir	87,88	As is, 20%, 10% and 1% in petrolatum (commercialized form?)[31] Acyclovir 10% in petrolatum[40] C*: 10% in petrolatum	—
Allylisopropylacetylurea	89	—	—
5-aminosalicylic acid	80	3% in petrolatum	—
Amoxicillin	2,9–11,13,31, 33,46,49	10% in petrolatum seems to be specific C*: 10% in petrolatum	Immediate reactions in case of anaphylaxis
Betalactam antibiotics	2,31,33,83,84	C*: penicillin G, potassium salt 10% in petrolatum, dicloxacillin sodium salt hydrate 10% in petrolatum, cefotaxim sodium salt 10% in petrolatum; cefradine 10% in petrolatum, cefalexin 10% in petrolatum	Immediate reactions in case of anaphylaxis
Azathioprine	47,48	—	—
Captopril	2,90	At 1% and 10% in petrolatum[91] False positive results.[2,18] C*: 5% in petrolatum	—
Carbamazepine	3,66,68,82	10% in petrolatum C*: 1% in petrolatum	3
Cefcapene pivoxil	92	10% and 1% in petrolatum	—
Celecoxib Frequent false positive reactions	16,65,93	Has to be tested at 10% or 1%. Higher concentrations can induce false positive results[16]	—
Chloroquine No true positive reaction	—	False positive reactions The threshold of specificity has to be determined[18]	
Chlorphenamine	94	20% in petrolatum (commercialized form?) 15 negative controls	

Drug	Ref.	Notes	
Clindamycin	—	C*: 10% in petrolatum	—
Ciprofloxacin	51,100		—
Clarithromycin	—	C*: 10% in petrolatum	—
Clindamycin	31,52		—
Clobazam	95		96
Codeine	96	Diluted at 1% and 5% in petrolatum (Two negative controls)	—
Colchicine False positive results	18	Diluted at 10% in petrolatum, 80% of 29 negative controls developed false-positive results[18]	—
Corticosteroids	2,53,97	If negative, have to be diluted in ethyl alcohol[1]	—
Cotrimoxazole: sulfamethoxazole/ Trimethoprim	21,23,25	10%, 20% or 50% in dimethyl sulfoxide (DMSO) but frequently negative when diluted in petrolatum[3] C*: 10% in petrolatum	—
Cyamemazine	2	30% petrolatum (commercialized form)	—
Cyclines	68	0.1% and 1% in a DRESS C*: doxycycline 10% in petrolatum; minocycline 10% in petrolatum	—
Desloratadine	17	Diluted at 10% in petrolatum in 8/10 volunteers, seems to be specific when tested diluted at 1% in petrolatum (7 negative controls)[17]	—
Diazepam	12		—
Diclofenac	98	1% in petrolatum[99] C*: 1% in petrolatum	At 1% pet in an anaphylactic shock[4]
Diltiazem	2,54,99	10% in petrolatum C*: 10% in petrolatum	—
Enoxoparin	2	Pure	—
Erythromycin	—	C*: 10% in petrolatum	—
Esomeprazole	70		—
Estrogens	3	If negative, tested diluted in alcohol	—
Famciclovir	88	50% in petrolatum (commercialized form)	—

(continued on next page)

Table 1
(continued)

Drug or Drug Class	References	Concentrations Used and Controls (when available)	Relapse of the CADR Caused by Drug Patch Tests
Fluindione	71	5% and 30% in petrolatum (commercialized form), doubtful in water	—
Fluoroquinolones	2,51,99,100	30% in petrolatum or water (commercialized form) C*: norfloxacine 10% in petrolatum; ciprofloxacine hydrochloride 10% in petrolatum	—
Fusafungine	2	30% in petrolatum (commercialized form)	—
Ganciclovir	21	As is, 20% in petrolatum To study cross reactions with aciclovir	—
Gentamycin	31	—	—
Heparin derivatives	18,43	Nonspecific results do to sensitization to excipients (benzyl alcohol)[18]	—
Hydantoin	—	C*: 10% in petrolatum	—
Hydrochlorothiazide	—	10% in petrolatum	—
Hydroxyzine	1,2	10% in petrolatum C*: 1% in petrolatum	2
Ibuprofen	—	C*: 10% in petrolatum	—
Isoniazide	33,68	at 50% in petrolatum (10 negative controls)[68]	—
Ketoprofene	—	C*: 1% in petrolatum	—
Lamisil (terbinafine)	2	As is; detail of the test remained negative[2]	—
Meprobamate	2	30% in petrolatum (commercialized form)	—
Metamizole	55,70	1% and 10% in petrolatum	55
Methoxalene	56		—
Metronidazole	54,102		—
Mexiletine hydrochloride	103	Diluted at 10% and 20% in petrolatum[104]	—
Misoprostol No true positive reaction	18	False positive results in 9/10 negative controls at the day 2 reading, no false positive results at the day 4 reading or when Cytotec was diluted at 1% in petrolatum[18]	—

Drug	Ref	Concentration/excipient	Relapse Ref
Morphine	57	—	—
Nimesulide	58,104	10% in petrolatum (commercialized form?)[95]	—
Neomercazole	47	—	—
Nystatin	105	10% in petrolatum (10 negative controls)	—
Omeprazole	18	30% in petrolatum or water (commercialized form)	—
No true positive reaction			
Oxicams	106–108	1% in petrolatum[107] or 10% in petrolatum[109]; C*: piroxicam 1% in petrolatum	—
Paracetamol (acetaminophen)	109	C*: 10% in petrolatum	Relapse of an AGEP?[109]
Pristinamycin	2,36	C*: 10% in petrolatum	2
Pseudoephedrine	2,59,60,81	Tested at 1% in petrolatum to avoid any relapse of the CADR	2,81,111
Radio contrast medium (RCM)	39–42,79	Pure	—
Ranitidine	61	—	—
Rifampicin	110	—	—
Spironolactone	72	Can induce false positive reactions[18]	—
Spiramycin	—	C*: 10% in petrolatum	—
Teicoplanin	34	4% water (20 negative controls)	34
Tetrazepam	2,22,62,111	30% in commercialized form, 10% in petrolatum	—
Triamcinolone	2	30% in petrolatum (commercialized form)	2
Valaciclovir	87,88	30% in petrolatum, water or alcohol,[88] commercialized form; as is, 20%, 10%, 1% commercialized form?[87]	—
Vancomycin	34	0.005% in water (20 negative controls)	34
Vitamin K1	112	10 mg/mL in olive oil	—
Vitamin K3	112	10 mg/mL in olive oil	—

Concentrations and excipients used in preparing the material for these positive tests are reported. In the last columns, references in which drug patch tests induced a relapse of the CADR are reported.

Abbreviation: C*, Chemotechnique Laboratory, Malmö, Sweden antibiotics, 36% had positive patch tests and IDT, but eight patients had positive IDT with negative patch tests.[33]

However, in a CADR caused by vancomycin, prick tests—as well as IDT with glycopeptide antibiotics—remained negative even on delayed readings, while drug patch tests were positive and specific (20 negative controls).[34] This study emphasizes that delayed reactions to IDT are not always sufficient to investigate a CADR because of delayed hypersensitivity to drugs, but drug patch tests also have to be performed since they can be positive despite of a negative IDT.

The Usefulness of Drug Skin Tests Depends on the Clinical Features of the CADR

Patch tests are of value in determining the responsible drug in generalized eczema or systemic contact dermatitis (**Table 2**).

In patients who have maculopapular rashes, patch tests have been reported to be useful.[1,3,4,10,13,35] Even if they are rare, delayed positive results on prick tests have been reported.[2,36] In 165 patients suffering from a CADR, with a high imputability of one drug, patch tests were positive in 33/61 (54%) MPR, but in only 2/33 (6%) of urticarias and the difference was statistically significant (Chi 2 test).[3,4]

Recent studies have confirmed the value of IDT in investigating delayed hypersensitivity to drugs. In MPR, delayed positive reactions of IDT have been reported with betalactam antibiotics,[3,37] synergistins,[36] platinium salts[38] or radiocontrast medias.[39-42] Delayed positive results of IDT have also been reported in investigating localized eczema or MPR caused by heparins.[3,43,44] Even though they are not drugs, recent studies emphasize that radio contrast media (RCM) can induce delayed CADR. The value of patch tests in delayed hypersensitivity to RCM varied from 2/15[40] to 46/58,[45] but IDT have a better value as 8/15 patients had delayed positive reactions on IDT only.[40] Consequently, drug skin tests are of value in investigating MPR.

The sequence of testing depends on the clinical situation and severity of symptoms. A very cautious approach would be to begin the investigations with patch tests, followed, if negative, by prick tests (with delayed readings at 24 h hours) and, if the injectable form of the drugs are available, continue with IDT with immediate and delayed readings. However, in many clinical situations the testing is more concentrated: prick testing, application of patch tests, and, if negative, IDT.

In cell-mediated delayed hypersensitivity to heparins, the most sensitive test for diagnosis is the IDT[3,43,44] read after 24 hours and 72 hours. Tolerance to heparin derivatives is best proven with a subcutaneous test.[43,46] Attention has to be paid to avoid subcutaneously injecting too many heparin derivatives simultaneously because they could induce a strong anticoagulation. Because they are not useful and dangerous in case of heparin-induced necrosis, drug skin tests are contraindicated.

In AGEP, patch tests seems of value as they were positive in 7/14 patients with AGEP tested by Wolkenstein and colleagues.[32] Single cases have been published emphasizing the value of drug patch tests in AGEP with carbimazole,[47] azathioprine,[48] betalactam antibiotics,[2,49] bleomycin,[50] ciprofloxacin,[51] clindamycin,[52] corticosteroids (two cases),[53] diltiazem,[54] metamizole,[55] methoxalene,[56] metronidazole,[54] morphin,[57] nimesulide,[58] pseudoephedrin,[59,60] ranitidine[61] and tetrazepam.[62]

Some reports have been published on other tests in investigating AGEP. Komericki and colleagues[63] described positive results on provocation tests with different heparins but inducing a generalized rash occurring the day following the subcutaneous injections. Subcutaneous provocation testing showed cross-reactions to enoxaparin, certoparin, reviparin, nadroparin, danaparoid and fondaparinux. Lymphocyte activation tests have been reported with positive results in patients with AGEP who had

Table 2			
The value of drug skin tests according to the clinical features of the cutaneous adverse drug reaction			
	Patch Tests	Prick Tests	IDT
Maculopapular rash	Useful	+ before IDT and with delayed readings at 24 h	With immediate but especially delayed readings at 24 h and later if negative
Generalized eczema	Useful	+ before IDT and with delayed readings at 24 h	With immediate but especially delayed readings at 24 h and later if negative
Localized eczema caused by heparins	Useful	No value but done before IDT	With immediate but especially delayed readings at 24 h and later if negative (frequently positive only after 3 days)
SDRIFE (Baboon syndrome)	Useful	Unknown value	Unknown value
Acute generalized exanthematous pustulosis	Useful	Unknown value	Unknown value
Fixed drug eruption	Useful on the residual area	Unknown value	Unknown value
DRESS	Probably of value, but without any large reported series of patients	Unknown value, probably very low value	Unknown value. Has to be cautiously applied (flare-up reactions)
Vasculitis	No value	No value	No value and could be dangerous
TEN	Can be done but is rarely positive. Could be interesting to perform on the mostly affected area	No value	Are rarely done because they could be dangerous (flare-up) reactions
Photosensitivity	Photopatch tests (5 J)	No value	No value

SDRIFE, Symmetric drug-related intertriginous and flexural exanthema; DRESS, drug reaction with eosinophilia and systemic symptoms.
  Widely used drugs for IDT.
  Data from Barbaud A. Drug skin tests and systemic drug reactions: an update. Expert Rev Dermatol 2007; 2:481–95.

also positive patch tests with corticosteroids,[53] diltiazem,[54] metamizole,[55] metronidazole[54] and morphin[57] or negative patch tests with cotrimoxazole.[64]

In DRESS, there is no study with a large number of patients who have been tested for a DRESS. Patch tests could be of value because cases have been reported with positive results with antituberculosis drugs,[65] anticonvulsant drugs,[66,67] cyclines,[68] cefadroxil,[69] esomeprazole,[70] fluindione[71] or spironolactone.[72]

TEN and SJS: patch testing has a weak sensitivity in SJS or toxic epidermal necrolysis (TEN) as only two patients among the 22 SJS/TEN cases tested by Wolkenstein and colleagues[32] had a relevant positive test. However, a few case reports have been published with positive drug patch tests in patients with TEN. Positive patch tests in such patients have been reported with amoxicillin and penicillin,[73] ampicillin,[74] carbamazepine,[75] co-trimoxazole[21] or pseudoephedrine diluted at 3%.[76] According to the case reported by Klein and colleagues,[21] testing in the affected area could be of value in SJS/TEN patients.

Even if there are a few reports on IDT in SJS/TEN patients, the authors would like to emphasize that such tests are potentially dangerous in such patients. In investigating a patient with recurrent NSAID-induced erosions of the nipple, considered to be a FDE, the authors observed a generalized rash within the 3 hours following IDT done with the incriminated NSAIDs (A. Barbaud, unpublished data, 2007). The authors could obtain photographs taken during one of the previous onset of the adverse drug reaction, displaying erosions on the nipple but also on the lips that were suggestive of a SJS. This case emphasizes the risk of relapse of SJS in performing IDT in SJS/TEN patients. Patch tests with NSAIDs were negative and well tolerated by this patient.

In Baboon syndrome, which was recently renamed as symmetric drug-related intertriginous and flexural exanthema (SDRIFE), patch tests can be useful, with positive results reported with betalactam antibiotics, clindamycin, erythromycin, neomycin,[77,78] RCM,[79] 5-aminosalicylic acid diluted at 3% in petrolatum[80] or pseudoephedrin.[81] In this CADR, supposed to be a systemic contact dermatitis or more probably a recall phenomenon of an earlier dermatitis that had occurred in precisely the same areas, patch tests can remain negative as reported with betalactam antibiotics,[82] heparin,[83] intravenous immunoglobulins[78] or cetuximab.[84] Patch tests induced a flare up of a SDRIFE caused by pseudoephedrin.[81] One case has been reported with delayed positive reactions on a prick test done with amoxicillin.[85] A relapse can be elicited by a systemic exposure to the offending drug or cross reactive drugs,[78,86] possibly with a more severe generalized reaction.[78]

Usefulness of Drug Skin Tests According to the Tested Drug

The usefulness of drug skin tests also depends on the tested drug. Miscellaneous drugs have been reported as yielding CADR with positive drug patch tests.[2,3,9–12,16–18,21,22,31,33,34,36,39–43,47–49,51–62,65,66,69,71,73,74,81,87–112] They are reported in **Table 1**.

Most of the papers published on the usefulness of prick tests and IDT concern CADR caused by betalactam antibiotics.[3,30,32,33,91,113,114] On 998 skin tests done with betalactams, 14.7% of the patients had positive results.[28] Among 166 subjects with associated aminopenicillin-associated MPR, patch tests and delayed-reading intradermal tests with amoxicillin and ampicillin were positive in 52.4% and 54.2% respectively.[33] In delayed CADR, prick tests and IDT have also been performed with other drugs (**Table 3**).[3,4,11,13,18,30,32,33,36–44,46,110,111,114–124]

Usefulness of Drug Skin Tests to Study Cross-Reactivity Between Drugs

Skin tests can help to study the ability of drugs to elicit symptoms caused by cross-reactivity, such as between betalactam antibiotics (eg, penicillins and

Table 3	
Main drugs reported with positive intradermal tests in investigating delayed cutaneous adverse drug reactions	
Drug Classes	**References**
Betalactam antibiotics	3,11,13,18,30,32,33,37,114–116
Local anesthetics	111
Corticosteroids	118
Estradiol	3
Heparin derivatives	3,4,43,44,46,119–121
Insulin	122,123
Platin salts	38
Quinolones	124
Radiocontrast media	39–42
Rifampicin	110
Synergistins	36

cephalosporins).[33] In MPR caused by diltiazem, patch tests with other calcium channel blockers are rarely positive, and no cross-reactions between dihydropyridine calcium channel blockers (CCB) and "non-dihydropyridine" CCB is found (verapamil, diltiazem).[99]

No or rare cross-reactivity between tetrazepam and diazepam was detected.[111] With patch tests and drug re-administration, cross-reactions between acyclovir, valacyclovir and famciclovir are frequent in patients suffering from CADR caused by acyclovir.[87,88] It could be caused by a common chemical structure because the 2-aminopurine nucleus is also found in ganciclovir but not in foscarnet or cidofovir.[88] Cross-reactions between synergistins are very frequent as demonstrated in 29 cases of CADR caused by pristinamycin.[36] Cross-reactions between synergistins occurred in patients sensitized to pristinamycin, in 9/22 cases with virginiamycin and in 7/8 cases with dalfopristin-quinupristin.

In piroxicam reactions, the profile of cross-sensitization may differ in distinct clinical features of the CADR.[106–108] In photosensitization, photopatch tests with piroxicam were positive in 27/31. However, there was no cross-reaction with tenoxicam and lenoxicam and only 1/31 had positive photopatch tests with meloxicam. On the other hand, in one case of a photosensitization to piroxicam, all photopatch tests with piroxicam, tenoxicam, droxicam and meloxicam were positive.[107] However, in eight patients who had FDE, cross-reactions between oxicams were very frequent.[108] There is cross-reactivity among pseudoephedrin and different sympathomimetic drugs, such as phenylephrine or ephedrine.[125] Drug patch tests can also be used to study reactions between the native drug and its metabolites, as done for carbamazepine and its main metabolite carbamazepine oxide.[91]

Between unfractionated heparins (UHF), low-molecular weight heparins (LMWH), heparinoid (danaparoid) and the pentasaccharide (fondaparinux) cross reactions have been studied.[3,4,43,46,119–121] They have been studied with prick tests and mainly IDT in cell-mediated type IV reactions (localized eczema and MPR). Cross-reactions are frequent between UFH and LMWH. They are rarer with danaparoid and seldomly occur with fondaparinux.[44,46,119] These tests have no value in cases of heparin-induced thrombocytopenia or necrosis and are actually dangerous in these reactions.

With patch tests, prick tests, and IDT, cross reactions have also been demonstrated between radiocontrast medias.[40] The reactivity pattern differs from one patient to another and no general rule of cross-reactivity can be given. Therefore, a broad testing is recommended to find a replacement within the same therapeutic class.

Negative predictive value of drug patch tests

The predictive value of a negative drug skin test is unknown. There are many published cases of CADR with negative drug patch tests but positive delayed IDT.[3,4] It was also reported with rifampicin.[110]

In a recent study[126] the authors re-exposed patients with CADR and negative patch, prick, and intradermal tests either to the same drug (drug rechallenge [DR]) or an alternative drug, but still belonging to the same drug class (substituted drug [ST]). Of 260 patients, 27 reacted to the same drug (10, 4%) and of 143 patients exposed to a different, but related drug, 15 reacted (10, 5%). Considering only delayed CADR, DR results were positive in 15/175 cases (8.6%) and ST in 7/76 cases (9.2%). Lammintausta and Kortekangas-Savolainen[31] performed drug challenges in 229 patients who had negative patch tests or prick tests. They had a positive challenge in 22/229 patients (9.6%).

Considering challenges in betalactam hypersensitivity, Romano and colleagues[115] did not observe any positive challenge in 49 patients having negative patch tests, prick tests, IDT and specific IgE against betalactams. In a study by Waton and colleagues,[126] 4/30 (13%) of the patients with negative skin tests had a positive DR and 2/48 (4%) of the patients had a positive ST. In 93 children retreated by betalactam antibiotics, after having had negative responses in skin and challenge tests to these antibiotics, only one child developed a rash. This latter study emphasizes the good predictive negative value of drug skin testing followed by oral challenge and does not support the notion that skin testing should be repeated in children diagnosed nonallergic to betalactams.[116]

With corticosteroids 5/19 cases (26%) had a positive ST,[126] as Padial and colleagues[118] observed 19 positive reactions among 30 patients (63%) with a CADR caused by corticosteroids. In delayed reactions occurring with RCM, the negative predictive value seems to be low. Indeed, even with negative patch tests, prick tests, and IDT, 5/12 patients that had negative skin tests to the readministered RCM, had a relapse during the re-administration of this RCM.[40]

Consequently, negative drug skin tests do not exclude the responsibility of one drug in the onset of a CADR. However, because the skin tests have in general a high specificity (see below), skin testing reduces the need of provocation testing. This finding is important because provocation testing in delayed reactions are not standardized and it is currently not clear which dose and for how many days a re-exposure should be done.

Nevertheless, in nonsevere CADR, negative drug skin tests with the responsible drug or with related drugs belonging to the same class as the suspected drug should be followed by an oral provocation test with the incriminated drug or a related drug with at least the full daily dose under surveillance.

Safety of drug skin tests

Drug patch tests can re-induce the delayed CADR as reported with miscellaneous drugs (see **Table 1**). The relapse of the CADR is more frequent with IDT,[3] occurring in almost 10% of the cases.

Even with negative results, a relapse of a pruritic rash occurred following a prick test with pristinamycin.[36] The relapse of an AGEP has been provoked with patch tests with acetaminophen (paracetamol) while these tests remained negative.[109] Thus, patch tests, prick tests, and IDT can induce a systemic reaction even though their results were negative.

Relevance and specificity of drug patch tests

One crucial point is the interpretation of the results of skin tests with drugs. As negative control, the vehicle used to dilute the material for patch tests should be tested. False positive drug patch tests are very rare but can be observed when caused by a sensitization to ethyl alcohol but also to petrolatum.[127]

False positive results are more frequent in performing IDT,[18] but false positive or nonrelevant results can also be obtained in drug patch testing, namely with the commercialized form of drugs containing sodium laurylsulfate in their formulation or colchicines, misoprostol, captopril, chloroquine, omeprazole,[18] celecoxib[16] or desloratadine.[17]

This finding emphasizes the necessity to compare skin test results of patients with those obtained in negative controls.[3,18] Because of individual differences, at least 20 controls should be tested with the same preparation.

A drug patch test may be positive because of a contact dermatitis to a drug or excipient with no relevance to the CADR.[18] Drug patch tests can also be positive with a commercialized form of a drug but not because the patient is sensitized to the drug but because of a contact allergy to another component of the commercialized form. Such nonrelevant positive drug patch tests, done with commercialized forms of drugs, have been reported where preservatives or stabilizers were causative but not the drug itself, eg, iodine in antiflu pills, avocado oil, sodium sulfite in certain formulations, or benzyl alcohol in patients with heparin–intolerance.[18] With most of the drugs, the usual dosage leads to irritating immediate reactions in performing IDT,[18] however, because the practices used for performing IDT and their readings are not standardized, it is impossible at the moment to compare the thresholds for specificity from one study to another.

SUMMARY

Drug skin tests can be helpful in determining the cause of a CADR caused by a delayed hypersensitivity, but they still represent experimental procedures, which are best done in larger centers collecting and exchanging their experience and controlling positive test results in healthy controls. Drug skin tests can induce adverse reactions; however, severe adverse reactions are very rare. Patch tests and prick tests can, in principle, be done with any commercialized form of a drug, but they need to be controlled by testing healthy control patients. IDT can be done if an injectable form of the drug is commercialized; they have a greater sensitivity but lower specificity because of more false positive reactions and more difficult readings of the results. The results of drug skin tests depend on the clinical features of the CADR and on the tested drug. The negative predictive value of drug skin tests will have to be studied in more detail in the near future.

REFERENCES

1. Barbaud A. Drug patch testing in systemic cutaneous drug allergy. Toxicology 2005;209:209–16.
2. Barbaud A, Reichert-Penetrat S, Trechot P, et al. The use of skin testing in the investigation of cutaneous adverse drug reactions. Br J Dermatol 1998;139: 49–58.
3. Barbaud A, Gonçalo M, Bruynzeel D, et al. Guidelines for performing skin tests with drugs in the investigation of cutaneous adverse drug reactions. Contact Dermatitis 2001;45:321–8.

4. Barbaud A. Drug skin tests and systemic drug reactions: an update. Expert Rev Dermatol 2007;2:481–95.

5. Osawa J, Naito S, Aihara M, et al. Evaluation of skin test reactions in patients with non-immediate type drug eruptions. J Dermatol 1990;17:235–9.

6. Bruynzeel DP, Van Ketel WG. Patch testing in drug eruptions. Semin Dermatol 1989;8:196–203.

7. Posadas SJ, Pichler WJ. Delayed drug hypersensitivity reactions - new concepts. Clin Exp Allergy 2007;37:989–99.

8. Barbaud A. Tests cutanés dans l'investigation des toxidermies: de la physiopathologie aux résultats des investigations. Therapie 2002;57:258–62 [in French].

9. Alanko K, Stubb S, Reitamo S. Topical provocation of fixed drug eruption. Br J Dermatol 1987;116:561–7.

10. Bruynzeel DP, Van Ketel WG. Skin tests in the diagnosis of maculopapular drug eruptions. Semin Dermatol 1987;6:119–24.

11. Romano A, Di Fonso M, Pietrantonio F, et al. Repeated patch testing in delayed hypersensitivity to beta-lactam antibiotics. Contact Dermatitis 1993;28:190.

12. Felix RH, Comaish JS. The value of the patch tests and other skin tests in drug eruptions. Lancet 1974;1:1017–9.

13. Barbaud A, Bene MC, Schmutz JL, et al. Role of delayed cellular hypersensitivity and adhesion molecules in maculopapular rashes induced by amoxicillin. Arch Dermatol 1997;133:481–6.

14. Britschgi M, Steiner UC, Schmid S, et al. T-cell involvement in drug-induced acute generalized exanthematous pustulosis. J Clin Invest 2001;107:1433–41.

15. Brockow K, Romano A, Blanca M, et al. General considerations for skin test procedures in the diagnosis of drug hypersensitivity. Allergy 2002;57:45–51.

16. Kleinhans M, Linzbach L, Zedlitz S, et al. Positive patch test reactions to celecoxib may be due to irritation and do not correlate with the results of oral provocation. Contact Dermatitis 2002;47:100–2.

17. Barbaud A, Bursztejn AC, Schmutz JL, et al. Patch tests with desloratadine at 10% induce false-positive results: test at 1%. J Eur Acad Dermatol Venereol 2008;22:1504–5.

18. Barbaud A, Trechot P, Reichert-Penetrat S, et al. Relevance of skin tests with drugs in investigating cutaneous adverse drug reactions. Contact Dermatitis 2001;45:265–8.

19. Conilleau V, Dompmartin A, Michel M, et al. Photoscratch testing in systemic drug-induced photosensitivity. Photodermatol Photoimmunol Photomed 2000;16:62–6.

20. Wilkinson DS, Fregert S, Magnusson B, et al. Terminology of contact dermatitis. Acta Derm Venereol (Stockholm) 1970;50:287–92.

21. Klein CE, Trautmann A, Zillikens D, et al. Patch testing in an unusual case of toxic epidermal necrolysis. Contact Dermatitis 1995;33:448–9.

22. Barbaud A, Trechot P, Reichert-Penetrat S, et al. Drug patch testing: the usefulness in testing on the most previously affected site in a systemic cutaneous adverse drug reaction to tetrazepam. Contact Dermatitis 2001;44:259–60.

23. Ozkaya-Bayazit E, Bayazit H, Ozarmagan G. Topical provocation in 27 cases of cotrimoxazole-induced fixed drug eruption. Contact Dermatitis 1999;41:185–9.

24. Schick E, Weber L, Gall H. Topical and systemic provocation of fixed drug eruption due to phenazone. Contact Dermatitis 1996;35:58–9.

25. Mahboob A, Haroon TS, Iqbal Z, et al. Fixed drug eruption: topical provocation and subsequent phenomenon. J Coll Physicians Surg Pak 2006;16:747–50.

26. Sehgal VN, Srivastava G. Fixed drug eruption (FDE): changing scenario of incriminating drugs. Int J Dermatol 2006;45:897–908.

27. Gupta R. Drugs causing fixed drug eruptions: confirmed by provocation tests. Indian J Dermatol Venereol Leprol 2003;69:120–1.
28. Co Minh HB, Bousquet PJ, Fontaine C, et al. Systemic reactions during skin tests with beta-lactams: a risk factor analysis. J Allergy Clin Immunol 2006;117:466–8.
29. Romano A, Guéant-Rodriguez RM, Viola M, et al. Diagnosing immediate reactions to cephalosporins. Clin Exp Allergy 2005;35:1234–42.
30. Torres M-J, Sanchez-Sabate E, Alvarez J, et al. Skin test evaluation in nonimmediate allergic reactions to penicillins. Clin Exp Allergy 2004;59:219–24.
31. Lammintausta K, Kortekangas-Savolainen O. The usefulness of skin tests to prove drug hypersensitivity. Br J Dermatol 2005;152:968–74.
32. Wolkenstein P, Chosidow O, Flechet M-L, et al. Patch testing in severe cutaneous adverse drug reactions, including Stevens-Johnson syndrome and toxic epidermal necrolysis. Contact Dermatitis 1996;35:234–6.
33. Romano A, Viola M, Mondino C, et al. Diagnosing nonimmediate reactions to penicillins by in vivo tests. Int Arch Allergy Immunol 2002;129:169–74.
34. Bernedo N, Gonzalez I, Gastaminza G, et al. Positive patch test in vancomycin allergy. Contact Dermatitis 2001;45:43.
35. Padial A, Antunez C, Blanca-Lopez N, et al. Non-immediate reactions to beta-lactams: diagnostic value of skin testing and drug provocation test. Clin Exp Allergy 2008;38:822–8.
36. Barbaud A, Trechot P, Weber-Muller F, et al. Drug skin tests in cutaneous adverse drug reactions to pristinamycin: 29 cases with a study of cross-reactions between synergistins. Contact Dermatitis 2004;50:22–6.
37. Romano A, Di Fonso M, Papa G, et al. Evaluation of adverse cutaneous reactions to aminopenicillins with emphasis on those manifested by maculopapular rashes. Allergy 1995;50:113–8.
38. Leguy-Seguin V, Jolimoy G, Coudert B, et al. Diagnostic and predictive value of skin testing in platinum salts hypersensitivity. J Allergy Clin Immunol 2007;119:726–30.
39. Brockow K, Becker EW, Worret WI, et al. Late skin test reactions to radiocontrast medium. J Allergy Clin Immunol 1999;104:1107–8.
40. Vernassiere C, Trechot P, Schmutz JL, et al. Results and negative value of skin tests in investigating delayed reactions to radio-contrast media. Contact Dermatitis 2004;50:359–66.
41. Brockow K, Christiansen C, Kanny G, et al. ENDA; EAACI interest group on drug hypersensitivity. Management of hypersensitivity reactions to iodinated contrast media. Allergy 2005;60:150–8.
42. Gueant-Rodriguez RM, Romano A, Barbaud A, et al. Hypersensitivity reactions to iodinated contrast media. Curr Pharm Des 2006;12:3359–72.
43. Scherer K, Tsakiris DA, Bircher AJ. Hypersensitivity reactions to anticoagulant drugs. Curr Pharm Des 2008;14:2863–73.
44. Ludwig RJ, Beier C, Lindhoff-Last E, et al. Tolerance of fondaparinux in a patient allergic to heparins and other glycosaminoglycans. Contact Dermatitis 2003;49:158–9.
45. Akiyama M, Nakada T, Sueki H, et al. Drug eruption caused by non-ionic iodinated X-ray contrast media. Acad Radiol 1998;5:S159–61.
46. Jappe U, Juschka U, Kuner N, et al. Fondaparinux: a suitable alternative in cases of delayed-type allergy to heparins and semisynthetic heparinoids? A study of 7 cases. Contact Dermatitis 2004;51:67–72.
47. Grange-Prunier A, Roth B, Kleinclaus I, et al. Pustulose exanthématique aigue generalisee due au carbimazole (Neomercazole): premier cas et valeur des patch tests. Ann Dermatol Venereol 2006;133:708–10 [in French].

48. Elston GE, Johnston GA, Mortimer NJ, et al. Acute generalized exanthematous pustulosis associated with azathioprine hypersensitivity. Clin Exp Dermatol 2007;32:52–3.

49. Harries MJ, McIntyre SJ, Kingston TP. Co-amoxiclav-induced acute generalized exanthematous pustulosis confirmed by patch testing. Contact Dermatitis 2006; 55:372.

50. Altaykan A, Boztepe G, Erkin G, et al. Acute generalized exanthematous pustulosis induced by bleomycin and confirmed by patch testing. J Dermatolog Treat 2004;15:231–4.

51. Hausermann P, Scherer K, Weber M, et al. Ciprofloxacin-induced acute generalized exanthematous pustulosis mimicking bullous drug eruption confirmed by a positive patch test. Dermatology 2005;211:277–80.

52. Valois M, Phillips EJ, Shear NH, et al. Clindamycin-associated acute generalized exanthematous pustulosis. Contact Dermatitis 2003;48:169.

53. Buettiker U, Keller M, Pichler WJ, et al. Oral prednisolone induced acute generalized exanthematous pustulosis due to corticosteroids of group a confirmed by epicutaneous testing and lymphocyte transformation tests. Dermatology 2006; 213:40–3.

54. Girardi M, Duncan KO, Tigelaar RE, et al. Cross-comparison of patch test and lymphocyte proliferation responses in patients with a history of acute generalized exanthematous pustulosis. Am J Dermatopathol 2005;27:343–6.

55. Gonzalo-Garijo MA, Pérez-Calderón R, De Argila D, et al. Metamizole-induced acute generalized exanthematous pustulosis. Contact Dermatitis 2003;49:47–8.

56. Morant C, Devis T, Alcaraz I, et al. Pustulose exanthématique aigue généralisée au méthoxalène (Méladinine) avec positivité des tests épicutanés. Ann Dermatol Venereol 2002;129:234–5 [in French].

57. Kardaun SH, de Monchy JG. Acute generalized exanthematous pustulosis caused by morphine, confirmed by positive patch test and lymphocyte transformation test. J Am Acad Dermatol 2006;55:S21–3.

58. Teixeira M, Silva E, Selores M. Acute generalized exanthematous pustulosis induced by nimesulide. Dermatol Online J 2006;12:20.

59. Mayo-Pampín E, Flórez A, Feal C, et al. Acute generalized exanthematous pustulosis due to pseudoephedrine with positive patch test. Acta Derm Venereol 2006;86:542–3.

60. Padial MA, Alvarez-Ferreira J, Tapia B, et al. Acute generalized exanthematous pustulosis associated with pseudoephedrine. Br J Dermatol 2004;150:139–42.

61. Martínez MB, Salvador JF, Aguilera GV, et al. Acute generalized exanthematous pustulosis induced by ranitidine hydrochloride. Arch Dermatol 2003;139: 1181–3.

62. Thomas E, Bellón T, Barranco P, et al. Acute generalized exanthematous pustulosis due to tetrazepam. J Investig Allergol Clin Immunol 2008;18:119–22.

63. Komericki P, Grims R, Kränke B, et al. Acute generalized exanthematous pustulosis from dalteparin. J Am Acad Dermatol 2007;57:718–21.

64. Anliker MD, Wüthrich B. Acute generalized exanthematous pustulosis due to sulfamethoxazol with positive lymphocyte transformation test (LTT). J Investig Allergol Clin Immunol 2003;13:66–8.

65. Lee JH, Park HK, Heo J, et al. Drug Rash with Eosinophilia and Systemic Symptoms (DRESS) syndrome induced by celecoxib and anti-tuberculosis drugs. J Korean Med Sci 2008;23:521–5.

66. Aouam K, Bel Hadj Ali H, Youssef M, et al. Carbamazepine-induced DRESS and HHV6 primary infection: the importance of skin tests. Epilepsia 2008;49:1630–3.

67. Gaig P, García-Ortega P, Baltasar M, et al. Drug neosensitization during anticonvulsant hypersensitivity syndrome. J Investig Allergol Clin Immunol 2006;16:321–6.
68. Antunes A, Davril A, Trechot P, et al. Syndrome d'hypersensibilité à la minocycline. Ann Dermatol Venereol 1999;126:518–21 [in French].
69. Suswardana, Hernanto M, Yudani BA, et al. DRESS syndrome from cefadroxil confirmed by positive patch test. Allergy 2007;62:1216–7.
70. Caboni S, Gunera-Saad N, Ktiouet-Abassi S, et al. Esomeprazole-induced DRESS syndrome. Studies of cross-reactivity among proton-pump inhibitor drugs. Allergy 2007;62:1342–3.
71. Frouin E, Roth B, Grange A, et al. Syndrome d'hypersensibilité à la fluindione (Préviscan®). Positivité des tests épicutanés. Ann Dermatol Venereol 2005; 132:1000–2 [in French].
72. Ghislain PD, Bodarwe AD, Vanderdonckt O, et al. Drug-induced eosinophilia and multisystemic failure with positive patch-test reaction to spironolactone: DRESS syndrome. Acta Derm Venereol 2004;84:65–8.
73. Romano A, Di Fonso M, Pocobelli D, et al. Two cases of toxic epidermal necrolysis caused by delayed hypersensitivity to beta-lactam antibiotics. J Investig Allergol Clin Immunol 1993;3:53–5.
74. Tagami H, Tatsuta K, Iwatski K, et al. Delayed hypersensitivity in ampicillin-induced toxic epidermal necrolysis. Arch Dermatol 1983;119:910–3.
75. Friedmann PS, Strickland I, Pirmohamed M, et al. Investigation of mechanisms in toxic epidermal necrolysis induced by carbamazepine. Arch Dermatol 1994; 130:598–604.
76. Nagge JJ, Knowles SR, Juurlink DN, et al. Pseudoephedrine-induced toxic epidermal necrolysis. Arch Dermatol 2005;141:907–8.
77. Goossens C, Sass U, Song M. Baboon syndrome. Dermatology 1997;194: 421–2.
78. Barbaud A, Trechot P, Granel F, et al. A baboon syndrome induced by intravenous human immunoglobulins: report of a case and immunological analysis. Dermatology 1999;199:258–60.
79. Arnold AW, Hausermann P, Bach S, et al. Recurrent flexural exanthema (SDRIFE or baboon syndrome) after administration of two different iodinated radio contrast media. Dermatology 2007;214:89–93.
80. Gallo R, Parodi A. Baboon syndrome from 5-aminosalicylic acid. Contact Dermatitis 2002;46:110.
81. Sánchez TS, Sánchez-Pérez J, Aragüés M, et al. Flare-up reaction of pseudoephedrine baboon syndrome after positive patch test. Contact Dermatitis 2000; 42:312–3.
82. Wolf R, Orion E, Matz H. The baboon syndrome or intertriginous drug eruption. a report of eleven cases and a second look at its pathomechanism. Dermatol Online J 2003;9:2.
83. Herfs H, Schirren CG, Przybilla B, et al. Das "baboon-syndrom". Hautarzt 1993; 44:466–9.
84. Sans V, Jouary T, Hubiche T, et al. Baboon syndrome induced by cetuximab. Arch Dermatol 2008;144:272–4.
85. Kick G, Przybilla B. Delayed prick test reaction identifies amoxicillin as elicitor of baboon syndrome. Contact Dermatitis 2000;43:366–7.
86. Handisurya A, Stingl G, Wöhrl S. SDRIFE (baboon syndrome) induced by penicillin. Clin Exp Dermatol 2009;34:355–7.
87. Lammintausta K, Mäkela L, Kalimo K. Rapid systemic valaciclovir reaction subsequent to aciclovir contact allergy. Contact Dermatitis 2001;45:181.

88. Vernassiere C, Barbaud A, Trechot PH, et al. Systemic acyclovir reaction subsequent to acyclovir contact allergy: which systemic antiviral drug should then be used? Contact Dermatitis 2003;49:155–7.
89. Sakakibara T, Hata M, Numano K, et al. Fixed-drug eruption caused by allylisopropylacetylurea. Contact Dermatitis 2001;44:189–90.
90. Gaig P, San Miguel-Moncin MM, Bartra J, et al. Usefulness of patch tests for diagnosing selective allergy to captopril. J Investig Allergol Clin Immunol 2001;11:204–6.
91. Lee AY, Choi J, Chey WY. Patch testing with carbamazepine and its main metabolite carbamazepine epoxide in cutaneous adverse drug reactions to carbamazepine. Contact Dermatitis 2003;48:137–9.
92. Kawada A, Aragane Y, Maeda A, et al. Drug eruption induced by cefcapene pivoxil hydrochloride. Contact Dermatitis 2001;44:197.
93. Verbeiren S, Morant C, Charlanne H, et al. Toxidermie due au celecoxib avec tests épicutané positif. Ann Dermatol Venereol 2002;129:203–5 [in French].
94. Brown VL, Orton DI. Cutaneous adverse drug reaction to oral chlorphenamine detected with patch testing. Contact Dermatitis 2005;52:49–50.
95. Machet L, Vaillant L, Dardaine V, et al. Patch testing with clobazam: relapse of generalized drug eruption. Contact Dermatitis 1992;26:347–8.
96. Estrada JL, Alvarez Puebla MJ, Ortiz de Urbina JJ, et al. Generalized eczema due to codeine. Contact Dermatitis 2001;44:185.
97. Kilpio K, Hannuksela M. Corticosteroid allergy in asthma. Allergy 2003;58:1131–5.
98. Jonker MJ, Bruynzeel D. Anaphylactic reaction elicited by patch testing with diclofenac. Contact Dermatitis 2003;49:114–5.
99. Cholez C, Trechot P, Schmutz JL, et al. Maculopapular rash induced by diltiazem: allergological investigations in four patients and cross reactions between calcium channel blockers. Allergy 2003;58:1207–9.
100. Rodriguez-Morales A, Alonso Llamazares A, Palacios Benito R, et al. Fixed drug eruption from quinolones with a positive lesional patch test to ciprofloxacin. Contact Dermatitis 2001;44:255.
101. Rebello S, Sanchez P, Vega JM, et al. Hypersensitivity syndrome from isoniazid with positive patch test. Contact Dermatitis 2001;45:306.
102. Quinones Estevez D, Fernandez Schmitz C. Exanthema to metamizole. Allergy 2001;56:262–3.
103. Sasaki K, Yamamoto T, Kishi M, et al. Acute exanthematous pustular drug eruption induced by mexiletine. Eur J Dermatol 2001;11:469–71.
104. Malheiro D, Cadinha S, Rodrigues J, et al. Nimesulide-induced fixed drug eruption. Allergol Immunopathol (Madr) 2005;33:285–7.
105. Barranco R, Tornero P, De Barrio M, et al. Type IV hypersensitivity to oral nystatin. Contact Dermatitis 2001;45:60.
106. Montoro J, Diaz M, Genis C, et al. Non-pigmenting cutaneous-mucosal fixed drug eruption due to piroxicam. Allergol Immunopathol 2003;31:53–5.
107. Trujillo MJ, de Barrio M, Rodriguez A, et al. Piroxicam-induced photodermatitis. Cross-reactivity among oxicams. A case report. Allergol Immunopathol (Madr) 2001;29:133–6.
108. Gonçalo M, Figueiredo A. Cross-reactions among oxicams in cutaneous adverse drug reactions. Contact Dermatitis 2002;46:S31.
109. Mashiah J, Brenner S. A systemic reaction to patch testing for the evaluation of acute generalized exanthematous pustulosis. Arch Dermatol 2003;139:1181–3.

110. Strauss RM, Green ST, Gawkrodger DJ. Rifampicin allergy confirmed by an intradermal test, but with a negative patch test. Contact Dermatitis 2001;45:108.
111. Pirker C, Misic A, Brinkmeier T, et al. Tetrazepam drug sensitivity - usefulness of the patch test. Contact Dermatitis 2002;47:135–8.
112. Wong DA, Freeman S. Cutaneous allergic reaction to intramuscular vitamin K1. Australas J Dermatol 1999;40:147–52.
113. Antunez C, Martin E, Cornejo-Garcia JA, et al. Immediate hypersensitivity reactions to penicillins and other betalactams. Curr Pharm Des 2006;12:3327–33.
114. Bonadonna P, Schiappoli M, Senna G, et al. Delayed selective reaction to clavulanic acid: a case report. J Investig Allergol Clin Immunol 2005;15:302–4.
115. Romano A, Quaratino D, Papa G, et al. Aminopenicillin allergy. Arch Dis Child 1997;76:513–7.
116. Ponvert C, Weilenmann C, Wassenberg J, et al. Allergy to betalactam antibiotics in children: a prospective follow-up study in retreated children after negative responses in skin and challenge tests. Allergy 2007;62:42–6.
117. Berkun Y, Ben-Zvi A, Levy Y, et al. Evaluation of adverse reactions to local anesthetics: experience with 236 patients. Ann Allergy Asthma Immunol 2003;91: 342–5.
118. Padial A, Posadas S, Alvarez J, et al. Nonimmediate reactions to systemic corticosteroids suggest an immunological mechanism. Allergy 2005;60:665–70.
119. Ludwig RJ, Schindewolf M, Alban S, et al. Molecular weight determines the frequency of delayed type hypersensitivity reactions to heparin and synthetic oligosaccharides. Thromb Haemost 2005;94:1265–9.
120. Ludwig RJ, Schindewolf M, Utikal J, et al. Management of cutaneous type IV hypersensitivity reactions induced by heparin. Thromb Haemost 2006;96:611–7.
121. Gerhardt A, Zotz RB, Stockschlaeder M, et al. Fondaparinux is an effective alternative anticoagulant in pregnant women with high risk of venous thromboembolism and intolerance to low-molecular-weight heparins and heparinoids. Thromb Haemost 2007;97:496–7.
122. Adachi A, Fukunaga A, Horikawa T. A case of human insulin allergy induced by short-acting and intermediate-acting insulin but not by long-acting insulin. Int J Dermatol 2004;43:597–9.
123. Lee AY, Chey WY, Choi J, et al. Insulin-induced drug eruptions and reliability of skin tests. Acta Derm Venereol 2002;82:114–7.
124. Schmid DA, Depta JP, Pichler WJ. T cell-mediated hypersensitivity to quinolones: mechanisms and cross-reactivity. Clin Exp Allergy 2006;36:59–69.
125. Barranco R, Rodriguez A, de Barrio M, et al. Sympathomimetic drug allergy: cross-reactivity study by patch test. Am J Clin Dermatol 2004;5:351–5.
126. Waton J, Tréchot P, Loss-Ayav C, et al. Negative predictive value of drug skin tests in investigating cutaneous adverse drug reactions. Br J Dermatol 2009; 160:786–94.
127. Ulrich G, Schmutz JL, Trechot P, et al. Sensitization to petrolatum: an unusual cause of false positive drug patch tests. Allergy 2004;59:1006–9.

In Vitro Tests in Drug Hypersensitivity Diagnosis

Priska Lochmatter, MSc, Anna Zawodniak, MD, Werner J. Pichler, MD*

KEYWORDS

- Drug hypersensitivity • In vitro tests
- Lymphocyte transformation test • CD69 upregulation
- Cytokines • Cytotoxicity

Drug hypersensitivity reactions (DHRs) account for approximately 15% of adverse drug reactions.[1] The clinical symptoms of DHRs are various and of variable severity. The exact pathophysiology of DHRs is mostly unknown; nevertheless, DHRs can be classified in a scheme proposed by Gell and Coombs,[2] which correlates the clinical phenotype to the immunologic mechanism involved. In this scheme, drug-induced IgE-mediated type I reactions (urticaria, bronchoconstriction, angioedema, and anaphylaxis), IgG-mediated type II reactions (hemolytic anemia and thrombocytopenia), immune-complex–mediated type III reactions (vasculitis and purpura) and T-cell–mediated type IV reactions (allergic contact dermatitis; fixed drug eruptions; and maculopapular exanthema [MPE], bullous exanthema, or pustular exanthema) have been differentiated.

The delayed-appearing T-cell–mediated (type IV) reactions have recently been further subclassified to correlate the heterogeneous T-cell functions to the clinically distinct pictures.[3] Hence, type IV reactions can be subclassified into type IVa, IVb, IVc, and IVd according to the effector phenotype of the involved T cells. Type IVa and IVb correspond to T helper (Th) 1 and Th2 cytokine-driven reactions, respectively. Type IVc refers to cytotoxic reactions, whereas type IVd represents T-cell–induced neutrophilic inflammations, whereby interleukin (IL)-8 and possibly IL-17 are involved.

A diagnosis of delayed-type drug hypersensitivity has two aims: first, to confirm that the symptoms correspond to a DHR and, second, to identify the causative drug. It is still an area of much uncertainty, but recent progress in the understanding of these reactions opens new possibilities.

In vivo tests include skin tests and drug provocation tests. Patch, prick, and intracutaneous tests have an overall low sensitivity, even in patients with a well-documented history of DHR.[4–8] Drug provocation tests may help to rule out immediate

Division of Allergology, Clinic of Rheumatology and Clinical Immunology/Allergology, Inselspital, Bern University Hospital and University of Bern, CH-3010 Bern, Switzerland
* Corresponding author.
E-mail address: werner.pichler@insel.ch (W.J. Pichler).

Immunol Allergy Clin N Am 29 (2009) 537–554
doi:10.1016/j.iac.2009.04.009
0889-8561/09/$ – see front matter © 2009 Elsevier Inc. All rights reserved.

immunology.theclinics.com

reactions but are not well standardized in delayed reactions regarding dose, duration of symptoms, and definition of positivity, and are therefore difficult to perform. In some cases, an entire treatment period would be necessary because some reactions clearly depend on dose and may start after 4 to 5 days of treatment only. Moreover, they do not reveal the pathomechanism and may still bear the risk for severe reactions. Thus, they are not well accepted by physicians and patients.

In vitro tests would be safe for patients and can provide deeper insight into the pathomechanisms involved in a certain type of DHR. The nonphysiologic environment is one of the main disadvantages of in vitro tests, however. The clinical symptoms are influenced by cofactors that are not present in vitro, such as certain hepatic enzymes necessary for metabolizing inert drugs into immunogenic compounds or infections that were enhancing immune reactions at the time of the DHR. In addition, most in vitro tests are not yet standardized and still represent mainly a research tool.

In spite of these disadvantages, in vitro tests are of great interest because they guarantee absolute safety for patients and allow simultaneous assessment of T-cell responses to multiple drugs. At present, even a test with relatively low sensitivity but still good specificity would be considered helpful in many clinical situations. In this article, the best investigated in vitro tests are discussed, which aim to identify the causative drug by detecting drug-reacting cells in the peripheral blood of patients with delayed-type drug hypersensitivities (**Fig. 1**). Nevertheless, one has to be aware that such tests, like other immunologic tests, can only reflect a sensitization, which is a relevant risk factor for a DHR, but can never prove that a complete immune reaction with inflammation would take place on re-exposure.

PATHOMECHANISMS OF T-CELL–MEDIATED DRUG HYPERSENSITIVITY

T cells have been shown to play a central role in mediating DHRs and are practically involved in all types of immune reactions to drugs. On antigen-specific stimulation, T cells secrete various cytokines and can orchestrate different effector mechanisms of immune response. Immediate IgE-mediated reactions are stimulated by secretion of IL-4 and IL-13; monocyte- or macrophage-rich inflammations are stimulated by secretion of interferon-γ (IFNγ) and tumor necrosis factor-α (TNFα); eosinophilic inflammation is stimulated by secretion of IL-5; and neutrophilic inflammation is stimulated by secretion of IL-8, granulocyte-macrophage colony-stimulating factor, and possibly IL-17.[3,9,10] Moreover, drug-induced cytotoxic effector T cells were shown to infiltrate and kill tissue cells in the skin and liver of patients with severe forms of drug hypersensitivity.[11–13] The number of in vitro (eg, lymphocyte transformation test [LTT], ELISA,

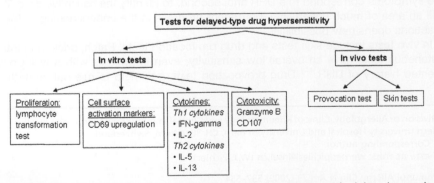

Fig. 1. Tests for the detection of drug-specific T cells in patients with delayed-type drug hypersensitivity.

enzyme-linked immunospot [ELISPOT] assay, CD69 measurement) and in vivo (de-layed reading of intradermal and patch tests) tests and, in particular, the generation of drug-specific T-cell lines (TCLs) and T-cell clones (TCCs) from tissue lesions and peripheral blood of patients with different forms of drug hypersensitivity have confirmed the central role of T cells in the complex pathomechanism of drug hypersensitivity.

Two main models have been proposed to explain how T cells recognize small chem-ical substances, namely, the hapten or prohapten model and the p-i concept based on pharmacologic interaction of drugs with immune receptors. According to the hapten or prohapten model, chemically reactive drugs or their metabolites may covalently bind to certain proteins and initiate immune responses by transmitting a danger signal to the innate immune system. The modified haptenated proteins would be then pro-cessed and presented on major histocompatibility complex (MHC) molecules to hapten- or drug-specific T cells activating the specific immune system.[14–18]

In contrast, the p-i concept postulates that inert drugs unable to act as haptens may bind directly and reversibly to immune receptors, particularly to the T-cell receptor (TCR) and possibly also to the MHC. This noncovalent drug interaction with the MHC-TCR complex leads to the activation and proliferation of drug-specific T cells, as illustrated by analysis of drug-specific TCCs to various drugs (lidocaine, mepiva-caine, sulfamethoxazole, lamotrigine, carbamazepine, p-phenylenediamine, and ci-profloxacin).[19–25] This concept is similar to stimulation of cells by pharmacologic activation by means of other receptors, and is hence called pharmacologic interaction with immune receptors (p-i concept).[26,27]

Some of these drug-activated T cells can persist as memory cells in peripheral blood of drug-allergic patients, even several years after disease outcome. A recent study of Beeler and colleagues[28] showed that the frequency of drug-reactive T cells in peripheral blood of some allergic patients in remission is in the range of 1:250 to 1:10,000. It is thus even higher than the frequency of T cells able to react with tetanus toxoid in the same tetanus-immunized subject. It is not known how this relatively large pool of drug-specific memory T cells is maintained in spite of strict avoidance of the drug. It is possibly related to some cross-reactivity of the drug-specific T cells with other peptide antigens or even self-peptides. Indeed, approximately 30% of drug-reactive clones showed cross-reactivity with allogeneic MHC-peptide complexes.[29]

This long-lasting persistence of drug-reactive memory T cells in peripheral blood of drug-allergic patients has a crucial impact on in vitro diagnosis of drug hypersensitivity because all available in vitro tests rely on measurement of specific effector function of drug-reactivated memory T cells. Thus, such a test is only informative if it measures the same effector mechanisms as involved in an in vivo reaction. For instance, the result of a test evaluating IgE to a drug is negative in MPE because this disease does not involve IgE formation to the drug; similarly, the result of a test for proliferation might be negative if the delayed immune reaction involved mainly cytotoxicity. These features have to be considered in interpreting test results and demonstrate why prog-ress in diagnosis of drug allergy relies primarily on a better understanding of immuno-logic pathomechanisms involved.

KINETICS OF T-CELL ACTIVATION

The full activation of a T cell is assumed to require multiple sequential engagements of the TCR by the antigen presented on the MHC on antigen-presenting cells. This leads to the recruitment of costimulatory, adhesion, and signaling molecules to the antigen-TCR contact site and results in activation of the T cell. After being triggered by a specific antigen, T cells enter a maturation process of several days, which can be divided into three phases: commitment, proliferation, and functional differentiation (**Fig. 2**).

Commitment follows rapidly after the triggering of a TCR by a specific antigen presented on MHC I or II; within a few minutes, the Ras-mitogen-activated protein kinase signaling pathway and the calcium- and protein kinase C-mediated signaling pathway get activated. This leads to the activation of three critical transcription factors (nuclear factor of activated T cells, activator protein-1, and nuclear factor-κB) within half an hour after antigen recognition, which enhance the transcription of genes encoding for various cytokines, such as IL-2, IL-4, IFNγ, TNFα, and the early activation markers CD40L and CD69 within 1 to 2 hours. After 1 to 2 days, CD25 (IL-2 receptor),[30] CD71, human leukocyte antigen–D-related (HLA-DR), and various adhesion molecules are expressed. IL-2 has an autocrine effect on the T cells and induces the proliferation of the activated T cells, which goes along with DNA synthesis (see **Fig. 2**).

Approximately 3 to 5 days after activation, some T cells undergo functional differentiation. The CD4+ T cells differentiate into two major subsets of effector cells, Th1 and Th2 cells, which secrete distinct cytokine patterns. These cytokine patterns determine the effector functions of activated cells. They do not only mediate the expansion of one subset but inhibit the expansion of the reciprocal subset. Therefore, once an immune response develops in one direction, it gets progressively polarized. Th1 cells are characterized by the secretion of proinflammatory cytokine IFNγ, which stimulates the microbicidal activity of phagocytes, and the production of complement-fixing and opsonizing IgG antibodies, which promote phagocytosis. In contrast, Th2 cells typically secrete IL-4, IL-5, IL-13, and IL-10, which inhibit macrophage activation but activate eosinophils and induce antibody isotype switch to mast cell-activating IgE. In 2005, Th17 cells were proposed as a third distinct Th cell subset. This subset is characterized by the secretion of IL-17 and most probably functions to eliminate specific pathogens that are not efficiently cleared by the Th1- or Th2-mediated immune response.[31–33]

Naive T cells can also differentiate into regulatory T cells in peripheral lymphoid organs. These so-called "adaptive T-regulatory cells" produce high levels of IL-10 and transforming growth factor-β, which have an immunosuppressive function.[34]

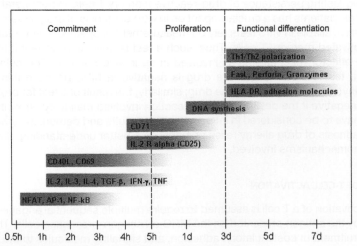

Fig. 2. Gene expression profile of antigen-activated T cells.

Antigen-activated T lymphocytes can differentiate into cytotoxic effector cells that recognize and kill target cells presenting the antigen on MHC molecules. These cells are characterized by the production of cytotoxic proteins like perforin and granzymes and proinflammatory cytokines, namely, IFNγ and TNFα. They can also express Fas ligand, which binds to Fas molecules on target cells, inducing apoptosis.

The measurement of these events in T-cell activation could theoretically serve to detect drug-reacting T cells in vitro. Because of technical limitations and the nonphysiologic in vitro environment, however, not all these events are suited for diagnosis of T-cell–mediated drug allergy. In the following sections of this article, in vitro tests that aim to detect various events in the T-cell activation induced by drugs are discussed.

LYMPHOCYTE TRANSFORMATION TEST

The LTT is the most widely used test to detect T-cell sensitization to drugs in the diagnosis of drug allergy. The principle of the LTT follows the rules of a simple proliferation test with a protein antigen. It measures proliferation and expansion of T cells after stimulation with the specific antigen (drug), which is the common effector function of different types of T-cell immune reactions (eg, Th1, Th2, Th0, Th17). Generation of drug-specific TCLs and TCCs from LTT-positive patients and the finding that peripheral blood cells from healthy drug-exposed donors do not normally show enhanced proliferation to the drug prove that the T-cell proliferation detected in the LTT is a drug-specific response found only in symptomatic patients.[35–38] This test has been shown to be useful in patients with delayed T-cell–mediated forms of drug hypersensitivity like MPE, pustular exanthema, and bullous exanthema;[10,23] drug rash with eosinophilia and systemic symptoms (DRESS);[22] and immediate IgE-mediated reactions, including severe anaphylaxis.[36] Rarely, the LTT has been evaluated in other forms of drug hypersensitivity: positive reactions were reported in isolated drug fever[39] followed by vasculitis, in drug-induced pancreatitis (found positive with pyritinol[40]), for interstitial and eosinophilic lung diseases,[41] or even in some drug-induced autoimmune diseases.[42] Often, these are case reports, and there is not enough information regarding sensitivity and specificity. In drug-induced hepatitis, the result of the LTT can occasionally be positive[43,44] and has then been found useful in discriminating immune hepatitis from toxic reactions caused by antituberculous drugs.[45] Recently, it has also been shown useful in determination of cross-reactivity patterns in T-cell–mediated allergic reactions to iodine contrast media.[46]

In the LTT, peripheral blood mononuclear cells (PBMCs) obtained from drug-sensitized patients and separated over a density gradient are cultured in the presence of suspected drug for 6 days. The drug should be available as a pure substance. If the pure substance form of the drug is not available, one can use the contents of a capsule or an injectable form of the drug. Drugs tested as tablets are mostly unsuited for an LTT. All drugs must be tested in a group of controls, and toxic concentrations have to be defined by toxicity tests (for details, see the article by Pichler and Tilch[47]).

Memory T lymphocytes persist in the circulation of patients with DHRs. After antigen encounter, these memory T cells undergo blastogenesis and generate cytokines, such as IL-2. The proliferative response can be measured by incorporation of ^{3}H-thymidine during DNA synthesis and given as the count per minute. The result is usually expressed as the stimulation index (SI), which is the ratio of cell proliferation with antigen divided by the background proliferation (without antigen). Because the spontaneous proliferation obtained with various donors differs, SI values are more comparable and easier to communicate than count-per-minute results. An SI greater than 2m and greater than 3 for β-lactams, is considered to be a cutoff value for a positive response. An SI between 2 and 3 is considered to be weakly positive. The relevance of such a low proliferation is hard to judge without additional clinical information or other tests. Drug-specific TCCs could be also generated from cell cultures with only a moderate SI of 2.1, which suggests that this weak response in the LTT could already indicate sensitization.[10] Drug-exposed but not allergic individuals do not mount a proliferative reaction to a drug.

High SI values in the LTT are not necessarily associated with the severity of clinical symptoms. Analysis of rather harmless MPE might reveal strong T-cell proliferation, whereas patients with severe forms of drug hypersensitivity, such as Stevens-Johnson syndrome (SJS) or toxic epidermal necrolysis (TEN), show only a marginally positive or even negative response.[48] This is attributable to the fact that the LTT reflects only the reactivation and proliferation of memory cells that are present in the peripheral blood of allergic patients, and the high precursor frequency of these cells is not necessarily associated with more severe clinical symptoms. In fact, the clinical severity of a DHR seems to be more closely related to the effector function of the reactive T cells. Thus, in some forms of drug hypersensitivity, cytotoxicity or a cytokine-based in vitro assay could be more useful than proliferation-based assays like the LTT.

The clinical sensitivity of a diagnostic test indicates to what extent it can detect clinically relevant sensitization. In several studies performed to date, the LTT had a general sensitivity of 60% to 70% and was often superior to skin testing for nonimmediate-type reactions.[35,36,49–52] A lower sensitivity rate of 33% was reported by Barna and colleagues,[53] and a rate of 38% was reported by Berg and colleagues.[54] A prominent retrospective analysis that included 923 patients with various adverse drug reactions indicated that the sensitivity of the LTT depends on the drug tested.[49] All patients in this study were classified based on their medical history into three groups: patients with definite, highly probable, or not probable immune-mediated drug reactions. Seventy-eight of 100 patients classified as definitely drug allergic showed positive reactions in the LTT; thus, the LTT sensitivity was 78%. When only allergies to β-lactam antibiotics were analyzed, the LTT sensitivity was approximately 74%, and thus higher than that of skin tests (62%). Patients from the high-probability group and low-probability group were positive in the LTT at rates of 47% and 33%, respectively. Fifteen of 102 presumably non–drug-allergic patients had positive LTT results; thus, the authors could define the specificity of the LTT as being no higher than 85%. This relatively low specificity was attributed to the fact that all positive LTT results to nonsteroid anti-inflammatory drugs (NSAIDs) were calculated as false-positive. NSAIDs are known to cause mainly pseudoallergic (non–immune-mediated) reactions and may also slightly enhance proliferation in in vitro tests, which is explained by their ability to inhibit prostaglandin E2 synthesis.[55] This effect is not seen consistently, however, and some compounds, such as diclofenac and pyrazolones, might even cause "real" immune-mediated reactions and true-positive LTT results. Other studies indeed showed far better specificity for the LTT using various drugs.[35–38,56] Recent analyses of LTTs to antiepileptic drugs eliciting DRESS revealed a sensitivity of 97% and a specificity of 100% for carbamazepine and lamotrigine hypersensitivity. This high specificity (93%) was recently also confirmed for β-lactam hypersensitivity.[36–38]

Some drugs are able to elicit enhanced proliferation even in nonsensitized individuals. Examples are vancomycin, possibly paracetamol, and certain radiocontrast media, which might elicit slightly enhanced proliferation (SI of 2–4) in PBMCs of certain individuals previously not exposed. The mechanism of this is not known at the present time. In contrast, certain drugs, such as abacavir,[57] may elicit severe generalized hypersensitivity reactions and positive delayed-type skin test results but a negative proliferation test result.

Different modifications of the LTT have been proposed. One example is the memory lymphocyte immunostimulation assay (MELISA). In this assay, PBMCs from allergic donors are depleted of monocytes before antigen stimulation. The MELISA is mainly applied to test sensitization to metals, with rather controversial results.[58,59] Recently, Lopez and colleagues[60] postulated that a lymphocyte proliferation test with monocyte-derived dendritic cells was a more appropriate diagnostic tool in delayed hypersensitivity reactions to heparins than a classic LTT.

In conclusion, the LTT has an overall sensitivity of 60% to 70% under optimal conditions. It is thus suitable as a complement to other tests. Nevertheless, it is still a controversial method because of several disadvantages: it requires sterile cell cultures; it takes a long time and is cumbersome; the drug-specific proliferation depends on the quality of the culture medium; and it involves radioactivity, and thus expensive equipment. In the hands of an experienced technician, however, it can help to define the incriminating drug in the DHR. A positive LTT result helps to define the culprit drug, but a negative test result cannot rule out drug hypersensitivity.

CD69 UP-REGULATION AS A MARKER FOR T-CELL–MEDIATED DRUG HYPERSENSITIVITY

Different surface molecules are expressed on T cells after stimulation, such as CD25, CD69, CD71, and HLA-DR. The CD69 molecule is one of the earliest markers expressed on T cells, B cells, and natural killer (NK) cells after stimulation by various mitogenic substances.[61–63] CD69 is a membrane type II C-type lectin, which belongs to the family of NK receptors and is transiently expressed on activated lymphocytes. The surface expression of this molecule allows its flow cytometric detection on different T-cell subsets by fluorescence-conjugated antibodies. Maino and colleagues[64] reported that CD69 is a valuable marker for early T-cell activation after stimulation of whole blood with pokeweed mitogen, CD2/CD2R monoclonal antibodies, superantigen staphylococcal enterotoxin B, or the specific antigen Candida albicans. CD69 was rapidly unregulated on CD3+ T cells within 4 hours after stimulation and could be measured by multicolor flow cytometry. Various other studies reported CD69 as an in vitro marker for T-cell activation by mitogenic substances or superantigens.[65,66] Also, in T-cell–mediated DHRs, CD69 has been shown to be an in vitro marker for drug-induced T-cell activation. CD69 was up-regulated in T cells from patients who had drug-induced MPE, erythema multiforme, SJS, and DRESS when assessed by flow cytometry.[67,68] A study by Beeler and colleagues[69] addressed the suitability of CD69 up-regulation as a tool for diagnosis of delayed-type drug hypersensitivity. It showed that CD69 measurement is a promising tool for diagnosing delayed-type drug hypersensitivity. Compared with other activation markers, such as CD71 or CD25, CD69 was the most suitable because of its rapid up-regulation and stronger increase in surface expression after drug stimulation.[69] In this study, PBMCs from 15 patients with previous DHRs were stimulated with the culprit drug. After 48 hours, substantial CD69 up-regulation on CD4+ and CD8+ T cells of all 15 patients was observed. This CD69 up-regulation was drug-specific because no drug-induced CD69 up-regulation was detected in control subjects. In 15 patients, a positive CD69 test result correlated to a positive LTT result, which was performed in parallel to the CD69 test.[69] These findings suggest that CD69 measurement is comparable to the LTT. The same study also suggested that the drug activates only few drug-specific T cells, which produce cytokines that activate many "bystander" T cells. This amplification occurred only in presence of drug-specific T cells, and therefore substantially increases the sensitivity but does not decrease the specificity of this assay.[69] In conclusion, flow cytometric CD69 measurement seems to be suitable for routine diagnosis, similar to the LTT, but with the advantage that it does not require radioactive substances and is less time-consuming (**Fig. 3**). It is, however, a flow cytometry-based test, which is difficult to standardize. A large prospective study is required to evaluate this test and to determine sensitivity and specificity in drug hypersensitivity diagnosis. This prospective study is currently being performed by the authors' drug allergy research group in Bern.

MEASUREMENT OF DRUG-INDUCED CYTOKINE PRODUCTION FROM EX VIVO PERIPHERAL BLOOD MONONUCLEAR CELLS

Cytokines are secreted by the cells of the innate and adaptive immune system, and they mediate cell activation, proliferation, and differentiation during an immune response. The cytokine pattern induced by a certain antigen determines the type of immune response; therefore, cytokines play a key role in the effector phase of the immune response.

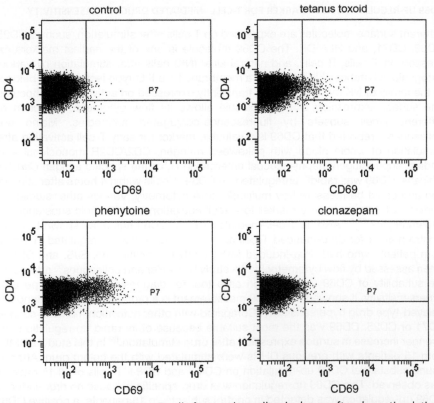

Fig. 3. CD69 expression on CD4+ T cells from a drug-allergic donor after drug stimulation. PBMCs from a phenytoin-allergic donor were stimulated for 48 hours with culture medium alone (negative control), tetanus toxoid (positive control), the culprit drug phenytoin, and the unrelated drug clonazepam. Flow cytometric analysis showed CD69 up-regulation on CD4+ T cells in response to tetanus toxoid and phenytoin but not in response to clonazepam (A. Zawodniak, P. Lochmatter, unpublished data, 2008).

Many researchers have focused on correlation of a clinical picture with a Th1- or Th2-type immune reaction in various DHRs. Ex vivo studies with PBMCs have revealed a controversial picture: some showed a polarized pattern with more Th1 cytokines (IL-2, IFNγ, and TNFα) in patients with delayed-type reactions and the Th2 cytokine IL-4 in patients with immediate reactions.[70,71] In another in vitro study, immediate-type hypersensitivity reactions to penicillin or amoxicillin could not be associated with a clear Th2- or Th1-type cytokine pattern but showed a mixed Th1/Th2 pattern, whereas delayed-type reactions were restricted to a Th1 cytokine pattern.[72] A more recent in vitro study showed no association of delayed-type DHR with sulfonamides and amoxicillin with a Th1 pattern but revealed a mixed Th1/Th2 cytokine pattern.[73] Other studies with TCCs and TCLs from drug-allergic patients with immediate- or delayed-type reactions have shown a heterogeneous cytokine pattern, which could not be related to a clear Th1 or Th2 phenotype and is best described as a Th0 pattern.[19,22,74] It seems that the drug-induced cytokine pattern observed in vitro does not correlate with the ex vivo cytokine pattern observed in the acute phase of the DHR.

There have also been attempts to associate a certain cytokine with a clinical phenotype. Allergic cutaneous drug reactions, such as MPE, acute generalized exanthematous pustulosis, and DRESS, and severe forms, such as SJS or TEN, have been associated with IFNγ release in different studies.[37,75–79] IFNγ seems to be a predominant cytokine in allergic cutaneous drug reactions and may play an important role in their pathophysiology. Different studies have shown that in vitro drug-stimulated PBMCs from patients with drug-induced cutaneous reactions secreted an increased amount of IFNγ. In a study that included 36 patients with various cutaneous adverse drug reactions tested for a wide panel of drugs, IFNγ secretion had a sensitivity of 77.8%.[75] In another study of 7 patients who had phenytoin-induced exanthema and 11 control individuals, the sensitivity of IFNγ secretion was 71.4% and the specificity was 100%.[78] In a study by Gaspard and colleagues,[72] 6 (75%) of 8 patients with amoxicillin- or penicillin G-induced delayed-type DHRs showed induction of IFNγ expression after drug stimulation. Therefore, IFNγ might be a suitable in vitro marker for delayed-type cutaneous drug reactions and a useful tool with which to identify the responsible drug.

Another cytokine described in different forms of DHRs is the Th2 cytokine IL-5. DRESS has been shown to be associated with in vivo release of IL-5[76,80] and, conversely, with a predominant release of IFNγ from drug-specific TCCs in vitro.[37] It has also been shown that IL-5 is released in vivo and ex vivo in patients who have drug-induced MPE.[11,76,81] The measurement of IL-5 has also been proposed as a useful in vitro method for detecting drug sensitization in a study that included 10 patients who had drug-induced MPE and 10 control individuals, with a sensitivity of 92% and a specificity of 100%. Further, the combination of IL-5 measurement and the LTT was demonstrated to be a better readout for drug sensitization than the LTT alone.[82–84]

Lately, two studies have been performed that aimed to find the most suitable cytokine for the diagnosis of delayed-type DHR. In these studies, supernatants from drug-stimulated patients' PBMC cultures were screened for a panel of different cytokines. In a study by Khalil and colleagues[79] in which 18 patients who had MPE in response to penicillins and 12 control subjects were screened for drug-specific in vitro secretion of IL-2, IL-5, and IFNγ. IFNγ and IL-2 were suggested as useful methods for the assessment of penicillin allergy, with a sensitivity of 87% and a specificity of 100%. In a recent study, PBMCs of 10 patients with delayed-type DHR to amoxicillin or sulfonamides and 5 control subjects were screened for the secretion of 17 cytokines and chemokines after drug stimulation in vitro so as to identify marker cytokines for delayed-type drug hypersensitivity. Cytokine secretion by healthy nonallergic controls after drug stimulation was used to set a cutoff point. Four cytokines, namely, IL-2, IL-5, IL-13, and IFNγ, were predominantly secreted after drug stimulation and were significantly increased compared with nonallergic controls. IL-2, IL-5, and IL-13 were secreted in 80% of patients and IL-5 was secreted in 60% of patients after a 3-day drug stimulation, whereas in the controls, cytokine secretion was lower than the cutoff for positivity.[73]

The gene expression level of cytokines can be measured by molecular techniques, such as quantification of mRNA by reverse transcription polymerase chain reaction (RT-PCR), which detects relative changes in transcription, or by competitive quantitative RT-PCR, which allows absolute quantification of transcript concentrations. At the protein level, cytokines can be measured intracellularly by flow cytometry with fluorescent-conjugated monoclonal antibodies. This method might not be sensitive enough, however. More sensitive methods for measuring secreted cytokines in the cell culture supernatant are enzyme-linked immunoassays, such as the ELISA or ELISPOT assay, or multiplexed bead-based flow cytometric assays, such as Bioplex (Biorad Laboratories, Reinach, Switzerland) or Luminex xMAP (Luminex, Toronto, Canada) assay, which allow the simultaneous measurement of a panel of cytokines.

In conclusion, the measurement of IL-2, IL-5, IL-13, and IFNγ cytokines might be a promising tool for detecting drug sensitization in delayed-type reactions (**Fig. 4**). Nevertheless, studies that include a large number of patients, such as those performed for evaluation of the LTT as a diagnostic tool, are necessary to evaluate an accurate cutoff for positivity and the exact sensitivity and specificity of these assays.

CYTOTOXICITY: GRANZYME B ENZYME IMMUNOSPOT ASSAY

Analyses of drug-induced skin diseases have indicated an important role for cytotoxic mechanisms in maculopapular, bullous, and pustular reactions.[3,11,81,85–87] In particular, histologic and immunohistologic analyses of affected skin lesions have revealed the presence of perforin- and granzyme B (GzB)-positive T-cell infiltrates.[11,35,87] Elution of skin-infiltrating T cells and characterization of drug-specific cytotoxic TCLs and TCCs from the peripheral blood of drug-allergic patients have confirmed that drug-dependent killing occurs.[12,88]

In maculopapular drug eruptions, perforin- and GzB-positive CD4+ and CD8+ T cells were found at the dermoepidermal junction zone or in the epidermis, along with signs of keratinocyte cell damage.[11] In more severe forms of DHR, predominant activation of cytotoxic CD8+ T cells, NK cells, and NK-like T cells may lead to a massive widespread apoptosis of epidermal cells mediated by perforin/GzB[13,89] or Fas ligand/Fas.[90,91] Recently, a role of granulysin, a cytotoxic protein secreted by T cells and NK

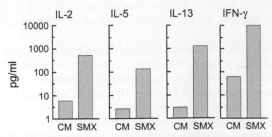

Fig. 4. Drug-induced cytokine secretion in a drug-allergic donor. Secretion of IL-2, IL-5, IL-13, and IFNγ was induced in PBMCs of a sulfamethoxazole (SMX)-allergic donor after a 72-hour stimulation by SMX compared with incubation with culture medium (CM) alone (P. Lochmatter, unpublished data, 2008).

cells, has been implied to be responsible for disseminated keratinocyte apoptosis and skin detachment in severe life-treating bullous skin lesions (eg, SJS, TEN).[92]

Over the past years, several approaches have been developed for the identification of antigen (peptide)-specific cytotoxic T cells on a single-cell basis.[48] A standard chromium release assay[93] and more recently used methods that monitor the release of fluorescent dyes from target cells are cumbersome and semiquantitative.[94,95] MHC multimers were not of practical application in identification of drug-specific cytotoxic T cells. Intracellular cytokine staining and the IFNα ELISPOT assay are commonly used, but none of these methods directly examine the cytotoxic effector function of T cells.[96] Recently, the authors' group adapted two methods to detect drug-reactive cytotoxic cells in peripheral blood of drug-allergic patients in remission, namely, the GzB ELISPOT assay and flow cytometry-based CD107a measurement.

Cytotoxic T lymphocytes mediate the killing of target cells by means of two major pathways: a granule-dependent mechanism (perforin/granzyme) and a death receptor-mediated mechanism (Fas/Fas ligand and TNF-related apoptosis–inducing ligand [TRAIL]).[97,98] Recently, the role of TRAIL has been described in paracetamol and virally induced liver failure.[99] However, the exact role of TRAIL in drug-induced liver disease is still unclear. Once cytotoxic T cells get activated, the lytic granules reach the plasma membrane, the content of cytotoxic granules (granzymes and perforin) is released into immunologic synapses, and the cumulative exposure of granular membrane proteins (CD107a) can be measured on the surface of responding cytotoxic cells, providing a positive marker for degranulation (**Fig. 5**).[96,100] Release of GzB measured by an ELISPOT assay can be used to detect the cytotoxic function of in vivo sensitized antigen-specific T cells.[101] The ELISPOT assay detects molecules secreted by individual cells present in low frequencies. It is highly sensitive because plate-bound antibodies directly capture the product secreted around the cell before it is diluted in the supernatant and absorbed by high-affinity receptors or degraded by proteases.[101] The GzB ELISPOT assay and the degranulation marker CD107a have been used successfully to detect peptide-specific cytotoxic T lymphocytes in patients who have chronic virus infections and in patients monitored in vaccine trials.[102–108] The GzB ELISPOT assay also seems to be the most sensitive and robust method to detect cytotoxic cells in the peripheral blood of drug-allergic patients. CD107a measurement might be useful to reveal the phenotype of reacting cytotoxic cells.

Because cytotoxicity-based in vitro tests measure effector cell function distinct from proliferation, such tests might be promising tools in drug hypersensitivity diagnosis and in supplementing proliferation-based assays. In contrast to the LTT, the GzB ELISPOT test gives results as early as 48 to 72 hours after stimulation and does not involve radioactivity.

WHEN SHOULD DIAGNOSTIC TESTS BE PERFORMED?

According to common opinion, in vitro tests to identify the drug involved in a hypersensitivity reaction should not be performed during the acute stage because the immune cells are still strongly activated, causing high background proliferation and activity.[35] For example, in LTTs, cells obtained ex vivo from patients in the acute stage are still activated and show high spontaneous proliferation. Thus, additional in vitro drug stimulation could lead to only marginal and difficult-to-detect enhancement of proliferation or even to stimulation-induced cell death.

This concept has recently been challenged by Kano and colleagues.[109] They observed that the correct timing of drug hypersensitivity diagnosis with the LTT

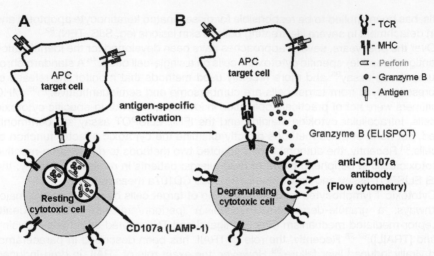

Fig. 5. Degranulation of cytotoxic cell after antigen-specific stimulation. (*A*) In the resting cell with cytotoxic potential, lytic molecules (granzymes and perforin) are stored in cytotoxic granules. The membrane of these granules is lined with membrane glycoproteins, including CD107a (LAMP-1). (*B*) Once the cell gets activated by the specific antigen, the lytic granules reach the plasma membrane, the cytotoxic molecules are released, and the cumulative exposure of granular membrane proteins (CD107a) can be measured on the surface of responding cytotoxic cells, providing a positive marker for degranulation. Granzyme B (GzB) released from the granules can be detected in the GzB ELISPOT assay. APC, antigen-presenting cell.

depends on the type of drug reaction. In patients who had DRESS, negative results were more frequently observed when the LTT was performed during the acute stage of the disease. In contrast, the culprit drug could be better identified when proliferation tests were performed during the acute stage, rather than the recovery stage, in maculopapular eruptions and SJS or TEN. Thus, the authors recommend performing the LTT within 1 week after the onset of skin rashes in patients who had maculopapular eruptions and SJS or TEN and more than 5 to 8 weeks after the event in patients who had DRESS.

In vitro diagnostic tests measure a memory T-cell response. At present, one cannot predict whether the reactivity of these drug-specific T cells in an individual patient is likely to persist for months or even years and whether these patients who lost their reactivity in in vitro tests are, in fact, likely to tolerate the drug again. The authors and others have observed a positive LTT reaction even 15 years after the original treatment with drugs that caused a delayed or even anaphylactic reaction.[28] Conversely, some patients lose reactivity within 1 to 3 years after the reaction. Thus, many groups carry out the tests after a minimal interval of 3 weeks but less than 3 to 6 months after the acute event. This interval is also used to wash out any immunosuppressive drugs, particularly corticosteroids, which are often used for the treatment of acute delayed reactions and may also suppress the immune response in vitro.

SUMMARY

The diagnosis of DHR is a challenging task because multiple and complex mechanisms are involved. The overall poor sensitivity of drug allergy tests has various reasons, with one being that a multitude of mechanisms are involved, not each of which might be covered by the tests applied. Therefore, at present, a practical approach to drug hypersensitivity diagnosis is needed, combining history, various skin tests, in vitro tests, and possibly provocation tests.

With regard to in vitro tests, the "old" proliferation-based assays have been supplemented by new and more rapid tests. The latter include evaluation of cytokine secretion, up-regulation of activation markers, and analysis of cytotoxic potential. These novel in vitro tests seem promising for drug allergy diagnosis and still need further evaluation.

In vitro tests offer the advantage of safety, simultaneous assessment of T-cell responses to multiple drugs, lack of risk for resensitization, and insight into the pathomechanism. This latter aspect may improve our understanding of particular immune mechanisms in different drug allergy diseases, which could open a more pathogenesis-tailored approach to drug allergy diagnosis, and consequently result in higher sensitivity.

REFERENCES

1. Hunziker T, Bruppacher R, Kuenzi UP, et al. Classification of ADRs: a proposal for harmonization and differentiation based on the experience of the comprehensive hospital drug monitoring Bern/St. Gallen, 1974–1993. Pharmacoepidemiol Drug Saf 2002;11(2):159–63.
2. Coombs PR, Gell PG. Classification of allergic reactions responsible for clinical hypersensitivity and disease. In: Gell RR, editor. Clinical Aspects of Immunology. Oxford: Oxford University Press; 1968. p. 575–96.
3. Pichler WJ. Delayed drug hypersensitivity reactions. Ann Intern Med 2003; 139(8):683–93.
4. Torres MJ, Romano A, Mayorga C, et al. Diagnostic evaluation of a large group of patients with immediate allergy to penicillins: the role of skin testing. Allergy 2001;56(9):850–6.
5. Torres MJ, Blanca M, Fernandez J, et al. Diagnosis of immediate allergic reactions to beta-lactam antibiotics. Allergy 2003;58(10):961–72.
6. Romano A, Blanca M, Torres MJ, et al. Diagnosis of nonimmediate reactions to beta-lactam antibiotics. Allergy 2004;59(11):1153–60.
7. Padial A, Antunez C, Blanca-Lopez N, et al. Non-immediate reactions to beta-lactams: diagnostic value of skin testing and drug provocation test. Clin Exp Allergy 2008;38(5):822–8.
8. Bousquet PJ, Pipet A, Bousquet-Rouanet L, et al. Oral challenges are needed in the diagnosis of beta-lactam hypersensitivity. Clin Exp Allergy 2008;38(1): 185–90.
9. Posadas SJ, Pichler WJ. Delayed drug hypersensitivity reactions—new concepts. Clin Exp Allergy 2007;37(7):989–99.
10. Britschgi M, Steiner UC, Schmid S, et al. T-cell involvement in drug-induced acute generalized exanthematous pustulosis. J Clin Invest 2001;107(11):1433–41.
11. Yawalkar N, Egli F, Hari Y, et al. Infiltration of cytotoxic T cells in drug-induced cutaneous eruptions. Clin Exp Allergy 2000;30(6):847–55.
12. Schnyder B, Frutig K, Mauri-Hellweg D, et al. T-cell-mediated cytotoxicity against keratinocytes in sulfamethoxazole-induced skin reaction. Clin Exp Allergy 1998;28(11):1412–7.
13. Nassif A, Bensussan A, Boumsell L, et al. Toxic epidermal necrolysis: effector cells are drug-specific cytotoxic T cells. J Allergy Clin Immunol 2004;114(5):1209–15.
14. Naisbitt DJ, Gordon SF, Pirmohamed M, et al. Immunological principles of adverse drug reactions: the initiation and propagation of immune responses elicited by drug treatment. Drug Saf 2000;23(6):483–507.

15. Padovan E, Bauer T, Tongio MM, et al. Penicilloyl peptides are recognized as T cell antigenic determinants in penicillin allergy. Eur J Immunol 1997;27(6):1303–7.

16. Lu L, Vollmer J, Moulon C, et al. Components of the ligand for a Ni++ reactive human T cell clone. J Exp Med 2003;197(5):567–74.

17. Gallucci S, Matzinger P. Danger signals: SOS to the immune system. Curr Opin Immunol 2001;13(1):114–9.

18. Park BK, Pirmohamed M, Kitteringham NR. Role of drug disposition in drug hypersensitivity: a chemical, molecular, and clinical perspective. Chem Res Toxicol 1998;11:969–87.

19. Brander C, Mauri-Hellweg D, Bettens F, et al. Heterogeneous T cell responses to beta-lactam-modified self-structures are observed in penicillin-allergic individuals. J Immunol 1995;155(5):2670–8.

20. Yawalkar N, Hari Y, Frutig K, et al. T cells isolated from positive epicutaneous test reactions to amoxicillin and ceftriaxone are drug specific and cytotoxic. J Invest Dermatol 2000;115(4):647–52.

21. Zanni MP, Mauri-Hellweg D, Brander C, et al. Characterization of lidocaine-specific T cells. J Immunol 1997;158(3):1139–48.

22. Mauri-Hellweg D, Bettens F, Mauri D, et al. Activation of drug-specific CD4+ and CD8+ T cells in individuals allergic to sulfonamides, phenytoin, and carbamazepine. J Immunol 1995;155(1):462–72.

23. Hertl M, Geisel J, Boecker C, et al. Selective generation of CD8+ T-cell clones from the peripheral blood of patients with cutaneous reactions to beta-lactam antibiotics. Br J Dermatol 1993;128(6):619–26.

24. Sieben S, Kawakubo Y, Al Masaoudi T, et al. Delayed-type hypersensitivity reaction to paraphenylenediamine is mediated by 2 different pathways of antigen recognition by specific alphabeta human T-cell clones. J Allergy Clin Immunol 2002;109(6):1005–11.

25. Schmid DA, Depta JP, Pichler WJ. T cell-mediated hypersensitivity to quinolones: mechanisms and cross-reactivity. Clin Exp Allergy 2006;36(1):59–69.

26. Pichler WJ, Beeler A, Keller M, et al. Pharmacological interaction of drugs with immune receptors: the p-i concept. Allergol Int 2006;55(1):17–25.

27. Pichler WJ. Lessons from drug allergy: against dogmata. Curr Allergy Asthma Rep 2003;3(1):1–3.

28. Beeler A, Engler O, Gerber BO, et al. Long-lasting reactivity and high frequency of drug-specific T cells after severe systemic drug hypersensitivity reactions. J Allergy Clin Immunol 2006;117(2):455–62.

29. von Greyerz S, Bultemann G, Schnyder K, et al. Degeneracy and additional alloreactivity of drug-specific human alpha beta(+) T cell clones. Int Immunol 2001;13(7):877–85.

30. Cerdan C, Martin Y, Courcoul M, et al. CD28 costimulation regulates long-term expression of the three genes (alpha, beta, gamma) encoding the high-affinity IL2 receptor. Res Immunol 1995;146(3):164–8.

31. Park H, Li Z, Yang XO, et al. A distinct lineage of CD4 T cells regulates tissue inflammation by producing interleukin 17. Nat Immunol 2005;6(11):1133–41.

32. Harrington LE, Hatton RD, Mangan PR, et al. Interleukin 17-producing CD4+ effector T cells develop via a lineage distinct from the T helper type 1 and 2 lineages. Nat Immunol 2005;6(11):1123–32.

33. Langrish CL, Chen Y, Blumenschein WM, et al. IL-23 drives a pathogenic T cell population that induces autoimmune inflammation. J Exp Med 2005;201(2):233–40.

34. Bluestone JA, Abbas AK. Natural versus adaptive regulatory T cells. Nat Rev Immunol 2003;3(3):253–7.

35. Hari Y, Frutig-Schnyder K, Hurni M, et al. T cell involvement in cutaneous drug eruptions. Clin Exp Allergy 2001;31(9):1398–408.
36. Luque I, Leyva L, Jose Torres M, et al. In vitro T-cell responses to beta-lactam drugs in immediate and nonimmediate allergic reactions. Allergy 2001;56(7):611–8.
37. Naisbitt DJ, Britschgi M, Wong G, et al. Hypersensitivity reactions to carbamazepine: characterization of the specificity, phenotype, and cytokine profile of drug-specific T cell clones. Mol Pharmacol 2003;63(3):732–41.
38. Naisbitt DJ, Farrell J, Wong G, et al. Characterization of drug-specific T cells in lamotrigine hypersensitivity. J Allergy Clin Immunol 2003;111(6):1393–403.
39. Osterwalder P, Koch J, Wuthrich B, et al. [Intermittent fever of unknown origin]. Dtsch Med Wochenschr 1998;123(24):761–5 [in German].
40. Straumann A, Bauer M, Pichler WJ, et al. Acute pancreatitis due to pyritinol: an immune-mediated phenomenon. Gastroenterology 1998;115(2):452–4.
41. Berger D, Pichler W, Savic S, et al. Fever pneumonia and eosinophilia. Praxis 2007;96(40):1543–7 [in German].
42. Pichler WJ. Drug-induced autoimmunity. Curr Opin Allergy Clin Immunol 2003; 3(4):249–53.
43. Marla VA, Victorino RM. Diagnostic value of specific T cell reactivity to drugs in 95 cases of drug induced liver injury. Gut 1997;41:534–40.
44. Tsutsui H, Terano Y, Sakagami C, et al. Drug-specific T cells derived from patients with drug-induced allergic hepatitis. J Immunol 1992;149(2):706–16.
45. Schreiber J, Zissel G, Greinert U, et al. Lymphocyte transformation test for the evaluation of adverse effects of antituberculous drugs. Eur J Med Res 1999; 4(2):67–71.
46. Lerch M, Keller M, Britschgi M, et al. Cross-reactivity patterns of T cells specific for iodinated contrast media. J Allergy Clin Immunol 2007;119(6):1529–36.
47. Pichler WJ, Tilch J. The lymphocyte transformation test in the diagnosis of drug hypersensitivity. Allergy 2004;59(8):809–20.
48. Roujeau JC, Albengres E, Moritz S. Lymphocyte transformation test in drug-induced toxic epidermal necrolysis. Int Arch Allergy Appl Immunol 1985;78:22–4.
49. Nyfeler B, Pichler WJ. The lymphocyte transformation test for the diagnosis of drug allergy: sensitivity and specificity. Clin Exp Allergy 1997;27(2):175–81.
50. Neukomm CB, Yawalkar N, Helbling A, et al. T-cell reactions to drugs in distinct clinical manifestations of drug allergy. J Investig Allergol Clin Immunol 2001; 11(4):275–84.
51. Everness KM, Gawkrodger DJ, Botham PA, et al. The discrimination between nickel-sensitive and non-nickel-sensitive subjects by an in vitro lymphocyte transformation test. Br J Dermatol 1990;122(3):293–8.
52. Warrington RJ, Tse KS. Lymphocyte transformation studies in drug hypersensitivity. Can Med Assoc J 1979;120:1089–94.
53. Barna BP, Gogate P, Deodhar SD, et al. Lymphocyte transformation and radioallergenosorbent tests in drug hypersensitivity. Am J Clin Pathol 1980;73(2): 172–6.
54. Berg PA, Brattig N, Diao G-J, et al. Diagnose arzneimittelbedingter Nebenwirkungen mit Hilfe des Lyphozytentransformationstests. Allergologie 1983;6: 77–81 [in German].
55. Walker C, Kristensen F, Bettens F, et al. Lymphokine regulation of activated (G1) lymphocytes. I. Prostaglandin E2-induced inhibition of interleukin 2 production. J Immunol 1983;130(4):1770–3.
56. Schnyder B, Pichler WJ. Skin and laboratory tests in amoxicillin- and penicillin-induced morbilliform skin eruption. Clin Exp Allergy 2000;30(4):590–5.

57. Phillips EJ, Sullivan JR, Knowles SR, et al. Utility of patch testing in patients with hypersensitivity syndromes associated with abacavir. AIDS 2002;16(16):2223–5.
58. Cederbrant K, Hultman P, Marcusson JA, et al. In vitro lymphocyte proliferation as compared to patch test using gold, palladium and nickel. Int Arch Allergy Immunol 1997;112(3):212–7.
59. Stejskal V, Hudecek R, Stejskal J, et al. Diagnosis and treatment of metal-induced side-effects. Neuro Endocrinol Lett 2006;27(Suppl 1):7–16.
60. Lopez S, Torres MJ, Rodriguez-Pena R, et al. Lymphocyte proliferation response in patients with delayed hypersensitivity reactions to heparins. Br J Dermatol 2009;160(2):259–65.
61. Lanier LL, Buck DW, Rhodes L, et al. Interleukin 2 activation of natural killer cells rapidly induces the expression and phosphorylation of the Leu-23 activation antigen. J Exp Med 1988;167(5):1572–85.
62. Testi R, Pulcinelli FM, Cifone MG, et al. Preferential involvement of a phospholipase A2-dependent pathway in CD69-mediated platelet activation. J Immunol 1992;148(9):2867–71.
63. Lopez-Cabrera M, Santis AG, Fernandez-Ruiz E, et al. Molecular cloning, expression, and chromosomal localization of the human earliest lymphocyte activation antigen AIM/CD69, a new member of the C-type animal lectin superfamily of signal-transmitting receptors. J Exp Med 1993;178(2):537–47.
64. Maino VC, Suni MA, Ruitenberg JJ. Rapid flow cytometric method for measuring lymphocyte subset activation. Cytometry 1995;20(2):127–33.
65. Pitsios C, Dimitrakopoulou A, Tsalimalma K, et al. Expression of CD69 on T-cell subsets in HIV-1 disease. Scand J Clin Lab Invest 2008;68(3):233–41.
66. Lina G, Cozon G, Ferrandiz J, et al. Detection of staphylococcal superantigenic toxins by a CD69-specific cytofluorimetric assay measuring T-cell activation. J Clin Microbiol 1998;36(4):1042–5.
67. Nishio D, Izu K, Kabashima K, et al. T cell populations propagating in the peripheral blood of patients with drug eruptions. J Dermatol Sci 2007;48(1):25–33.
68. Torres MJ, Mayorga C, Cornejo-Garcia JA, et al. Monitoring non-immediate allergic reactions to iodine contrast media. Clin Exp Immunol 2008;152(2):233–8.
69. Beeler A, Zaccaria L, Kawabata T, et al. CD69 upregulation on T cells as an in vitro marker for delayed-type drug hypersensitivity. Allergy 2008;63(2):181–8.
70. Cornejo-Garcia JA, Fernandez TD, Torres MJ, et al. Differential cytokine and transcription factor expression in patients with allergic reactions to drugs. Allergy 2007;62(12):1429–38.
71. Posadas SJ, Leyva L, Torres MJ, et al. Subjects with allergic reactions to drugs show in vivo polarized patterns of cytokine expression depending on the chronology of the clinical reaction. J Allergy Clin Immunol 2000;106(4):769–76.
72. Gaspard I, Guinnepain MT, Laurent J, et al. Il-4 and IFN-gamma mRNA induction in human peripheral lymphocytes specific for beta-lactam antibiotics in immediate or delayed hypersensitivity reactions. J Clin Immunol 2000;20(2):107–16.
73. Lochmatter P, Beeler A, Kawabata TT, et al. Drug-specific in vitro release of IL-2, IL-5, IL-13 and IFN-gamma in patients with delayed-type drug hypersensitivity. Allergy 2009 [Epub ahead of print].
74. Brugnolo F, Annunziato F, Sampognaro S, et al. Highly Th2-skewed cytokine profile of beta-lactam-specific T cells from nonatopic subjects with adverse drug reactions. J Immunol 1999;163(2):1053–9.
75. Halevy S, Cohen AD, Grossman N. Clinical implications of in vitro drug-induced interferon gamma release from peripheral blood lymphocytes in cutaneous adverse drug reactions. J Am Acad Dermatol 2005;52(2):254–61.

76. Yawalkar N, Shrikhande M, Hari Y, et al. Evidence for a role for IL-5 and eotaxin in activating and recruiting eosinophils in drug-induced cutaneous eruptions. J Allergy Clin Immunol 2000;106(6):1171–6.

77. Posadas SJ, Torres MJ, Mayorga C, et al. Gene expression levels of cytokine profile and cytotoxic markers in non-immediate reactions to drugs. Blood Cells Mol Dis 2002;29(2):179–89.

78. Tsuge I, Okumura A, Kondo Y, et al. Allergen-specific T-cell response in patients with phenytoin hypersensitivity; simultaneous analysis of proliferation and cytokine production by carboxyfluorescein succinimidyl ester (CFSE) dilution assay. Allergol Int 2007;56(2):149–55.

79. Khalil G, El-Sabban M, Al-Ghadban S, et al. Cytokine expression profile of sensitized human T lymphocytes following in vitro stimulation with amoxicillin. Eur Cytokine Netw 2008;19(3):131–41.

80. Choquet-Kastylevsky G, Intrator L, Chenal C, et al. Increased levels of interleukin 5 are associated with the generation of eosinophilia in drug-induced hypersensitivity syndrome. Br J Dermatol 1998;139(6):1026–32.

81. Yawalkar N. Drug-induced exanthems. Toxicology 2005;209(2):131–4.

82. Sachs B, Erdmann S, Malte Baron J, et al. Determination of interleukin-5 secretion from drug-specific activated ex vivo peripheral blood mononuclear cells as a test system for the in vitro detection of drug sensitization. Clin Exp Allergy 2002;32(5):736–44.

83. Sachs B, Erdmann S, Al-Masaoudi T, et al. In vitro drug allergy detection system incorporating human liver microsomes in clorazepate-induced skin rash: drug-specific proliferation associated with interleukin-5 secretion. Br J Dermatol 2001;144(2):316–20.

84. Merk HF. Diagnosis of drug hypersensitivity: lymphocyte transformation test and cytokines. Toxicology 2005;209(2):217–20.

85. Schmid S, Kuechler PC, Britschgi M, et al. Acute generalized exanthematous pustulosis: role of cytotoxic T cells in pustule formation. Am J Pathol 2002; 161(6):2079–86.

86. Le Cleach L, Delaire S, Boumsell L, et al. Blister fluid T lymphocytes during toxic epidermal necrolysis are functional cytotoxic cells which express human natural killer (NK) inhibitory receptors. Clin Exp Immunol 2000; 119(1):225–30.

87. Hertl M, Bohlen H, Jugert F, et al. Predominance of epidermal CD8+ T lymphocytes in bullous cutaneous reactions caused by beta-lactam antibiotics. J Invest Dermatol 1993;101(6):794–9.

88. Kuechler PC, Britschi M, Schmid S, et al. Cytotoxic mechanisms in different forms of T-cell-mediated drug allergies. Allergy 2004;59(6):613–22.

89. Nassif A, Bensussan A, Dorothee G, et al. Drug specific cytotoxic T-cells in the skin lesions of a patient with toxic epidermal necrolysis. J Invest Dermatol 2002; 118(4):728–33.

90. Viard I, Wehrli P, Bullani R, et al. Inhibition of toxic epidermal necrolysis by blockade of CD95 with human intravenous immunoglobulin. Science 1998; 282(5388):490–3.

91. Murata J, Abe R, Shimizu H. Increased soluble Fas ligand levels in patients with Stevens-Johnson syndrome and toxic epidermal necrolysis preceding skin detachment. J Allergy Clin Immunol 2008;122(5):992–1000.

92. Chung WH, Hung SI, Yang JY, et al. Granulysin is a key mediator for disseminated keratinocyte death in Stevens-Johnson syndrome and toxic epidermal necrolysis. Nat Med 2008;14(12):1343–50.

93. Brunner KT, Mauel J, Cerottini JC, et al. Quantitative assay of the lytic action of immune lymphoid cells on 51-Cr-labelled allogeneic target cells in vitro; inhibition by isoantibody and by drugs. Immunology 1968;14(2):181–96.

94. Sheehy ME, McDermott AB, Furlan SN, et al. A novel technique for the fluorometric assessment of T lymphocyte antigen specific lysis. J Immunol Methods 2001;249(1–2):99–110.

95. Liu L, Chahroudi A, Silvestri G, et al. Visualization and quantification of T cell-mediated cytotoxicity using cell-permeable fluorogenic caspase substrates. Nat Med 2002;8(2):185–9.

96. Betts MR, Brenchley JM, Price DA, et al. Sensitive and viable identification of antigen-specific CD8+ T cells by a flow cytometric assay for degranulation. J Immunol Methods 2003;281(1–2):65–78.

97. Andersen MH, Schrama D, Thor Straten P, et al. Cytotoxic T cells. J Invest Dermatol 2006;126(1):32–41.

98. Trapani JA, Smyth MJ. Functional significance of the perforin/granzyme cell death pathway. Nat Rev Immunol 2002;2(10):735–47.

99. Dunn C, Brunetto M, Reynolds G, et al. Cytokines induced during chronic hepatitis B virus infection promote a pathway for NK cell-mediated liver damage. J Exp Med 2007;204(3):667–80.

100. Alter G, Malenfant JM, Altfeld M. CD107a as a functional marker for the identification of natural killer cell activity. J Immunol Methods 2004;294(1–2):15–22.

101. Rininsland FH, Helms T, Asaad RJ, et al. Granzyme B ELISPOT assay for ex vivo measurements of T cell immunity. J Immunol Methods 2000;240(1–2):143–55.

102. Boon AC, de Mutsert G, Fouchier RA, et al. Functional profile of human influenza virus-specific cytotoxic T lymphocyte activity is influenced by interleukin-2 concentration and epitope specificity. Clin Exp Immunol 2005;142(1):45–52.

103. Burkett MW, Shafer-Weaver KA, Strobl S, et al. A novel flow cytometric assay for evaluating cell-mediated cytotoxicity. J Immunother 2005;28(4):396–402.

104. Devevre E, Romero P, Mahnke YD. LiveCount Assay: concomitant measurement of cytolytic activity and phenotypic characterisation of CD8(+) T-cells by flow cytometry. J Immunol Methods 2006;311(1–2):31–46.

105. Rock MT, Yoder SM, Wright PF, et al. Differential regulation of granzyme and perforin in effector and memory T cells following smallpox immunization. J Immunol 2005;174(6):3757–64.

106. Rubio V, Stuge TB, Singh N, et al. Ex vivo identification, isolation and analysis of tumor-cytolytic T cells. Nat Med 2003;9(11):1377–82.

107. Shafer-Weaver K, Rosenberg S, Strobl S, et al. Application of the granzyme B ELISPOT assay for monitoring cancer vaccine trials. J Immunother 2006;29(3):328–35.

108. van Besouw NM, Zuijderwijk JM, de Kuiper P, et al. The granzyme B and interferon-gamma enzyme-linked immunospot assay as alternatives for cytotoxic T-lymphocyte precursor frequency after renal transplantation. Transplantation 2005;79(9):1062–6.

109. Kano Y, Hirahara K, Mitsuyama Y, et al. Utility of the lymphocyte transformation test in the diagnosis of drug sensitivity: dependence on its timing and the type of drug eruption. Allergy 2007;62(12):1439–44.

The Basophil Activation Test in Immediate-Type Drug Allergy

Oliver V. Hausmann, MD[a],*, Thomas Gentinetta, MSc[a],
Chris H. Bridts, MLT[b], Didier G. Ebo, MD, PhD[b]

KEYWORDS

• Drug allergy • Basophil activation test • Passive sensitization
• CD63 • CD203c • p38 MAPK

Allergic adverse drug reactions (ADRs) are important and underestimated health issues leading to considerable comorbidity and additional health costs.[1] Diagnosis of drug allergy is difficult for several reasons:

Type of immune reaction—drugs can elicit a broad range of immune reactions, each of which may require different tests to prove an involvement.

Epitope—drugs can act as haptens, and they may bind to different proteins. The exact epitope (hapten–carrier complex) causing the reaction is frequently unknown.

Clinical correlation—the outcome of in vitro or in vivo tests with different drug concentrations might not correlate with situations in clinical routine.

Comedication and comorbidity—the eliciting drug often is given in combination with other drugs in patients with different diseases. This comedication and the underlying disease may influence an immune reaction to a drug or the clinical picture.

Drug challenge—the gold standard or reference diagnostic test is a time-consuming and potentially dangerous endeavor limited to specialized centers.

In view of these limitations, many efforts have been made to enlarge the armamentarium to diagnose drug allergic reactions, one of them being the basophil activation test (BAT). This article summarizes the use of BAT as a functional in vitro test in immediate-type drug allergy. These immediate-type hypersensitivity reactions are orchestrated by T cells and mediated by specific IgE (sIgE) antibodies on the surface of

[a] Department of Allergology, Department of Rheumatology, Allergology and Clinical Immunology, Inselspital, Freiburgstrasse, 3010 Bern, University of Bern, Switzerland
[b] Allergology Unit, Department of Immunology, Allergology and Rheumatology, University Hospital Antwerp, University of Antwerp, Belgium
* Corresponding author.
E-mail address: oliver.hausmann@insel.ch (O.V. Hausmann).

Immunol Allergy Clin N Am 29 (2009) 555–566
doi:10.1016/j.iac.2009.04.011　　　　　　　　　　　　immunology.theclinics.com
0889-8561/09/$ – see front matter © 2009 Elsevier Inc. All rights reserved.

two related but autonomous groups of effector cells: the basophils in peripheral blood and the tissue-resident mast cells. They show similar activation pathways by means of membrane-bound IgE (via FcεRI) produced by plasma cells in the bone marrow. These plasma cells were stimulated by allergens in the periphery with the help of T cells (TH2 cells).[2] Even if basophils and mast cells might share a common bone marrow progenitor,[3,4] mast cells are no simple tissue counterparts of the basophils. Basophils can migrate into different tissues (eg, peribronchial basophils in asthma) and drive the inflammatory process side by side with mast cells and eosinophils.[5] Mast cells are more abundant than basophils, which are actually the smallest leukocyte species by number in peripheral blood. But in contrast to mast cells, basophils are easily accessible in the peripheral blood and therefore are favored for experimental approaches and future routine diagnostics.

BAT relies on flow cytometric quantification of alterations of specific activation markers[6–8] on the surface (CD63, CD203c) or inside the basophils (phosphorylated p38 mitogen-activated protein kinase, P-p38MAPK) as illustrated in **Fig. 1**. These changes can be detected and quantified on a single-cell basis by flow cytometry using specific monoclonal antibodies coupled to a fluorochrome. Obviously, BAT is only applicable in those cases where the final effector function relies on activation of basophils (eg, IgE-mediated immediate type hypersensitivity).

BAT may depend on bridging of adjacent allergen-specific membrane-bound IgE molecules on the surface of basophils. One has to be aware, however, that other mechanisms of cell activation (complement system or even nonimmunologic, pharmacologic basophil activation) may occur. Consideration of this fact is particularly important in BAT with drugs. Actually, the use of BAT for drug reaction to nonsteroidal anti-inflammatory drugs (NSAIDs) may rely on a heightened sensitivity of in vivo activated basophils to NSAID and is not a sign of IgE-mediated reactions.

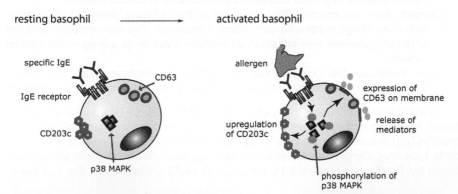

Fig. 1. Upon cross-linking of membrane-bound IgE, basophils not only secrete particular mediators, but also up-regulate the expression of specific activation markers such as CD63 and CD203c. A main difficulty of basophil activation test for drugs may be an insufficient IgE cross-linking by drugs with small molecular weight, so they are only able to bind to one IgE molecule; crosslinking and basophil activation may only occur, if the drug molecule is bivalent like eg, chlorhexidine and certain neuromuscular blocking agents or if more than two drug molecules bind to a larger protein, which then cross-links two adjacent IgE molecules. The exact mechanisms that govern basophil degranulation remain elusive, but it has been demonstrated that phosphorylation of p38 MAPK exerts a pivotal role in cell activation. (*From* Ebo DG, Hagendorens MM, Bridts CH, et al. The basophil activation test in immediate drug allergy. Acta Clin Belg 2009;64:129–35; with permission.)

In the context of an allergic reaction for drugs or related compounds, BAT has been validated in the diagnosis of an IgE-mediated allergy from neuromuscular blocking agents (NMBAs), beta-lactam antibiotics, and clavulanic acid as β-lactamase inhibitor, iodinated radiocontrast media (RCM), the antiseptic chlorhexidine, gelatine-based plasma expanders, and the infusion-excipient carboxymethylcellulose.

In some of these studies, BAT has proven to complement skin tests in assessing clinical relevant cross-reactivity and tailoring individual safe alternative therapeutic or diagnostic regimens. In an increasing number of case reports, BAT constituted the sole or a valuable additional test for agents such as the solvent Cremophor, low molecular weight heparins, the dye patent blue, starch colloids, platinum salts, the enzyme hyaluronidase, recombinant hepatitis B vaccine, the antiviral agent valacyclovir, and methylprednisolone.

PRINCIPLE OF THE BASOPHIL ACTIVATION TEST

Activation of basophils is a stepwise process starting with intracellular changes (signal transduction from FcεRI by means of phosphorylation of p38MAPK and calcium influx) followed by changes on the cell membrane (CD203c) with final degranulation of the basophils (CD63 detectable after fusion of intracellular granules with cell membrane and mediator release).[6]

BAT measures an in vitro activation of patients' basophils in the test tube. After blood sample preparations (whole-blood assay versus leukocyte isolation) and preincubation with interleukin (IL)-3 (depending on the allergen of interest) or prewarming of blood samples and reagents to 37°C, allergen is added, and basophils are incubated for 15 minutes to 1 hour at 37°C in the water bath (again depending on the allergen of interest). BAT is only applicable for drugs or excipients existing in a galenic formulation that is soluble in the stimulation buffer. After testing for cytotoxicity, usually one is not using a single concentration of the substance of interest but a concentration range spanning 3 to 7 log scales to demonstrate dose dependence of basophil activation. Afterwards, staining with monoclonal antibodies coupled to fluorochromes and lysis of contaminating erythrocytes follows. To select basophils from the whole leukocyte population, several positive and negative selection strategies are possible (eg, anti-CCR3/anti-CD3, anti-CD123/anti-HLA-DR). To determine the activation state, different markers, such as CD63, CD203c, or P-p38MAPK, are used. The minimal number of basophils to be analyzed should be 200 per test tube for accurate quantification of basophil activation, but it is preferred that 600 to 1000 basophils are evaluated to minimize variation of results caused by equipment measurement error alone.[9] In the past, thresholds for positivity often were set arbitrarily (greater than 5% activated basophils with a stimulation index greater than 2, eg, less than 2.5% stimulation in negative control), These have been replaced by accurate receiver operating characteristics (ROC) analysis for the different allergens including nonallergic exposed controls.[6]

BAT is an established diagnostic test for different IgE-mediated allergies, including inhalant (eg, pollen, house dust mite, cat dander), food, hymenoptera venom, drug, and latex allergy.[6–8] A major observation from these studies is that in contrast to protein allergens, chemicals such as drugs elicit less-pronounced in vitro basophil activation, resulting in a lower sensitivity of BAT for drugs as compared with inhalant and food allergens. New gating strategies and the combined use of extra- and intracellular activation markers such as phosphorylated p38 MAPK,[10] however, might increase the sensitivity of BAT in this respect. For example, **Fig. 2** displays the BAT results for the different activation markers in a patient who had anaphylactic shock during intravenous therapy with cefuroxime.

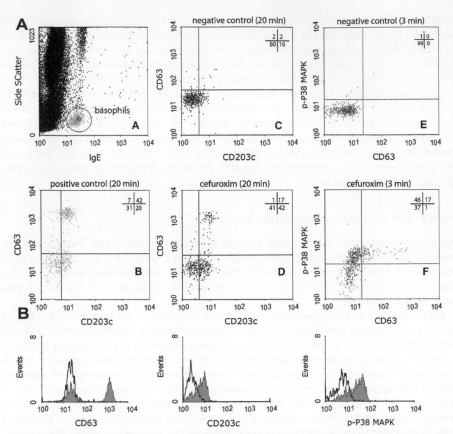

Fig. 2. Flow cytometric analysis using a dot plot (side scatter and fluorescence). Alexa 488-conjugated anti-IgE positive basophils are gated out in a circular region (*top left*). Pre-warmed basophils are stimulated for 3 or 20 minutes at 37°C with anti-IgE as positive control (*middle left*), washing solution to measure spontaneous CD63, CD203c, and phosphorylated p38 MAPK expression (negative control, *top middle* and *top right*) and cefuroxime (*central panel* and *middle right*). Note the clear bimodal up-regulation of CD63 and the more homogenous up-regulation of CD203c and phosphorylation of p38 MAPK in a larger proportion of the cells. A combination of these activation markers might increase the sensitivity of the test, particularly when only a low number of basophils can be analyzed. This is also clear from the histograms in the lower panel (open histogram spontaneous expression by resting cells, closed histogram expression after stimulation of cells with cefuroxime). (*From* Ebo DG, Hagendorens MM, Bridts CH, et al. The basophil activation test in immediate drug allergy. Acta Clin Belg 2009;64:129–35; with permission.)

The European Interest Group for the Evaluation of BAT in clinical routine (EuroBAT, part of the European Academy of Allergy and Clinical Immunology [EAACI] working group on allergy diagnosis) focuses on harmonization of the existing different BAT protocols (maybe even establishing a reference BAT protocol) to render results internationally comparable, so that as a final goal, multicenter studies are easier to conduct. This is especially important in the field of drug allergy, where the number of patients allergic to a specific drug or drug group per center is usually low, and conclusions of single-center studies are limited. Current limitations of and open questions in BAT, together with possible solutions, are shown in **Table 1**.

Table 1	
Limitations and open questions in the basophil activation test	
Open Questions	**Possible Solutions**
Optimal drug concentration	Dose–response curve with patients and healthy (exposed) controls for exclusion of unspecific stimulation
Thresholds for positivity	Receiver operating characteristics analysis for the different drugs in question with confirmed drug-allergic patients and healthy (exposed) controls instead of arbitrarily chosen thresholds
Minimal basophil number to be analyzed (600–1000 per tube)	Multicenter studies for the different drugs in question
Drug solubility	Contact experienced centers and test for unspecific stimulation by solvent (eg,EtOH) if needed
Blood sample storage and preparation (whole blood versus isolated leukocytes)	EDTA as anticoagulant at 4°C for a maximum of 24 h or passive sensitization of donor basophils with patient sera (IgE stabile for months)
Optimal preincubation conditions (interleukin 3 addition versus prewarming) and incubation time (10–40 min)	Multicenter studies for the different drugs in question

PRINCIPLE OF PASSIVE SENSITIZATION OF DONOR BASOPHILS WITH PATIENT SERUM

The proof of an IgE-mediated mechanism in drug allergy is of utmost importance for the individual patient concerning prognosis and avoidance strategies. BAT, in combination with passive sensitization of donor basophils, offers an in vitro correlate to the famous in vivo Prausnitz-Kuestner reaction or so-called passive cutaneous anaphylaxis (PCA).[11] This wheal-and-flare reaction on the forearm of a nonallergic subject (eg, Carl Prausnitz) 24 hours after intradermal injection of the serum of his fish-allergic colleague Kuestner at the same site, was the first proof of a serum factor transferring hypersensitivity, which later became known as IgE.[12] Because of the obvious risk of infection, this test was abandoned from clinical practice. Nevertheless, an in vitro Prausnitz-Kuestner approach using the BAT in combination with passive sensitization of healthy donor basophils would prove an IgE-mediated mechanism. Especially if the sensitizing capacity of patient's serum is lost after heating to 56°C for 30 minutes (with disintegration of immunoglobulins) or immunoglobulin elimination by affinity column, the IgE dependence of the reaction is proven.[13,14]

The principle steps of passive sensitization are:

Peripheral blood mononuclear cells (PBMC) isolation of a healthy donor, whose basophils are well-characterized in the ability of stimulation
Removal of receptor-bound IgE with lactic acid (pH 3.9), so-called stripping
Incubation with patient serum (1 hour, 37°C)
Regular BAT as described previously, including negative control (eg, unstripped and stripped), but unsensitized donor basophils

This multistep procedure represents an in vitro Prausnitz-Kuestner or in vitro passive anaphylaxis test. It depends on the exact and cautious handling of the basophils to avoid unspecific stimulation or cell death. A protocol elaborated by Pruzansky and colleagues,[15] which has been modified by different groups,[16,17] is working well in the authors' hands.

CURRENT APPLICATIONS
Neuromuscular Blocking Agents

Six larger studies have investigated the diagnostic performance of BAT in allergy from curarising neuromuscular blocking agents (NMBAs) (**Table 2**).[18–23] The widely varying sensitivity (36% to 92%, specificity greater than 90%) reported in some of these publications merits reflection. First, the lowest sensitivity was observed in surveys that failed to enroll well-characterized control individuals who were exposed but did not react to the drug(s) under investigation. Therefore, a ROC analysis for discriminative cut-off calculation between patients and controls was not possible, and an arbitrarily chosen decision threshold was set relative to spontaneous CD63 expression by resting basophils. These thresholds were based upon experience with potent protein allergens that are known to elicit stronger in vitro basophil responses than drugs. Second, the optimal concentration for basophil activation might differ considerably from one NMBA to another,[18] rendering the proposal to adopt a universal decision threshold for all NMBAs difficult to justify and probably obsolete. Finally, sensitivity of the test might decrease over time.[21]

In contrary to the in vivo drug challenge, BAT allows simultaneous testing of different potentially cross-reactive drugs (with subsequent drug challenge to document

Table 2
Basophil activation test in drug allergy

Stimulus	Reference Test	Sens	Spec	N	Reference
Neuromuscular blocking agents (NMBA)					
NMBA	H	64	93	62	18
NMBA	H ± ST	54	100	60	19
NMBA	H	79	100	31	20
NMBA	H + ST	36–86	93	92	21
Rocuronium (NMBA)	H + ST	92	100	22	22
NMBA	H ± ST ± IgE	68	100	49	23
Antibiotics					
β-lactam	H + ST	50	93	88	27
β-lactam	H ± ST ± IgE ± PT	49	91	110	28
β-lactam (amoxicillin)	H + ST	67 (CD203c) 33 (CD63)	100 (CD203c) 79 (CD63)	41	30
Nonsteroidal anti-inflammatory drugs (NSAID)					
Metamizol	H ± PT	42	100	55	36
Aspirin and NSAID	H ± PT	15–55	74–100	90	37
NSAID	H	43	100	72	38

Abbreviations: H, history; N, total number of patients and control individuals; PT, provocation tests; Sens, sensitivity; Spec, specificity; ST, skin test.

Data from Ebo DG, Sainte-Laudy J, Bridts CH, et al. Flow-assisted allergy diagnosis: current applications and future perspectives. Allergy 2006;61(9):1028–39.

tolerance) to find safe alternative regimens for future anesthesia. This is another advantage of this in vitro test.[18,20,22,24] The authors demonstrated that BAT[22] (not sIgE-inhibition assays)[25] is complementary to skin tests in identifying clinically relevant cross-reactivity between different NMBA.

Beta-lactam Antibiotics

The diagnostic approach for immediate allergic reactions to beta-lactam antibiotics recently was standardized under the aegis of the European Network for Drug Allergy (ENDA) and the European Academy of Allergy and Clinical Immunology (EAACI) interest group on drug hypersensitivity.[26] This position paper highlights the impor- tance of drug challenge for diagnosis in a considerable number of patients as quanti- fication of sIgE and skin test yields equivocal, contradictory, or false-negative results. In a comparison between quantification of sIgE and basophilic CD63 expression including 58 patients suffering from skin test-proven beta-lactam allergy and 30 healthy control individuals, sensitivity and specificity of the assays approximated 38% and 87% for sIgE and 50% and 94% for the basophil activation test, respec- tively.[27] Comparable results were observed in a survey by Torres and colleagues,[28] as shown in **Table 2**. Whether other (more upstream-located) activation markers such as down-regulation of membrane-bound IgE will increase sensitivity of the BAT[29] and whether CD203c is a more sensitive and specific marker than CD63 to diagnose allergy from beta-lactam antibiotics remains to be established.[30] It is of note that again in all these studies on antibiotics, as for NMBA, decision thresholds were set arbitrarily or relative to spontaneous expression of the applied activation marker.

Radiocontrast Material

RCM application generally is tolerated well. Besides the pharmacologic adverse effects (flush, nausea, vomiting), the associated risk of a severe anaphylactic reaction (angioedema, bronchospasm, hypotension) has been estimated to be between 0.02% (nonionic RCM) and 0.4% (ionic RCM).[31,32] Around 4% of these are highly suggestive of an IgE-mediated mechanism (positive skin test and BAT), which is therefore not the general rule in RCM allergy.[14,33] Direct histamine release by means of nonspecific RCM binding to membrane receptors on mast cells or basophils and indirect mast cell or basophil activation by means of the complement or kinin cascade outweigh the genuine IgE-mediated reactions.[34] Taking into account that in the United States RCM is applied in more than 10 million radiologic procedures, the relevance of these seemingly small percentages becomes obvious.[35] Especially because preventive medication with antihistamines and steroids does not avoid systemic reactions in these cases, IgE-mediated reactions need to be identified.[33] Besides identifying the culprit RCM and cross-reactive substances, BAT in combination with skin test results can help define a safe alternative for future radiologic diagnostics while rendering the choice for preventive provocation tests as safe as possible.

Aspirin and Nonsteroidal Anti-inflammatory Drugs

Besides case reports, three larger studies from Spain have assessed BAT in the diag- nosis of hypersensitivity to aspirin, metamizol, and other NSAIDs.[36–38] The sensitivity for the different NSAIDs varied from 15% for metamizol to 55% for naproxen, whereas specificity exceeded 90%. With positive predictive values up to 100%, authors clas- sified BAT a reliable instrument for diagnosing hypersensitivity from NSAIDs. In contrast, Erdmann and colleagues (20 patients, different NSAID)[39] and Malbran and colleagues (14 patients, diclofenac)[40] concluded that the value of CD63-based BAT in NSAID intolerance remains unclear, and especially with a negative BAT result, a drug challenge cannot be omitted. Currently, the authors do not recommend BAT in immediate hypersensitivity because of NSAIDs and believe that additional studies with consistent correlation to provocation tests are mandatory to confirm the Spanish data, particularly because NSAID-induced respiratory and cutaneous reactions are generally IgE-independent adverse events resulting from inhibition of cyclooxygenase-1 (COX-1), which results in depletion of prostaglandin E2 with unrestrained synthesis of cysteinyl leukotrienes and mediator release from mast cells and eosinophils.[41]

Chlorhexidine

Chlorhexidine is a cationic bisguanide antiseptic and can trigger irritant dermatitis, allergic contact dermatitis, and IgE-mediated reactions (including life-threatening anaphylaxis). For a long time, diagnosis of IgE-mediated chlorhexidine allergy has relied only upon skin prick tests, and additional confirmatory in vitro test were awaited. Recently, BAT[42] and quantification of sIgE[42,43] for chlorhexidine proved to be valuable and safe alternative diagnostic instruments, particularly for severe cases.[44]

Gelatine

Anaphylaxis to gelatine in vaccines and gelatine-based colloids is known[45] and generally can be established on quantification of sIgE and/or appropriate skin tests. In certain cases with unequivocal or even contradictory results, BAT has been proven to constitute a valuable additional diagnostic tool.[46]

Carboxymethylcellulose

Different groups have identified carboxymethylcellulose (CMC),[47–51] a common infusion excipient, as the elicitor of anaphylactic reactions following minimally invasive interventions (eg, joint infiltration with local anesthetic and steroids) by means of skin testing, ELISA and BAT. Especially in situations where multiple drugs are given simultaneously and repetitive procedures are needed, a clarification of the elicitor is of paramount importance. When infusion excipients like CMC are involved, repetitive anaphylaxis during following interventions with structurally unrelated alternative drugs can occur, as they might contain the same excipient (CMC). Even some steroids (for intramuscular injection) that might be used to treat anaphylaxis contain CMC and can aggravate the patient's critical state.

Miscellaneous

In an increasing number of cases, BAT helped to identify the plasma expander hydroxyl ethyl starch,[52] cremophor (the emulsifier of the intravenous cyclosporine formulation),[53] bovine serum albumin present in a semen culture medium for artificial insemination,[54] omeprazole,[55] different low-molecular-weight heparins,[56,57] viscotoxins of mistletoe (*Viscum album*),[58] the dye patent blue,[59] the enzyme hyaluronidase,[60] platinum salts,[61,62] recombinant hepatitis B vaccine,[63] clavulanic acid mimicking amoxicillin allergy,[64] and the antiviral valacyclovir[65] as the causative compound in patients with sometimes life-threatening allergic reactions. Moreover, in some of these patients, BAT has contributed to establish the individual therapeutic alternative or allowed identification of potentially cross-reactive structures.

SUMMARY

BAT provides the physician with a novel instrument in the diagnostic management of immediate-type drug allergy that involves IgE-dependent mast cell and basophil activation. It is of particular interest in those cases where current in vitro routine diagnostics do not provide alternative tests, and confirmation of clinical suspicion (despite negative skin test results) would require a potential dangerous drug provocation test. Currently, however, BAT mostly is applied for research settings, and additional clinical studies are mandatory to allow its entrance into clinical routine. Attempts to harmonize BAT protocols on an international scale under the aegis of the EAACI are ongoing. Correct selection of patients and appropriate exposed, nonallergic control groups are important prerequisites to establish optimal drug-specific positivity thresholds, replacing arbitrarily chosen decision thresholds, and should allow correct determination of sensitivity, specificity, and predictive values. Passive sensitization of donor basophils with patients' serum is another advantage of BAT, as this cannot be done in vivo (theoretical risk of infection) and provides an instrument to prove the IgE dependence of a drug reaction in question. This is important for prognosis and avoidance measurements, as IgE-mediated reactions are generally more dangerous and potentially life-threatening. The possibility to test several drugs at the same time helps in tailoring drug challenge for safe therapeutic alternatives. Additionally, novel basophil gating strategies and activation markers such as p38 MAPK might improve the diagnostic performance of BAT. Moreover, as these novel markers might become activated through alternative routes, it seems theoretically justified to anticipate that the BAT might be applicable for diagnosing IgE-independent basophil-mediated adverse drug reactions.

REFERENCES

1. Hayward RA, Hofer TP. Estimating hospital deaths due to medical errors: preventability is in the eye of the reviewer. JAMA 2001;286(4):415–20.
2. Abbas A, Lichtman A. Immediate hypersensitivity. In: Abbas A, Lichtman A, editors. Cellular and molecular immunology. 5th edition. Philadelphia: Saunders; 2003. p. 432–52.
3. Wang J, Qi JC, Konecny P, et al. Hemopoietic cells with features of the mast cell and basophil lineages and their potential role in allergy. Curr Drug Targets Inflamm Allergy 2003;2(4):293–302.
4. Kocabas CN, Yavuz AS, Lipsky PE, et al. Analysis of the lineage relationship between mast cells and basophils using the c-kit D816V mutation as a biologic signature. J Allergy Clin Immunol 2005;115(6):1155–61.
5. Bochner BS, Schleimer RP. Mast cells, basophils, and eosinophils: distinct but overlapping pathways for recruitment. Immunol Rev 2001;179:5–15.
6. Ebo DG, Hagendorens MM, Bridts CH, et al. In vitro allergy diagnosis: should we follow the flow? Clin Exp Allergy 2004;34(3):332–9.
7. Ebo DG, Sainte-Laudy J, Bridts CH, et al. Flow-assisted allergy diagnosis: current applications and future perspectives. Allergy 2006;61(9):1028–39.
8. de Weck AL, Sanz ML, Gamboa PM, et al. Diagnostic tests based on human basophils: more potentials and perspectives than pitfalls. Int Arch Allergy Immunol 2008;146(3):177–89.
9. Lorenz I, Schneider EM, Stolz P, et al. Sensitive flow cytometric method to test basophil activation influenced by homeopathic histamine dilutions. Forsch Komplementarmed Klass Naturheilkd 2003;10(6):316–24.

10. Ebo DG, Dombrecht EJ, Bridts CH, et al. Combined analysis of intracellular signaling and immunophenotype of human peripheral blood basophils by flow cytometry: a proof of concept. Clin Exp Allergy 2007;37(11):1668–75.
11. Prausnitz C, Kuestner H. [Studies on hypersensitivity]. Zentralblatt Bakteriologie 1921;86:160–9 [in German].
12. Cohen SG, Zelaya-Quesada M. Prausnitz and Kustner phenomenon: the P-K reaction. J Allergy Clin Immunol 2004;114(3):705–10.
13. Demeulemester C, Weyer A, Peltre G, et al. Thermoinactivation of human IgE: antigenic and functional modifications. Immunology 1986;57(4):617–20.
14. Kanny G, Maria Y, Mentre B, et al. Case report: recurrent anaphylactic shock to radiographic contrast media. Evidence supporting an exceptional IgE-mediated reaction. Allerg Immunol (Paris) 1993;25(10):425–30.
15. Pruzansky JJ, Grammer LC, Patterson R, et al. Dissociation of IgE from receptors on human basophils. I. Enhanced passive sensitization for histamine release. J Immunol 1983;131(4):1949–53.
16. Kleine Budde I, de Heer PG, van der Zee JS, et al. The stripped basophil histamine release bioassay as a tool for the detection of allergen-specific IgE in serum. Int Arch Allergy Immunol 2001;126(4):277–85.
17. Moneret-Vautrin DA, Sainte-Laudy J, Kanny G, et al. Human basophil activation measured by CD63 expression and LTC4 release in IgE-mediated food allergy. Ann Allergy Asthma Immunol 1999;82(1):33–40.
18. Abuaf N, Rajoely B, Ghazouani E, et al. Validation of a flow cytometric assay detecting in vitro basophil activation for the diagnosis of muscle relaxant allergy. J Allergy Clin Immunol 1999;104:411–8.
19. Monneret G, Benoit Y, Debard AL, et al. Monitoring of basophil activation using CD63 and CCR3 in allergy to muscle relaxant drugs. Clin Immunol 2002; 102(2):192–9.
20. Sudheer PS, Hall JE, Read GF, et al. Flow cytometric investigation of peri-anaesthetic anaphylaxis using CD63 and CD203c. Anaesthesia 2005;60(3):251–6.
21. Kvedariene V, Kamey S, Ryckwaert Y, et al. Diagnosis of neuromuscular blocking agent hypersensitivity reactions using cytofluorimetric analysis of basophils. Allergy 2006;61(3):311–5.
22. Ebo DG, Bridts CH, Hagendorens MM, et al. Flow-assisted diagnostic management of anaphylaxis from rocuronium bromide. Allergy 2006;61(8):935–9.
23. Sainte-Laudy J, Orsel I. [Interest of a new flow cytometric protocol applied to diagnosis and prevention of per anaesthetic accidents induced by neuromuscular blockers]. Revue francaise d'allergologie at d'immunologie clinique 2008; 48:470–5 [in French].
24. Sudheer PS, Appadurai IR. Anaphylaxis to vecuronium: the use of basophil CD63 expression as a possible screening tool to identify a safe alternative. J Clin Anesth 2007;19(7):555–7.
25. Ebo DG, Venemalm L, Bridts CH, et al. Immunoglobulin E antibodies to rocuronium: a new diagnostic tool. Anesthesiology 2007;107(2):253–9.
26. Aberer W, Bircher A, Romano A, et al. Drug provocation testing in the diagnosis of drug hypersensitivity reactions: general considerations. Allergy 2003;58(9):854–63.
27. Sanz ML, Gamboa PM, Antepara I, et al. Flow cytometric basophil activation test by detection of CD63 expression in patients with immediate-type reactions to betalactam antibiotics. Clin Exp Allergy 2002;32(2):277–86.
28. Torres MJ, Padial A, Mayorga C, et al. The diagnostic interpretation of basophil activation test in immediate allergic reactions to betalactams. Clin Exp Allergy 2004;34(11):1768–75.

29. Sainte-Laudy J, Boumediene A, Touraine F, et al. Use of both CD63 up-regulation and IgE down-regulation for the flow cytometric analysis of allergen induced basophil activation. Definition of an activation index. Inflamm Res 2007;56(7):291–6.

30. Abuaf N, Rostane H, Rajoely B, et al. Comparison of two basophil activation markers CD63 and CD203c in the diagnosis of amoxicillin allergy. Clin Exp Allergy 2008;38(6):921–8.

31. Caro JJ, Trindade E, McGregor M. The risks of death and of severe nonfatal reactions with high- vs low-osmolality contrast media: a meta-analysis. AJR Am J Roentgenol 1991;156(4):825–32.

32. Lieberman PL, Seigle RL. Reactions to radiocontrast material. Anaphylactoid events in radiology. Clin Rev Allergy Immunol 1999;17(4):469–96.

33. Trcka J, Schmidt C, Seitz CS, et al. Anaphylaxis to iodinated contrast material: nonallergic hypersensitivity or IgE-mediated allergy? AJR Am J Roentgenol 2008;190(3):666–70.

34. Morcos SK. Review article: acute serious and fatal reactions to contrast media: our current understanding. Br J Radiol 2005;78(932):686–93.

35. Szebeni J. Hypersensitivity reactions to radiocontrast media: the role of complement activation. Curr Allergy Asthma Rep 2004;4(1):25–30.

36. Gamboa PM, Sanz ML, Caballero MR, et al. Use of CD63 expression as a marker of in vitro basophil activation and leukotriene determination in metamizol allergic patients. Allergy 2003;58(4):312–7.

37. Gamboa P, Sanz ML, Caballero MR, et al. The flow-cytometric determination of basophil activation induced by aspirin and other non-steroidal anti-inflammatory drugs (NSAIDs) is useful for in vitro diagnosis of the NSAID hypersensitivity syndrome. Clin Exp Allergy 2004;34(9):1448–57.

38. Rodriguez-Trabado A, Camara-Hijon C, Ramos-Cantarino A, et al. Basophil activation test for the in vitro diagnosis of nonsteroidal anti-inflammatory drug hypersensitivity. Allergy Asthma Proc 2008;29(3):241–9.

39. Erdmann SM, Ventocilla S, Moll-Slodowy S, et al. [Basophil activation tests in the diagnosis of drug reactions]. Hautarzt 2005;56(1):38–43 [in German].

40. Malbran A, Yeyati E, Rey GL, et al. Diclofenac induces basophil degranulation without increasing CD63 expression in sensitive patients. Clin Exp Immunol 2007;147(1):99–105.

41. Mastalerz L, Setkowicz M, Sanak M, et al. Hypersensitivity to aspirin: common eicosanoid alterations in urticaria and asthma. J Allergy Clin Immunol 2004; 113(4):771–5.

42. Ebo DG, Bridts CH, Stevens WJ. IgE-mediated anaphylaxis from chlorhexidine: diagnostic possibilities. Contact Dermatitis 2006;55(5):301–2.

43. Garvey LH, Kroigaard M, Poulsen LK, et al. IgE-mediated allergy to chlorhexidine. J Allergy Clin Immunol 2007;120(2):409–15.

44. Pham NH, Weiner JM, Reisner GS, et al. Anaphylaxis to chlorhexidine. Case report. Implication of immunoglobulin E antibodies and identification of an allergenic determinant. Clin Exp Allergy 2000;30(7):1001–7.

45. Laxenaire MC, Charpentier C, Feldman L. [Anaphylactoid reactions to colloid plasma substitutes: incidence, risk factors, mechanisms. A French multicenter prospective study]. Ann Fr Anesth Reanim 1994;13(3):301–10 [in French].

46. Apostolou E, Deckert K, Puy R, et al. Anaphylaxis to gelofusine confirmed by in vitro basophil activation test: a case series. Anaesthesia 2006;61(3):264–8.

47. Beaudouin E, Kanny G, Gueant JL, et al. [Anaphylaxis caused by carboxymethylcellulose: report of 2 cases of shock from injectable corticoids]. Allerg Immunol (Paris) 1992;24(9):333–5 [in French].

48. Patterson DL, Yunginger JW, Dunn WF, et al. Anaphylaxis induced by the carboxymethylcellulose component of injectable triamcinolone acetonide suspension (Kenalog). Ann Allergy Asthma Immunol 1995;74(2):163–6.
49. Montoro J, Valero A, Elices A, et al. Anaphylactic shock after intra-articular injection of carboxymethylcellulose. Allergol Immunopathol (Madr) 2000;28(6):332–3.
50. Oppliger R, Hauser C. [Anaphylaxis after injection of corticosteroid preparations–carboxymethylcellulose as a hidden allergen]. J Dtsch Dermatol Ges 2004;2(11): 928–30 [in German].
51. Rival-Tringali AL, Gunera-Saad N, Berard F, et al. [Tolerability of oral administration of carboxymethylcellulose in two patients presenting anaphylactic reaction after carboxymethylcellulose injection]. Ann Dermatol Venereol 2008;135(5): 402–6 [in French].
52. Ebo DG, Schuerwegh A, Stevens WJ. Anaphylaxis to starch. Allergy 2000;55(11): 1098–9.
53. Ebo DG, Piel GC, Conraads V, et al. IgE-mediated anaphylaxis after first intravenous infusion of cyclosporine. Ann Allergy Asthma Immunol 2001;87(3):243–5.
54. Orta M, Ordoqui E, Aranzabal A, et al. Anaphylactic reaction after artificial insemination. Ann Allergy Asthma Immunol 2003;90(4):446–51.
55. Gamboa PM, Sanz ML, Urrutia I, et al. CD63 expression by flow cytometry in the in vitro diagnosis of allergy to omeprazole. Allergy 2003;58(6):538–9.
56. Caballero MR, Fernandez-Benitez M. Allergy to heparin: a new in vitro diagnostic technique. Allergol Immunopathol (Madr) 2003;31(6):324–8.
57. Ebo DG, Haine SE, Hagendorens MM, et al. Hypersensitivity to nadroparin calcium: case report and review of the literature. Clin Drug Investig 2004;24(7): 421–6.
58. Bauer C, Oppel T, Rueff F, et al. Anaphylaxis to viscotoxins of mistletoe (Viscum album) extracts. Ann Allergy Asthma Immunol 2005;94(1):86–9.
59. Ebo DG, Wets RD, Spiessens TK, et al. Flow-assisted diagnosis of anaphylaxis to patent blue. Allergy 2005;60(5):703–4.
60. Ebo DG, Goossens S, Opsomer F, et al. Flow-assisted diagnosis of anaphylaxis to hyaluronidase. Allergy 2005;60(10):1333–4.
61. Touraine F, Sainte Laudy J, Boumediene A, et al. [Investigation of allergic reactions to platinum salts]. Rev Mal Respir 2006;23:458–62 [in French].
62. Viardot-Helmer A, Ott H, Sauer I, et al. [Basophil activation test as in vitro assay for cisplatin allergy]. Hautarzt 2008;59(11):883–4 [in German].
63. Ebo DG, Bridts CH, Stevens WJ. IgE-mediated large local reaction from recombinant hepatitis B vaccine. Allergy 2008;63(4):483–4.
64. Longo N, Gamboa PM, Gastaminza G, et al. Diagnosis of clavulanic acid allergy using basophil activation and leukotriene release by basophils. J Investig Allergol Clin Immunol 2008;18(6):473–5.
65. Ebo DG, Bridts CH, De Clerck LS, et al. Immediate allergy from valacyclovir. Allergy 2008;63(7):941–2.

Provocation Tests in Drug Hypersensitivity

Werner Aberer, MD*, Birger Kränke, MD

KEYWORDS

- Drug hypersensitivity • Drug allergy • Provocation test
- Challenge test • Diagnosis

A drug provocation test (DPT) is defined as controlled administration of a drug to diagnose immune-mediated and non–immune-mediated drug hypersensitivity. Its advantage is that it permits testing of a patient with his or her individual metabolism and immunogenetic background. A DPT reproduces not only symptoms of allergy but other adverse clinical manifestations, irrespective of their mechanism.[1] A DPT is currently the "gold standard," but its use is limited by the possibility of severe and uncontrollable relapse of the reaction. Therefore, a DPT should be reserved for specific situations when a significant drug is suspected to have provoked an intolerance reaction and alternative test methods have failed to yield conclusive results. The patient being tested has to be in stable condition, and an anticipated positive reaction must be controllable by adequate measures. Because of these restrictions, only physicians experienced in drug allergy should perform this test. The two main indications for a DPT with the suspected drug are the following: to exclude hypersensitivity in the presence of unconvincing histories of drug hypersensitivity or in patients with nonspecific conditions, such as subjective symptoms under local anesthesia, or to establish a distinct diagnosis in suggestive histories of drug hypersensitivity with inconclusive, negative, or nonavailable allergy test results. A positive DPT result optimizes the avoidance of certain drugs, whereas a negative one permits the clinician to rule out a false diagnosis of drug hypersensitivity.[2]

Despite being regarded as the gold standard, DPTs are controversial. Many test procedures are yet to be validated. Protocols for every drug, or at least every group of drugs, with specific indications, contraindications, substances, dosing, grading of the reaction, and test and scoring criteria would be helpful. The development of individual DPT protocols is hindered by the countless number of drugs that may cause various types of hypersensitivity reactions (allergic and nonallergic) involving different time courses, severities, and outcomes; the individual patient's condition; and other factors that might influence the test reaction, however.[2] The European Network for

Department of Dermatology and Venerology, Medical University of Graz, Auenbruggerplatz 8, A-8036 Graz, Austria
* Corresponding author.
E-mail address: werner.aberer@medunigraz.at (W. Aberer).

Immunol Allergy Clin N Am 29 (2009) 567–584
doi:10.1016/j.iac.2009.04.008
0889-8561/09/$ – see front matter © 2009 Elsevier Inc. All rights reserved.

Drug Allergy (ENDA) (ie, the interest group on drug hypersensitivity of the European Academy of Allergy and Clinical Immunology [EAACI]) has therefore established general guidelines for DPTs that can be adapted to the specific problem under investigation.[1] The present report provides a summary of the recommended procedures concerning DPTs and specific protocols that have been published for specific drugs or groups of drugs.

PRINCIPLES OF TESTING FOR DRUG HYPERSENSITIVITY

Adverse drug reactions (ADRs) affect more than 7% of the general population.[3] Between 17% and 25% of patients at outpatient primary care centers reported ADRs.[4] Based on a recent meta-analysis, the overall incidence of ADRs in hospitalized patients was reported to be 15.1%. Nearly one half of these reactions were serious.[4,5] Underdiagnosis (because of underreporting) and overdiagnosis (because of the overuse of the term *allergy*) are potential problems. Misclassification based on the drug allergy history may have consequences on individual treatment choices and can lead to the use of more expensive and less effective drugs.[6] Any drug is liable to induce ADRs. Only approximately 6% to 10% of these are mediated by an immunologic mechanism, however.[5] In view of the high number of self-reported rates of hypersensitivity,[3] it is impossible to test the entire population for a supposed "allergic" drug reaction.[2]

A suspicion of drug hypersensitivity should be confirmed based on the concept of the underlying pathogenetic mechanism. An exact history and description of the clinical manifestations is mandatory to select adequate test procedures.[7] History taking should include all drugs taken by the patient before the reaction in addition to potential cofactors. The diagnosis of drug hypersensitivity reactions continues to be a challenge because the pathogenesis of certain reactions is unknown, the optimal skin test concentrations for several drugs are yet to be determined, and the few in vitro tests have not yet been validated for many drug reactions.[8] A positive skin or in vitro test result is an indication of hypersensitivity to a particular drug or drug allergen. The clinical relevance is then established on the basis of the patient's medical history, the clinical manifestation, the chronology, and the likelihood of the drug eliciting a hypersensitivity reaction of the specific type. A negative skin or in vitro test result does not necessarily justify exclusion of hypersensitivity to the drug or drug allergen in question because these tests mostly have a relatively low sensitivity. Therefore, in case of doubt, the potential drugs must be withdrawn from further pharmacotherapy or, alternatively, a DPT has to prove or disprove the clinical relevance of test results obtained with other in vivo or in vitro test methods. A DPT should only be performed if other less dangerous or less strenuous test methods fail to yield conclusive results or the outcome might help to clarify an otherwise obscure pathologic condition. Thus, a DPT should only be considered after balancing the risk-benefit ratio in the individual patient.

A DPT is performed by controlled administration of the substance under medical surveillance to establish or exclude a drug hypersensitivity reaction and, in selected cases, to provide alternative drugs for the patient. If the original reaction is delayed or not dangerous, a DPT may be performed on an outpatient basis.[9] Patients with more severe reactions ought to be hospitalized for a DPT, however.

A distinction must be made between a diagnostic DPT and therapeutic desensitization or tolerance induction procedures. Desensitization is performed when a sensitized patient has to take a drug and no alternatives are available. This measure produces a state of unresponsiveness that continues as long as the drug is given but resolves within a few days after cessation of drug delivery.[10] Graded challenge, also known as test dosing, refers to cautious administration of a medication to a patient who is unlikely to be truly allergic to it. Unlike desensitization, graded challenge does not modify or attempt to dupe the immune system into accepting a medication to which the individual is allergic.[4] Graded challenges are most commonly used when diagnostic testing is not adequate to rule out an allergy and the clinician has reason to believe that the patient is unlikely to be allergic. Whereas the protocol for desensitization should be followed even if a moderate reaction occurs during the process, DPT protocols and graded challenges must be stopped as soon as objective adverse reactions occur.[2]

PREREQUISITES FOR DRUG PROVOCATION TESTS

A three-step strategy has been deemed useful to identify drug hypersensitivity reactions (**Fig. 1**). The first step is a compatible history. Standardized questionnaires, such as that published by the ENDA in several languages, may be used.[11] The clinical assessment should include a full description of the reaction, delay between drug intake and symptoms, and association with other risk factors. It is important to distinguish between immediate and nonimmediate reactions. The former occur within 1 hour after the last drug administration and their clinical manifestations include urticaria, angioedema, rhinitis, bronchospasm, or anaphylactic shock. Nonimmediate reactions occur more than 1 hour after the last drug intake. The most common nonimmediate reactions are maculopapular eruptions and delayed appearance of urticaria or angioedema. In addition, drugs may elicit fixed eruptions, exfoliative dermatitis, acute generalized exanthematous pustulosis (AGEP), drug reaction with eosinophilia and systemic symptoms (DRESS), Stevens-Johnson syndrome (SJS), or toxic epidermal necrolysis.[12]

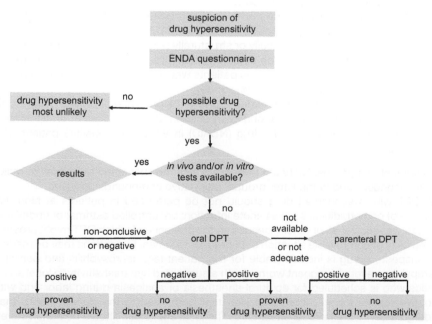

Fig. 1. Assessing drug allergy or hypersensitivity by a three-step strategy.

The second step consists of any relevant in vivo skin test or in vitro allergy test. Skin-prick tests and immediate-reading intradermal tests are the most readily available tools with which to diagnose immediate reactions.[13] Determination of specific IgE levels to a limited number of drug allergens is still the most common in vitro method for evaluating such reactions despite its many limitations.[14] Delayed-reading intradermal tests and patch tests are in vivo methods to diagnose nonimmediate reactions.[13,15] Tests like the lymphocyte transformation test (LTT)[16] or the basophil activation test[17] have been developed as in vitro diagnostic tools and are under clinical testing for the purpose of validation. Routine application of these tests might enhance the sensitivity of diagnostic workups, thus reducing the need for DPTs.[2]

In the event of a positive allergy test result, the patient may be tested for an alternative drug. In selected cases, the patient may undergo a DPT as the third step.

Indications and Contraindications

Any DPT must be preceded by an individual risk-benefit assessment.[1] Caution and surveillance are imperative in all cases. Severe reactions in the patient's medical history and patients in a poor state of health or at increased risk during emergency treatment require guarded and careful evaluation. A DPT should be avoided when the patient is unlikely to require the drug in the future. The indications for a DPT may be divided into five partly overlapping groups:[1]

1. To exclude hypersensitivity in the presence of a nonsuggestive history of drug hypersensitivity and in patients with nonspecific symptoms, such as vagal symptoms under local anesthesia[18]
2. To establish a conclusive diagnosis in the presence of a suggestive history of drug hypersensitivity with negative, inconclusive, or unavailable diagnostic test results, for example, a maculopapular eruption during aminopenicillin treatment with negative skin or in vitro allergy test results
3. To rule out an immediate-type allergy (eg, in a patient who has prior exanthema after aminopenicillins and negative skin and in vitro test results)
4. To provide safe pharmacologically or structurally nonrelated drugs in the presence of proved hypersensitivity, such as other antibiotics in β-lactam–allergic patients. This may also be helpful for anxious patients who would refuse to take the recommended drug without proof of its tolerance.
5. To exclude cross-reactivity of related drugs in the presence of proved hypersensitivity, for instance, a cephalosporin in a penicillin-allergic subject or an alternative nonsteroidal anti-inflammatory drug (NSAID) in an aspirin-sensitive patient who has asthma

In the first two groups, DPTs are performed with the suspected drug itself to make a final diagnosis, and in the latter groups, alternative compounds are used.

A DPT with a suspected drug should not be performed in patients at high risk because of comorbidities, such as acute infection; uncontrolled asthma; or underlying cardiac, hepatic, renal, or other diseases, in the presence of which DPT might provoke a medically uncontrollable situation or in pregnant women. Exceptions may be made if the suspected drug is indispensable for the patient (eg, neurosyphilis and penicillin therapy), however. A pregnant woman with a suspected hypersensitivity to local anesthetics who is scheduled for epidural anesthesia or analgesia during labor and with negative results for an intradermal skin test performed in the delivery room may undergo a DPT with the local anesthetic. The local anesthetic should be administered by the anesthetist in the delivery room before insertion of the epidural catheter.[1]

A DPT should never be performed in patients who have experienced severe reactions (**Box 1**).[12] The recommendations for some skin conditions in the published literature are diverse. In fixed-drug eruptions, oral provocation testing seems to be safe even in children if the patient had only one or a few lesions.[19] An oral DPT should not be attempted in patients who have experienced generalized bullous reactions, however, which may sometimes be difficult to distinguish from SJS. Reactions (including severe ones) that can be managed effectively, such as anaphylaxis, may be investigated in selected cases, however.[1]

The culprit drug must be substantially more effective than the alternatives or irreplaceable. A DPT should be performed only if other less potentially harmful tests do not permit the physician to establish or exclude hypersensitivity to a certain drug and if its outcome might contribute to making a conclusive diagnosis.[2]

A DPT is frequently performed when skin and in vitro diagnostic methods have been ineffective (eg, hypersensitivity reactions to NSAIDs), in vitro tests are not available or skin tests are not admissible because of local irritation (eg, quinolones), the sensitivity of the tests is limited (eg, for heparins and glucocorticosteroids), or other allergy tests with a high negative predictive value yield negative test results (eg, immediate or non-immediate hypersensitivity reactions after β-lactams).[2] In most cases, however, it is difficult to justify a DPT with drugs that are largely obsolete today, such as sulfonamides (except in HIV-positive persons), or substances of doubtful value, such as herbal products or "lifestyle drugs."

SPECIFIC RISK GROUPS

Persons infected with HIV need drugs for the treatment and prevention of opportunistic infections. Their frequent adverse reactions to these drugs increase morbidity

---

Box 1
Adverse drug reactions that represent no indication or, even more, contraindications for drug provocation testing

Autoimmune diseases

    Bullous pemphigoid

    Pemphigus vulgaris

    Systemic lupus erythematosus

Severe exfoliative skin reactions

    AGEP

    DRESS/Drug-induced hypersensitivity syndrome

    Exfoliative dermatitis

    SJS

    Toxic epidermal necrolysis

Severe vasculitis syndrome

Specific organ manifestations

    Blood cytopenia

    Hepatitis

    Nephritis

    Pneumonitis

and mortality.[20] Because the pathogenesis of these ADRs is not well defined, desensitization might be considered instead of a DPT protocol, particularly because the likelihood of a false-negative test outcome is rather high.[21]

In patients who have cystic fibrosis or tuberculosis, in which the (frequently long-term use of the anti-infective) drug concerned is more effective than the alternatives, drug desensitization rather than detailed allergy testing may be the initial measure. A compromise between the two would be a graded challenge.[22]

In patients who have cancer and develop immediate reactions directly associated with antineoplastic drugs, such as taxenes, an immediate desensitization procedure might be given preference because these patients frequently respond negatively to allergy tests.[23]

TESTING PROCEDURE
General Considerations

As a general rule, DPTs should be performed no earlier than 4 weeks after the drug hypersensitivity reaction. The drug elimination half-life should be awaited at least five times to ensure complete elimination. The reaction under investigation should have resolved completely, clinically, and according to laboratory data if it is found to be abnormal at the initial investigation. Any corrective medication or comedication that might influence the outcome of the test (**Table 1**) should be completely washed out. Whereas this happens within a few days with antihistamines or intravenous steroids for the treatment of systemic reactions, the washout period for topical steroids used to treat contact allergy might be as long as 4 weeks. There is no predefined limit and no general rule or consensus regarding the permitted maximal time delay between the adverse reaction and the DPT. Antibodies to penicillin may disappear from the serum within 6 to 12 months, whereas skin reactivity decreases over time but hypersensitivity remains. For these reasons, some researchers recommend repetition of the skin test or even a repeat challenge 2 to 4 weeks later, although this approach is not widely endorsed.[24]

An individual protocol must be prepared before any test, and the procedure must be supervised by an expert. A DPT should be regarded as a serious and potentially hazardous test procedure. The person receiving the DPT should be in a good state of health on the day of testing, with no sign of allergy or viral infection that could stimulate an immune response, although this might well have been a potential cofactor involved in the original reaction. The patient's personal details, medical history, and concomitant drug therapy before the DPT must be documented. Before and after the provocation, all relevant physical signs and changes in laboratory parameters, spirometry, and other parameters if relevant for the individual patient, such as changes on the electrocardiogram, must be recorded and filed. Comedication that may interfere with emergency treatment or augment ongoing reactions should be stopped and substituted adequately before any DPT when immediate reactions are anticipated (see **Table 1**). Because DPTs may induce life-threatening reactions, the tests should be performed under medical supervision. Well-trained medical staff should be immediately available in case of an emergency. Facilities for continuous monitoring of the patient's condition, intravenous access, and access to intensive care or emergency treatment should be available depending on the severity of the previous reaction and the type of drug. The emergence of life-threatening reactions may necessitate rapid access to intubation. Resuscitation facilities should be available. The monitoring procedure must be designed such that early signs of any relevant disorder secondary to the DPT can be detected immediately. Moreover, the recommendations of the

Table 1
Drugs to be avoided before performing a drug provocation test

Drug Class	Immediate Reaction	Nonimmediate Reaction	Free Interval	Consequence
H₁ antihistamines	+	−	3 to 7 days	Mask reaction
Antidepressants ("classic")	+	−	5 days	Mask reaction
β₂-agonists				
Short-acting	+	−	6 to 8 hours	Mask reaction
Long-acting	+	−	1 to 2 days	
Beta-blocking agents				
Per os	+	+	1 to 2 days	Aggravate reaction
Eye drops	+	−	1 to 2 days	Complicate emergency treatment
Corticosteroids				
Short-term, low-dose (<50 mg)	±	−	3 to 5 days	Mask reaction
Short-term, high-dose (>50 mg)	±	+	1 week	
Long-term	±	+	3 weeks	
Topicalᵃ	−	?	3 weeks	
Ipratropium bromide	+	−	6 to 8 hours	Mask reaction
Leukotriene modifiers	+	−	>1 week	Mask reaction
Long-acting theophylline	+	−	1 to 2 days	Mask reaction
Angiotensin-converting enzyme inhibitors	+	+	1 day	Aggravate reaction

ᵃ Prolonged external treatment (<5 days) may suppress provocative patch test reactions, repeated-open-application-tests and use-tests.

American Academy of Asthma, Allergy, and Immunology (AAAAI) and the American College of Allergy, Asthma, and Immunology (ACAAI) on anaphylaxis[25,26] and those of the EAACI-ENDA[1] should be followed.

Similar to skin testing, in which specific recommendations regarding observation time of the test areas are mandatory depending on the time course of the ADR under investigation, DPTs for immediate-type reactions should follow other rules than for delayed-type reactions. Whereas positive reactions in the former may occur rapidly and suddenly and be acutely life threatening, delayed reactions are usually milder but may appear late and might also respond less quickly to treatment. The latter reactions therefore need less strain after application but long observation times and hesitant interpretation—a positive reaction might even appear several days after exposure. There are no specific protocols regarding this topic, however.

A DPT should be performed in a single-blind placebo-controlled manner. In situations involving psychologic factors, a double-blind approach may be necessary. This is of utmost importance because as many as 41% of healthy volunteers and hospital staff receiving no medication other than placebo capsules reported (largely subjective) such symptoms as sedation, irritation, nasal congestion, fever, exanthema, and urticaria during a 3-day observation period.[27]

The test substance may be administered by various routes: oral, parenteral (intravenous, intramuscular, or subcutaneous), or topical (nasal, bronchial, conjunctival, or cutaneous). Preferentially, the drug should be administered in the same manner as it was given when the reaction occurred, and should eventually be given in future treatment. The oral route is favored,[28] however, because absorption is slower and adverse reactions can be treated earlier as compared with a DPT performed by the parenteral route.

Dosing and timing depend on several variables, including the characteristics of the drug itself, the severity of the hypersensitivity reaction under investigation, the route of administration, the expected time latency between application and reaction, the subject's state of health, and any comedication. Because the intensity of the reaction after a DPT is not absolutely predictable, a careful assessment of the dosage is mandatory. The medication should be introduced cautiously to reduce the risk for a severe reaction. According to the ENDA position paper, one should start with a low dose, increase it cautiously, and terminate the administration as soon as the first objective symptoms occur (**Table 2**).[1] If no symptoms appear, the clinician should achieve the maximum single dose of the specific drug. Administration of the defined daily dose is desirable. In case of a previous immediate reaction (ie, occurring less than 1 hour after administration of the drug),[29] the starting dose should range between 1:10,000 and 1:10 of the therapeutic dose, depending on the severity of the reaction. The time interval between doses should be at least 30 minutes, but many drugs and specific situations may require longer intervals. In case of previous nonimmediate reactions,[30] the starting dose should not exceed 1:100 of the therapeutic dose. Depending on the drug and the patient's response threshold, a DPT may be concluded within a few hours, days, or occasionally weeks.[28] A general rule is that immediate-type reactions under investigation need a short observation period, whereas delayed-type reactions in the history may necessitate similarly long observation periods after a DPT. Regarding the dosing, in immediate-type reactions, a defined daily dose should suffice, whereas after delayed-type reactions, prolonged testing may be necessary; however, again, no specific protocols exist that specify these questions.

If a DPT is performed to find an alternative drug, the maximum single therapeutic dose should be achieved. In some cases, it may be necessary to deliver a defined daily dose over a prolonged period; however, specific recommendations based on generally accepted protocols are not published yet.

Table 2
Sequence of increasing doses during a drug provocation test

Drug	Drug Class	Doses (mg)[a]	Route	Daily Dose for Adults[b]
Amoxicillin	Penicillin	1, 5, 25, 100, 500, 1000	Oral	1000–2000 mg
Cefaclor	Cephalosporin	1, 5, 25, 125, 500	Oral	750 mg
Cefixime	Cephalosporin	1, 5, 25, 100, 225	Oral	400 mg
Ceftriaxone	Cephalosporin	1, 5, 25, 100, 500, 1000	Intravenous	1000–2000 mg
Azithromycin	Macrolide	1, 5, 25, 75, 125, 250	Oral	500 mg
Ciprofloxacin	Quinolone	1, 5, 25, 100, 500	Oral	500–1500 mg
Acetylsalicylic acid	NSAID	1, 5, 20, 50, 100, 200, 500	Oral	500–3000 mg
Meloxicam	NSAID	1, 3, 7.5	Oral	7.5–15 mg
Prednisolone	Steroid	2, 10, 20, 40	Oral	20–80 mg
Omeprazole	PPI	1, 5, 10, 20	Oral	20–40 mg
Tetrazepam	Benzodiazepine	1, 2.5, 25, 50	Oral	50–100 mg
Any vaccine	Vaccine	0.1, 0.5	Subcutaneous	0.5 (1.0) mL
Lidocaine	Local anesthetic	0.1, 1, 2	Subcutaneous	1–3 mL

Abbreviation: PPI, proton pump inhibitor.
[a] Ten times less than the first dose for anaphylactic shock, individual approach.
[b] Recommendations may vary in different countries.

As a rule, commercial preparations are used. In case of drug combinations, as with some over-the-counter preparations, the single compounds should be tested separately. The proof of tolerance to a drug, however, should be assessed with the commercial preparation that is to be used in the future.

Separate testing of the active substances and additives must be considered because reactions may be caused by these compounds, although this may be a rare event.[31] Especially in patients who have experienced hypersensitivity reactions to several compounds, a DPT with excipients might be necessary. These include encapsulation agents (eg, carboxymethyl cellulose, gelatin), emulsifying agents or solvents (eg, dextran, egg albumin), synthetic sweeteners (eg, saccharin, aspartame), stabilizing agents or antioxidants (eg, sulfites, ethylenediamine), dyes (eg, tartrazine, xanthene dyes), preservatives (eg, benzoates, parabens), or adjuvants (eg, aluminum hydroxide, zinc oxide).[2]

If several drugs are suspected, each must be tested in sequence. If given together or too close to each other, with the time dependent on the expected reaction time, the clinician cannot identify the culprit drug. A DPT may be performed on the same day as diagnostic skin tests are performed if the reaction under investigation was an immediate one.

Patients should be observed as long as severe exposure-related reactions are anticipated. This depends on the type of previous drug reaction, the drug under investigation, and the patient's individual condition. If mild reactions occurred, the patient should be observed for at least 2 hours after stabilization. Hospitalization is mandatory after severe reactions because of the possibility of biphasic episodes that may be lethal if not identified early and treated adequately. After being discharged, the patient should be provided with adequate emergency treatment if further symptoms, such as urticaria, are anticipated (eg, antihistamines, β-mimetics, glucocorticosteroids).

In general, a "safety-first" policy should be followed. An observation period of 24 hours is desirable in many cases. Local regulations may influence these procedures.

Specific Test Protocols

Specific protocols with predefined indications, contraindications, substances, dosing, grading of the reaction, and scoring criteria for each drug, or at least each group of drugs, would be helpful. The development of individual DPT protocols is hindered by the countless drugs that may cause hypersensitivity reactions and the numerous factors that may influence the outcome. Nevertheless, a recent study provided useful information on the sequences of increasing doses of several drugs.[32]

β-lactams

DPTs are included in ENDA diagnostic algorithms to evaluate immediate[29] and nonimmediate[30] hypersensitivity reactions to β-lactams. Although the ENDA mentions a large number of indications, those stated by the AAAAI are fewer.[33] Although β-lactams are supposed to be the group of drugs for which skin and in vitro testing possesses the highest predictive value, several cases of allergy test negativity and challenge positivity have been reported in recent years, thus documenting the importance of DPTs even for this group of drugs.

Nonsteroidal anti-inflammatory drugs

A DPT is considered the gold standard to establish or exclude hypersensitivity to acetylsalicylic acid (ASA) and other NSAIDs. If positive, this test reproduces allergic and nonallergic hypersensitivity symptoms, whereas in case of a negative response, it may permit the clinician to rule out a hypersensitivity to the concerned NSAID. A recent review published jointly by the Global Allergy and Asthma European Network (GA^2 LEN) and the EAACI presented detailed protocols of oral, bronchial, and nasal ASA provocation tests.[34] The article also reviewed indications and contraindications for DPTs, rules for drug withdrawal, and the equipment used for DPTs. Challenge protocols for NSAIDs other than ASA, such as paracetamol, dipyrone, diclofenac, piroxicam, indomethacin, ibuprofen, ketoprofen, mefenamic acid, and salsalate, are available in the published literature.[2] Importantly, the patient's clinical history is not a reliable tool with which to diagnose NSAID hypersensitivity. The results of DPTs may be negative despite a quite convincing clinical history, probably because important cofactors, such as viral infection or inflammation, are missing.

Other drugs

DPT protocols have been published for non–β-lactam antibiotics, such as sulfonamides, quinolones, and macrolides.[2] Glucocorticosteroids, heparins, iodinated contrast media, local anesthetics, and other substances have also been investigated.[32]

Ethical Considerations

The risk-benefit ratio must be acceptable. The drug must be substantially more effective than the alternatives. The condition being treated must be serious. Further conditions would be the absence of alternative testing methods or inconclusive results. The patient should be informed about the consequences of using alternative treatments and the risks involved in a DPT. The patient should give his or her verbal (or preferably written) informed consent to the test. Additionally, approval by an ethics committee is mandatory if the provocation procedure is performed mainly for scientific or altruistic reasons (ie, other patients may benefit from the obtained knowledge); both of these aspects would exceed the scope of the present report.

Test Performance

Several factors influence the choice of the adequate procedure, with the most important being the drug or drug ingredient itself, the type of previous adverse reaction, the patient's constitution at the time of the DPT, and the availability or reliability of general clinical and specific in vitro and in vivo tests. Here, only general recommendations are given, with specific examples relating to the indications for testing as defined previously:

1. Exclude hypersensitivity in nonsuggestive history. Many patients are wrongly labeled as being allergic based on a suggestive history but not proved by tests or proved by tests with limited predictive value, such as skin tests with opiates, IgE detection in aspirin hypersensitivity, or other nonvalidated biologic tests. In such instances, a DPT might be the most valuable aid or even the only means of freeing the patient from his or her "allergy." For instance, several adverse reactions to local anesthetics are attributable to nonallergic factors that include vasovagal or adrenergic responses. To exclude the rare possibility of an immune-mediated reaction, graded exposure should be given preference. The patient may be emotionally upset because of past experience during severe clinical reactions or placebo testing, however. In fact, "reverse placebo provocation" may be required in some patients with prevailing subjective symptoms.[35]

2. Establish the diagnosis in cases of suggestive history by negative (skin or in vitro) test results. Skin tests are usually the first tests performed to clarify a suspected

drug hypersensitivity,[13,15] but frequently yield negative results. In these cases, the causative agent can only be identified by a DPT.[36]

3. Exanthematous nonurticarial reactions after ampicillin treatment are usually attributable to non–immune-mediated mechanisms but may also represent delayed-type immune reactions or even, in rare cases, immediate-type ADRs. Thus, not only do delayed mechanisms have to be excluded using patch and intradermal test with late readings but IgE-mediated processes have to be excluded by IgE testing and skin testing for immediate-type reactions. If all these test results are negative, a DPT is necessary to rule out any allergic reaction to β-lactams.

4. Provide safe alternatives in allergic patients and prove tolerance. Penicillin-allergic patients are claimed to have an approximately 10-fold higher risk for experiencing an allergic reaction to antimicrobial drugs of classes other than penicillins and cephalosporins. The general approach is to select an agent structurally distinct from the agent that caused the reaction and then to introduce the drug under close supervision. Exposure under controlled conditions might also be helpful for anxious persons, with distinct agents (eg, other classes of antibiotics after immune-mediated reactions), or with similar drugs under pretreatment regimens for the purpose of prevention (eg, radio contrast media).

5. Exclude cross-reactivity of related drugs in cases of proved hypersensitivity. Patients with a history of immediate-type allergy to penicillin and a positive skin test result are subject to a threefold higher risk if a cephalosporin is given. Therefore, a DPT under controlled conditions (after performing skin tests) is essential before rating cephalosporins as alternatives or classifying them as forbidden. The same is true for the frequently observed hypersensitivity reactions to NSAIDs. There is no definitive skin or in vitro test to identify patients who may react to aspirin, to other NSAIDs, or to 5-HT3 receptor antagonists. Thus, carefully performed DPTs with alternatives (mostly acetaminophen or celecoxib) are recommended to determine safe alternatives.

Assessment of Test Results

A DPT result may be called positive if it reproduces the original symptoms, or at least objective ones. If the original reaction is only manifested as subjective symptoms and challenge testing again induces similar nonverifiable symptoms, placebo challenge steps must be performed. If the placebo steps are negative, repetition of the previous dosing of the drug under investigation is highly recommended.

The clinician should always try to objectify the test result by exact surveillance of skin alterations (photographs are helpful) and other signs of the original drug reaction. In vivo tests that might be applicable are peak flow or spirometry for respiratory symptoms and determination of cardiovascular parameters for anaphylactic symptoms. The importance of in vitro testing is frequently overestimated by nonexpert physicians. General clinical tests, such as a complete blood cell count, total platelet count, or, for eosinophilia, determination of mediator release (histamine in blood or methylhistamine in urine, eosinophil cationic protein, and even serum tryptase),[37] are only rarely helpful. Measuring cytokines, immune complexes, complement components, complement split factors, and other parameters are still research tools with undetermined reliability for clinical use.

A negative DPT result is defined by the absence of any reaction during the test and after the observation period, which includes a certain delay after the end of the test (days or even weeks, depending on the drug and the immunologic pathway). When the clinical history is well defined and the result of the DPT is positive, the diagnosis of drug hypersensitivity may be confirmed. Likewise, if the test was performed to exclude a drug allergy, a negative test result indicates the absence of drug hypersensitivity. Test interpretation is more problematic if a negative test result is accompanied by a history strongly compatible with drug hypersensitivity or when a positive test result is obtained with a less compatible history of drug hypersensitivity. Reasons for false-negative or false-positive results should be taken into account. In the event of ambiguous results, it may be meaningful to perform a placebo-controlled test or repeat the DPT.

According to the ENDA position paper,[1] reasons for false-positive results of DPTs include the following: psychologic symptoms, preexisting symptoms (eg, urticaria), drug-induced aggravation of preexisting disease, or self-infliction. False-negative results might be attributable to several reasons: use of antiallergic drugs (eg, corticosteroids, antihistamines), missing cofactors (light, comedication, viral infections, and physical exercise), brief exposure or observation time, short time interval between the reaction and testing (refractory period), excessively long interval (natural desensitization) between the reaction and testing, tolerance induction or "desensitization" by testing, or erroneous attribution of responsibility to the tested substance.

Management and Documentation of Adverse Reactions

Treatment of adverse events during provocation testing depends on the type of reaction and its severity. The first step is to cease administration of the test drug. This should be followed by adequate general and specific procedures according to the treatment of anaphylactic reactions.[25,26] Introduction of suppressive therapy should, however, only be started when the symptoms are sufficiently specific to interpret the reaction as a conclusive positive test result. Corrective treatment is not administered in accordance with standardized procedures but must be decided individually, in keeping with general rules for emergency treatment. Corrective treatment of reactions to a DPT must also be documented in the test protocol.

Skin symptoms caused by a DPT should be documented in photographs. Histologic evaluation of a drug rash is not recommended as a general measure because it is not pathognomonic in most cases. In some instances, however, such as in lichenoid exanthemas, erythema multiforme, or cutaneous vasculitis, histology might support the clinical diagnosis.

Scoring Systems and Interpretation of Test Results

All clinical signs and symptoms, independent of their pathogenesis, must be documented in the test protocol, including the type and severity of reaction, any prodromi, the subjective and objective signs, the kinetics, the parameters for systemic involvement (eg, blood and liver parameters), and the eliciting substance and its dosing. Scoring systems might be helpful in some cases but are not generally accepted and not easily applicable in a clinical setting.

Whereas some methods, such as the French Pharmaco-Vigilance System,[38] are based on intrinsic patient-related and extrinsic literature-related criteria, which are evaluated separately, other methods are based on statistical models or standardized decision trees. Algorithms are not accurate for the diagnosis of drug hypersensitivity reactions,[39] but optimization of the current tools by using large case-control databases seems promising.[6]

The predictive value of a DPT mainly depends on the type or mechanism of reaction and the drug involved. Thus, urticarial reactions under penicillin therapy are frequently reproducible, whereas morbilliform eruptions after ampicillins are not, sometimes probably because of the absence of cofactors. A physician performing a DPT for drug hypersensitivity reactions must be familiar with the published literature on the subject and must have considerable experience to be able to distinguish among the many reasons for false-negative and false-positive test results. The reasons are numerous but can be evaluated and avoided in most cases.

Spontaneous desensitization or tolerance induction must be considered as an explanation for an unexpected negative DPT result, although this has not been reported in the published literature.

The patient needs adequate documentation of those drugs that he or she should no longer receive and those that have been tolerated in the test. The personal use of Medic-Alert tags or bracelets should be encouraged. It would be meaningful to issue an "allergy identity card" that the patient should be asked to show before receiving any drug prescription in the future. The card should contain the following minimum data:[1]

Generic and proprietary name of the drug and the active substance
Date and type of the reaction and its severity
Method used for assessment (eg, history, skin test, IgE detection, LTT, DPT), including date and comments
Recommended safe alternatives and the tolerated dose (in the DPT)

LIMITATIONS OF DRUG PROVOCATION TESTING

There are several limitations to the seemingly straightforward procedure of a DPT. Many individuals do not take only one drug at a time, and certain adverse events are sometimes indicative but rarely specific for a certain substance. A DPT helps to detect the cause but rarely ever the pathogenesis of the reaction. Less than 15% of undesirable drug reactions are attributable to immune-mediated mechanisms.[5]

When performing a DPT, one has to consider the considerable number of false-positive and false-negative results. A negative test result does not prove tolerance of the drug in the future, whereas a positive test result might not indicate lifelong hypersensitivity. Positive test reactions might be irrelevant when control patients cannot be studied because of ethical considerations.[40] A negative test result does not exclude a drug as being the culprit for a reaction because crucial cofactors might be absent during the test procedure. The setting during the test procedure may lack certain components prevailing when the drug is usually administered, such as the anxiety accompanying a dental procedure or an associated inflammatory disease like latent asthma, urticaria, or viral infections. In summary, there is no absolute certainty for future situations.

Because the intensity of a reaction after drug hypersensitivity reactions is not absolutely predictable, a careful assessment of the need for a DPT and the dosage is therefore essential. The predictive value of a DPT depends on the type of reaction and, more importantly, the type of drug. The limitations of a DPT are illustrated in a study on 204 patients with a history of anaphylactoid reactions after administration of radiocontrast media: only 24% with an unequivocal history reacted to a test dose; 67% of these developed symptoms despite antiallergic premedication, whereas 20% of those with a negative provocation test result reacted again on re-exposure.[41] Similarly, in penicillin allergy, skin test positivity has been observed in 2 (0.9%) of 216[42] and 26 (10.5%) of 247[43] children and adolescents retested more than 3 weeks after a negative DPT result, followed by a course of the suspected β-lactam. Thus, a DPT may resensitize or booster previously sensitized patients.

Defining specific test procedures for individual situations is rendered difficult by the heterogeneous side effects of a single drug and the enormous number of drugs on the market. Standardizing these procedures is even more difficult. Well-controlled protocols exist only for allergic contact dermatitis, fixed drug eruptions, maculopapular eruptions after aminopenicillins and cephalosporins, immediate and nonimmediate reactions to β-lactam antibiotics, urticaria and angioedema after NSAIDs, local anesthetics, and a few others.[2,32]

Despite the development of a series of serologic and cellular tests to clarify a patient's immunologic sensitization to penicillins, the tests do not, in most cases, permit an absolute prospective statement as to the risk associated with administering penicillin again. Provocation tests may narrow the gap but do not close it.

Establishment of the causality of a reaction requires stringent criteria. The value of a provocation test with all its variables regarding sensitivity and specificity depends on the diagnostic aim. A test with high sensitivity is needed when the clinician is looking for explanations of suspected drug hypersensitivity reactions, but evidence of causality would need tests of high specificity. In clinical practice, it might be more useful to look for safe alternatives rather than to prove that a drug was the definitive cause of the problem.

SUMMARY

Accurate identification of the agent inducing a patient's hypersensitivity reaction is essential.[44] The assessment should be based on the observation of clinical signs; their time course; their response to antiallergic treatment; and, most importantly, adequate test results, including a DPT in some instances. Confirmation of a presumptive diagnosis by a DPT is frequently the only reliable means of establishing a diagnosis when other diagnostic procedures, such as in vivo skin testing or in vitro laboratory tests, do not yield conclusive results. A DPT should be performed with great caution and only when it is absolutely necessary because it may cause severe or even fatal reactions.

Plans to avoid future adverse reactions and provide safe alternative drugs should be formulated as the final phase of the management of patients with suspected drug reactions. This process includes determination of the exact cause of hypersensitivity, which frequently involves a DPT. An individual risk-benefit calculation must be performed in every case, taking contraindications and ethical considerations into account.

The test should be performed in accordance with established criteria. The numerous limitations that may lead to false-positive or false-negative test results must be considered. The attribution of causality must follow certain predefined rules. The World Health Organization (WHO) Drug Monitoring Program suggests the following words: certain, probable or likely, possible, unlikely, conditional or unclassified, and unaccessible or unclassifiable.[45] Several algorithms have been defined, but none of them fulfills all expectations. Moreover, the algorithms are rarely used in clinical practice.

The general principles for DPTs as outlined in the position paper of the ENDA did help to establish specific protocols for different groups of drugs and various clinical signs of hypersensitivity. Regarding algorithms for drug testing, a DPT should prove or disprove ambiguous results obtained with other less potentially dangerous methods, such as skin or in vitro tests, and may therefore be regarded as the gold standard of drug testing in many clinical settings. Even a negative DPT result may neither predict tolerance to future exposure nor prove intolerance, however. Therefore, tests should be available to avoid provocation tests—a desirable yet unachieved condition thus far.

Currently, detailed recommendations for DPTs have been published only for β-lactams,[29,30] NSAIDs,[34] heparins,[46] radio contrast media,[47] and a few other drug groups.[2,32] Considerable effort is required to define protocols for major drugs that frequently trigger hypersensitivity reactions.[6] Research is also needed to prevent and manage drug hypersensitivity reactions.[48] Knowledge concerning genetic factors underlying a predisposition to drug-induced hypersensitivity has been significantly extended in recent years.[12,49] A promising quantitative approach has been used in employing genetic algorithms to design a probability scoring system for ADRs.[50] Currently, however, the diagnosis is based on DPTs, which might be replaced by less irksome procedures in the future.

REFERENCES

1. Aberer W, Bircher A, Romano A, et al. Drug provocation testing in the diagnosis of drug hypersensitivity reactions: general considerations. Allergy 2003;58:854–63.
2. Bousquet P-J, Gaeta F, Bousquet-Rouanet L, et al. Provocation tests in diagnosing drug hypersensitivity. Curr Pharm Des 2008;14:2792–802.
3. Gomes E, Cardoso MF, Praca F, et al. Self-reported drug allergy in a general adult Portuguese population. Clin Exp Allergy 2004;34:1597–601.
4. Solensky R. Drug hypersensitivity. Med Clin North Am 2006;90:233–60.
5. Lazarou J, Pomeranz BH, Corey PN. Incidence of adverse drug reactions in hospitalized patients: a meta-analysis of prospective studies. JAMA 1998;279: 1200–5.
6. Demoly P, Pichler W, Pirmohamed M, et al. Important questions in allergy: 1-drug allergy/hypersensitivity. Allergy 2008;63:616–9.
7. Weiss M, Adkinson N Jr. Diagnostic testing for drug hypersensitivity. Immunol Allergy Clin North Am 1998;18:731–44.
8. Bach S, Bircher AJ. Drug hypersensitivity reactions: from clinical manifestations to an allergologic diagnosis. Allerg Immunol (Paris) 2005;37:213–8.
9. Romano A, Quarantine D, Di Fonso M, et al. A diagnostic protocol for evaluating nonimmediate reactions to aminopenicillins. J Allergy Clin Immunol 1999;103: 1186–90.
10. Stark BJ, Earl HS, Gross GN, et al. Acute and chronic desensitization of penicillin-allergic patients using oral penicillin. J Allergy Clin Immunol 1987;79:523–32.
11. Demoly P, Kropf R, Bircher A, et al. Drug hypersensitivity: questionnaire. Allergy 1999;54:999–1003.
12. Aberer W, Kränke B. Clinical manifestations and mechanisms of skin reactions after systemic drug administration. Drug Discov Today Dis Mech 2008;5: e237–47 [Epub ahead of print].
13. Brockow K, Romano A, Blanca M, et al. General considerations for skin test procedures in the diagnosis of drug hypersensitivity. Allergy 2002;57:45–51.
14. Aberer W, Zidarn M, Kränke B. IgE antibodies to penicillin are indicative for but not conclusive proof of penicillin allergy. Br J Dermatol 2006;154:1209–10.
15. Barbaud A, Goncalo M, Bruynzeel D, et al. Guidelines for performing skin tests with drugs in the investigation of cutaneous adverse drug reactions. Contact Derm 2001;45:321–8.
16. Pichler WJ, Tilch J. The lymphocyte transformation test in the diagnosis of drug hypersensitivity. Allergy 2004;59:809–20.
17. DeWeck AL, Sanz ML, Gamboa PM, et al. Diagnostic tests based on human basophils: more potentials and perspectives than pitfalls. Int Arch Allergy Immunol 2008;146:177–89.

18. Baluga JC, Casmayou R, Carozzi E, et al. Allergy to local anaesthetics in dentistry. Myth or reality? Allergol Immunopathol (Madrid) 2002;30:14–9.
19. Mahboob A, Haroon TS, Iqbal Z, et al. Fixed drug eruption and intradermal provocation tests. J Coll Physicians Surg Pak 2008;18:736–9.
20. Guglielmi L, Guglielmi P, Demoly P. Drug hypersensitivity: epidemiology and risk factors. Curr Pharm Des 2006;12:3309–12.
21. Davis C, Shearer WT. Diagnosis and management of HIV drug hypersensitivity. J Allergy Clin Immunol 2008;121:826–32.
22. Bernstein ML, McCusker MM, Grant-Kels JM. Cutaneous manifestations of cystic fibrosis. Pediatr Dermatol 2008;25:150–7.
23. Feldweg AM, Lee CM, Matulonis UA, et al. Rapid desensitization for hypersensitivity reactions to paclitaxel and docetaxel: a new standard protocol used in 77 successful treatments. Gynecol Oncol 2005;96:824–9.
24. Solensky R, Earl HS, Gruchalla RS. Lack of penicillin resensitization in patients with a history of penicillin allergy after receiving repeated penicillin courses. Arch Intern Med 2002;162:822–6.
25. Lieberman P, Kemp S, Oppenheimer JJ, et al. The diagnosis and management of anaphylaxis: an update practice parameter. J Allergy Clin Immunol 2005; 115(Suppl):S483–523.
26. Sampson HA, Munoz-Furlong A, Campbell RL, et al. Second symposium on the definition and management of anaphylaxis: summary report. J Allergy Clin Immunol 2006;117:391–7.
27. Reidenberg MM, Lowenthal DT. Adverse nondrug reactions. N Engl J Med 1968; 279:678–9.
28. Bernstein L, Gruchalla RS, Lee Re, et al. Executive summary of disease management of drug hypersensitivity: a practice parameter. Ann Allergy Asthma Immunol 1999;83:665–700.
29. Torres MJ, Blanca M, Fernandez J, et al. Diagnosis of immediate allergic reactions to beta-lactam antibiotics. Allergy 2003;58:961–72.
30. Romano A, Blanca M, Torres MJ, et al. Diagnosis of nonimmediate reactions to beta-lactam antibiotics. Allergy 2004;59:1153–60.
31. Grims RH, Kränke B, Aberer W. Pitfalls in drug allergy skin testing: false-positive reactions due to (hidden) additives. Contact Derm 2006;54:290–4.
32. Messaad D, Sahla H, Benahmed S, et al. Drug provocation tests in patients with a history suggesting an immediate drug hypersensitivity reaction. Ann Intern Med 2004;140:1001–6.
33. Greenberger PA. Drug allergy. J Allergy Clin Immunol 2006;117(Suppl):S464–70.
34. Nizankowska-Mogilnicka E, Bochenek G, Mastalerz L, et al. EAACI/GA2LEN guideline: aspirin provocation tests for diagnosis of aspirin hypersensitivity. Allergy 2007;62:1111–8.
35. Przybilla B, Aberer W, Bircher AJ, et al. Allergological approach to drug hypersensitivity reactions. J Dtsch Dermatol Ges 2008;6:240–3.
36. Wöhrl S. Clinical work-up of adverse drug reactions. Expert Rev Dermatol 2007;2: 217–31.
37. Komericki P, Arbab E, Grims R, et al. Tryptase as severity marker in drug provocation tests. Int Arch Allergy Immunol 2006;140:164–9.
38. Moore N, Biour M, Paux G, et al. Adverse drug reaction monitoring: doing it the French way. Lancet 1985;2(8463):1056–8.
39. Benahmed S, Picot MC, Dumas F, et al. Accuracy of a pharmacovigilance algorithm in diagnosing drug hypersensitivity reactions. Arch Intern Med 2005;165: 1500–5.

40. Girard M. Conclusiveness of rechallenge in the interpretation of adverse drug reactions. Br J Clin Pharmacol 1987;23:73–9.
41. Yocum MW, Heller AM, Abels RI. Efficacy of intravenous pretesting and antihistamine prophylaxis in radiocontrast media-sensitive patients. J Allergy Clin Immunol 1978;62:309–13.
42. Mendelson LM, Ressler C, Rosen JP, et al. Routine elective penicillin allergy skin testing in children and adolescents: study of sensitization. J Allergy Clin Immunol 1984;73:76–81.
43. Pichichero ME, Pichichero DM. Diagnosis of penicillin, amoxicillin, and cephalosporin allergy: reliability of examination assessed by skin testing and oral challenge. J Pediatr 1998;132:137–43.
44. Wöhrl S, Vigl K, Stingl G. Patients with drug reactions—is it worth testing? Allergy 2006;61:928–34.
45. Venulet J. Role and place of causality assessment. Pharmacoepidemiol Drug Saf 1992;1:225–34.
46. Grims RH, Weger W, Reiter H, et al. Delayed-type hypersensitivity to low molecular weight heparins and heparinoids: cross-reactivity does not depend on molecular weight. Br J Dermatol 2007;157:514–7.
47. Brockow K, Romano A, Aberer W, et al. Skin testing in patients with hypersensitivity reactions to iodinated contrast media—a European multicenter study. Allergy 2009;64:234–41.
48. Adkinson NF Jr, Essayan D, Gruchalla R, et al. Task force report: future research needs for the prevention and management of immune-mediated drug hypersensitivity reactions. J Allergy Clin Immunol 2002;109(Suppl):S461–78.
49. Pirmohamed M. Genetic factors in the predisposition to drug-induced hypersensitivity reactions. AAPS J 2006;8:e20–6.
50. Koh Y, Yap CW, Li SC. A quantitative approach of using genetic algorithm in designing a probability scoring system of an adverse drug reaction assessment system. Int J Med Inf 2008;77:421–30.

Rapid Desensitization for Hypersensitivity Reactions to Medications

Mariana Castells, MD, PhD[a,b,c,d],*

KEYWORDS

- Desensitization • Antibiotics • Aspirin • Chemotherapy
- Monoclonal antibodies • Hypersensitivity reactions

The development of rapid desensitizations for the treatment of drug hypersensitivities is aimed at providing essential medications while protecting patients from IgE and non-IgE hypersensitivity reactions. Serious adverse drug reactions occur in 6.7% of hospitalized patients, and adverse drug reactions are the fourth to sixth leading cause of death in such patients.[1] Drug-induced type I hypersensitivity reactions, such as anaphylaxis, result from the release of mediators from IgE-sensitized mast cells and basophils. Drug-associated anaphylaxis can be triggered by β-lactam antibiotics, such as penicillin and cephalosporins, chemotherapy drugs, such as platins, therapeutic monoclonal antibodies, and others.[2–7] Cross-linking of IgE by drug antigens can lead to limited skin reactions (flushing, pruritus, urticaria, angioedema) or multiorgan system involvement (sneezing, sinus and nasal congestion, cough, shortness of breath, wheezing, abdominal pain, nausea, vomiting, diarrhea) with hypotension and cardiovascular collapse during anaphylaxis. Hypersensitivity reactions induced by drug antigens upon initial exposure, without prior sensitization and with symptoms similar to IgE-mediated reactions, are called "non-IgE hypersensitivity reactions," and can result from direct release of mediators from mast cells and basophils, such in vancomycin-induced red man syndrome, intravenous contrast dyes, or taxenes. In these reactions, nontypical symptoms can occur, such as the severe back and muscle pain seen in patients with taxene and monoclonals reactions.[8]

[a] Harvard Medical School, Boston, MA 02115, USA
[b] Adverse Drug Reactions and Desensitization Program, Brigham and Women's Hospital, 1 Jimmy Fund Way, Smith Building, Room 626D, Boston, MA 02115, USA
[c] Allergy and Immunology Training Program, Brigham and Women's Hospital, 1 Jimmy Fund Way, Smith Building, Room 626D, Boston, MA 02115, USA
[d] Division of Rheumatology, Allergy and Immunology, Department of Medicine, Brigham and Women's Hospital, 1 Jimmy Fund Way, Smith Building, Room 626D, Boston, MA 02115, USA
* Division of Rheumatology, Allergy and Immunology, Department of Medicine, Brigham and Women's Hospital, 1 Jimmy Fund Way, Smith Building, Room 626D, Boston, MA 02115.
E-mail address: mcastells@partners.org

Immunol Allergy Clin N Am 29 (2009) 585–606
doi:10.1016/j.iac.2009.04.012

PRINCIPLES AND CELLULAR AND MOLECULAR TARGETS OF DRUG DESENSITIZATION

Desensitization for type I hypersensitivity reactions in penicillin-allergic patients were first developed 50 years ago.[9] Successful cases of rapid-progressive penicillin re-administration led to the concept of temporary clinical tolerization.[10,11] The administration of suboptimal doses of drug antigens, followed by the full therapeutic dose was safely achieved in highly allergic patients, permitting the treatment of severe infections. Following the early success with antibiotics, other empiric protocols were developed to treat hypersensitivity reactions to essential drugs that could not be substituted in allergic patients, such as aspirin in the control and prevention of cardiac diseases,[5] insulin in diabetes,[6] chemotherapy drugs during cancer recurrence,[12,13] and, more recently, chimeric and humanized monoclonal antibodies in chronic inflammatory diseases.[14] Because rapid desensitizations reintroduce potentially lethal drugs into highly sensitized patients, the molecular mechanisms need to be elucidated to improve the efficacy and safety of these procedures. Recent studies of in vitro rapid antigen desensitizations implicate mast cells and basophils as cellular targets, as well as syk,[15] a signal transducing molecule, and signal transducer and activator of transcription 6 (STAT6),[16] which is responsible for the transcription of interleukin (IL)-4 and IL-13.

CLINICAL MANIFESTATIONS
Hypersensitivity Reactions Type I, Mast Cell/IgE Dependent

Drug-induced hypersensitivity reactions type I result from the release of mediators from IgE-sensitized mast cells or basophils and can affect all organ systems, leading to anaphylaxis and death. Drug antigens can sensitize patients after multiple courses, and repeated exposures are needed for the development of specific IgE.[17] Sensitizing drugs can act as complete antigens, such as insulin, or haptens, which are coupled to a carrier protein, such as penicillin.[18] Among chemotherapy drugs, platins, such as carboplatin, cisplatin, and oxaliplatin can induce IgE formation[19] by a mechanism similar to that of metal workers exposed to low molecular-weight platinum salts by inhalation and skin contact.[20] Symptoms are induced by a platinum salt's cross-linking of specific IgE bound to high-affinity IgE receptors, FcεRI (on mast cells or basophils), with the release of membrane and granule mediators. These mediators include vasoactive amines, such as histamine, proteases such as tryptase, and proinflammatory and vasoactive prostaglandins and leukotrienes.[21]

Cross-linking of IgE by drug antigens can lead to limited skin reactions (flushing, pruritus, urticaria, angioedema) or multiorgan system involvement (sneezing, sinus and nasal congestion, cough, shortness of breath, wheezing, abdominal pain, nausea, vomiting, diarrhea), with decreased blood pressure and cardiovascular collapse during anaphylaxis. Reactions can occur within minutes of exposure and minimal amounts of the drug can induce severe reactions in highly sensitized individuals, such as laryngeal edema with asphyxiation. Disseminated intravascular coagulation and seizure-like acitivity are rare complications of anaphylaxis.[22] Retrospectively, finding an elevated tryptase in serum[23] and histamine in urine[24] can confirm the diagnosis.

The diagnosis of type I hypersensitivity reactions to drugs relies on the demonstration of in vivo or in vitro drug-specific IgE. Skin testing to drug antigens, such as penicillin, has a very high negative-predictive value. Only 1.8% to 3% of patients with a negative skin test present mild skin-limited reactions upon drug re-exposure.[25] Using different reagents, recent European data indicate a lower predictive value (see article by authors elsewhere in this issue). In a population of 126 patients who received over six courses of carboplatin for recurrent ovarian cancer and were skin tested before each course, only 10 patients with negative skin test presented a hypersensitivity reaction, indicating that the rate of false-negative skin test is as low as 1.5%.[13] In the same population, 7 out of 41 patients with positive skin test were given carboplatin and all presented anaphylaxis. Eighty percent to 90% of patients reactive to present carboplatin have a positive skin test, indicating that the likelihood of a severe hypersensitivity reaction is very high in skin test-positive patients, and that rechallenging those patients is not indicated.

Hypersensitibity Reactions—Non-IgE Mediated

Hypersensitivity reactions induced by drug antigens upon initial exposure, without prior sensitization and with a similar clinical presentation and symptoms as IgE-mediated reactions are mostly considered non-IgE hypersensitivity reactions. Rarely, sensitization to a cross-reactive compound may occur (see article by authors elsewhere in this issue). They can result from the release of mediators from mast cells or basophils, without known IgE mechanism, and with a negative skin test.[26,27] Vancomycin-induced red man syndrome is caused by the direct release of histamine from mast cells and basophils.[28] Among chemotherapy drugs, taxenes can induce severe hypersensitivity symptoms, with cardiovascular collapse within few minutes of first exposure in patients who present a negative skin test. Mechanisms implicated in those reactions include the activation of complement by the diluent Cremophor[29] or the direct release of mediators. Reactions to aspirin and nonsteroidal anti-inflammatory medications include the inhibition of cyclooxygenase-1, decrease in bronchodilator prostaglandins E, and increased generation of inflammatory leukotrienes, as well as the release of tryptase from mast cell upon aspirin exposure in sensitive patients.[30–32]

CELLULAR AND MOLECULAR TARGETS

Although all clinical desensitization protocols are empiric and based on error and trial clinical experiences, in vitro desensitization of mast cells and basophils has provided some understanding of the mechanisms underlying successful in vivo desensitizations. Suboptimal doses of antigen, as low as one-tenth the optimal dose administered before an optimal dose, render mast cells and basophils unresponsive to antigens but not to other activating stimuli.[33] Suboptimal doses can induce unresponsiveness through excessive monomeric antigens, incapable of cross-linking surface FceRI receptors or through the rapid internalization of antigen cross-linked receptors depleting the cell surface.[34] Basophils can be desensitized in vitro to penicillin, but basophils isolated from a patient desensitized to penicillin were activated in vitro by penicillin antigens,[35] indicating that the presence of antigens at all times is critical to maintaining the desensitization state. In vitro rapid desensitization of human mast cells induces the decreased levels of signal-transducing molecules, such as syk, because of ubiquitinilation and degradation.[36,37] Naturally occurring syk-deficient basophils are unresponsive to drug antigens, indicating that syk is critical for activation and for desensitization.[15] In recent studies STAT6, which is responsible for the transcription of IL-4 and IL-13, has been involved in rapid desensitizations. STAT-6-deficient mast cells are capable of releasing mediators during the early phase of IgE cell activation but cannot release late cytokines, such as tumor necrosis factor (TNF)-α and IL-6, and cannot be desensitized to antigens.[16,38]

DESENSITIZATION TO ANTIBIOTICS

All antibiotics can induce IgE and non-IgE hypersensitivity reactions amendable to rapid desensitization, and the most common are β-lactams, including cephalosporins, vancomycin, and quinolones.

Penicillin and Cephalosporins

Patients allergic to penicillin are at risk when exposed to cephalosporins. Cross-reactivity between cephalosporins and penicillins is found in 4% to 11% of patients because of the related core β-lactam ring structure, mostly with first and second generation.[39] Specific cephalosporin IgE antibodies can be directed toward side-chain determinants that are not shared with β-lactam rings containing drugs,[40] posing less of a risk for penicillin-allergic patients. Other antibiotics containing β-lactam rings, such as monobactams (aztreonam), have no significant cross-reactivity with penicillins, and recently imipenem was shown to be tolerated by penicillin- and β-lactam-allergic patients.[41] Only immediate type I reactions to penicillin and β-lactams are amendable to rapid desensitization. Other reactions, such as maculopapular rashes, erythema multiforme, Stevens-Johnson syndrome, toxic epidermal necrolysis, bullous erythema, erythroderma, serum sickness, hemolytic anemia, neutropenia, thrombocytopenia, and acute interstitial nephropathy are not amendable to rapid desensitizations because outcomes are not available after drug re-exposure in these patients.

All patients with a history of IgE-mediated hypersensitivity and a positive skin test to either the minor or major penicillin determinants should avoid all β-lactam ring-containing medications, including penicillin, amoxicillin, ampicillin, and cephalosporins. Aztreonam and imipenem can be used as indicated by the infectious agents. If penicillin or cephalosporin treatment is mandated by the severity and nature of the infection, rapid desensitization is indicated.

Rapid Desensitization to β-Lactam antibiotics Including Penicillin and Cephalosporins

The first series of rapid penicillin desensitizations included escalating oral doses to treat 15 pregnant syphilis-infected women.[10] An intravenous protocol was later developed to treat 15 severely infected patients, which included 10-fold incremental doses[11] and induced 30% of nonlife-threatening side effects, including serum sickness. Since then, multiple case reports have been published with no series available to validate the efficacy and safety of the different protocols.

Up to 30% of cystic fibrosis patients develop hypersensitivity reactions after multiple exposures to β-lactams, which require rapid desensitizations.[42,43] A recent study indicated that 57 antibiotic desensitizations were done safely in 21 patients, 90% with cystic fibrosis. Most of the antibiotics were β-lactams and the success rate was 75%. Desensitization failures related to non-IgE mediated symptoms.[43]

A typical protocol for desensitization to intravenous penicillin and cephalosporins starts at one-ten-thousands to one-one-hundredth the target dose, and doubling doses are delivered every 15 to 20 minutes over the course of several hours until reaching the target dose.[44] Ceftazidime desensitization was done in seven cystic fibrosis patients to treat IgE-mediated hypersensitivity reactions,[45] with no major systemic reactions during desensitization. A recurrent rash occurred in two patients on the seventh and twelfth day after desensitization, one patient was successfully redesensitized, and one patient discontinued treatment. Cefotaxime desensitization was done in a 51-year-old man with bacterial spondylitis, and the treatment was continued for 4 weeks with no adverse events.[46] A series of eight patients with a positive skin test to penicillin and cephalosporins (cefepime, ceftriaxone, and cefazolin) were desensitized to β-lactam drugs using a 2-hour and 15-minute protocol in which tripling doses were administered every 15 minutes, without major side effects.[47] An imipenem- and penicillin-allergic patient was desensitized to intravenous imipenem for multiresistant *Acinobacter pneumoniae* and the treatment was continued for 21 days without adverse events.[48]

The author and colleagues have used a standardized protocol at the Brigham and Women's Hospital in Boston, which includes a three solution, 12-step infusion allowing the patients to receive full therapeutic doses after 5.8 h (**Tables 1** and **2**). The solutions were made by 10-fold dilutions of the full target concentration (solution 3). Each solution was administered in four different steps. The rate of each step was increased every 15 minutes to deliver approximately twice the dose of the previous step. This model is based on the chemotherapy standard-desensitization protocol.[49] The author and colleagues performed 42 antibiotic successful desensitizations in 2005 and 2006 with this protocol (**Table 3**).[50] Side effects during antibiotic desensitizations were mild and included flushing, warmth, tingling, pruritus, erythema, rash, and hives. No serious events occurred, all subjects were treated for their full courses, and no late reactions were observed. Subjects were maintained on their antibiotics during the course of their treatments without need for repeated desensitizations.

Other Antibiotics

Vancomycin is an antimicrobial agent that is often used as an alternative treatment for serious staphylococcal and streptococcal infections in patients with hypersensitivity reactions to β-lactam antibiotics or whose infection failed to respond to β-lactam antibiotics. The incidence of adverse reactions has been reported to be in the range of 5% to 14% in adults, with the most common manifestation as the red man syndrome associated to nonspecific histamine release.[51] The risk of an adverse reaction to vancomycin increases with concurrent use of narcotics because of non-IgE-mediated, direct release of histamine from mast cells.[52] Although red man syndrome can be treated with slow infusions, IgE-mediated hypersensitivity reactions resistant to slow infusions have been described in which desensitization has been done.[51] A series of seven patients with serious staphylococal infections resistant to β-lactams antibiotics underwent rapid continuous intravenous infusion with multiple small increases in vancomycin concentration with a syringe pump similar to the protocol described in **Tables 1** and **2**, without major side effects.[52]

IgE-mediated hypersensitivity reactions to quinolones have been reported with cross-reactivity among ciprofloxacin and levaquin. A 35-year-old woman with chronic granulomatous disease and *Burholderia cepacia* infection was desensitized to intravenous ciprofloxacin with no side effects, and the treatment was continued for 4 weeks uneventfully.[53]

Table 1			
Rapid intravenous desensitization to 1 g of ceftazidime in a cystic fibrosis patient			
Full Dose	1000.0 mg	mg/ml	Total mg to be Injected in Each Bottle
Solution 1	250 cc	0.040	10.000
Solution 2	250 cc	0.400	100.000
Solution 3	250 cc	3.969	992.130

Table 2 Steps for protocol shown in Table 1					
Step	Solution	Rate (cc/h)	Time (min)	Administered Dose (mg)	Cumulative Dose (mg)
1	1	2	15	0.0200	0.0200
2	1	5	15	0.0500	0.0700
3	1	10	15	0.1000	0.1700
4	1	20	15	0.2000	0.3700
5	2	5	15	0.5000	0.8700
6	2	10	15	1.0000	1.8700
7	2	20	15	2.0000	3.8700
8	2	40	15	4.0000	7.8700
9	3	10	15	9.9213	17.7913
10	3	20	15	19.8426	37.6339
11	3	40	15	39.6852	77.3191
12	3	75	186	922.6809	1000.0000
	Total time =		351 minutes		

DESENSITIZATION TO ASPIRIN AND NONSTEROIDAL ANTI-INFLAMMATORY DRUGS

Asperin (ASA) and nonsteroidal anti-inflammatory drugs (NSAIDs) include ibuprofen, indomethacin, sulindac, naproxen, tolmetin, fenoprofen, meclofenamate, ketoralac, etololac, oxaprozin, diclofenac, ketoprofen, flurbiprofen, piroxicam, nabumatone, and mefenamic acid, among others. Up to 20% of asthmatic patients develop broad ASA and NSAID intolerance manifested by upper and lower pulmonary symptoms

Table 3 Antibiotic desensitizations performed at Brigham and Women's Hospital 2005 to 2006 using the protocol from Tables 1 and 2	
Antibiotic	No. of Desensitizations
Ancef	1
Ceftaxidime	7
Ceftriaxone	4
Cefazolin	1
Ciprofloxacin	1
Ertapenem	1
Imipenem	9
Meropenem	1
Nafcillin	3
Penicillin	7
Piperacillin	3
Trimethoprim	1
Zosyn	3
TOTAL	42

There were no deaths or anaphylactic events during desensitization. Only mild side effects were observed (ie, pruritus, flushing). All patients completed the desensitization protocol, reached the target dose, and were able to receive the prescribed antibiotic course.

(asthma, rhino-conjunctivitis). Nonasthmatic patients can present cutaneous symptoms with chronic urticaria and angioedema when exposed to ASA and NSAIDS, and specific allergic reactions induced by one NSAID or ASA are also described, including anaphylaxis.[54] Desensitization to aspirin is considered in cardiac patients, asthmatic patients with recurrent polyps, and females with antiphospholipid syndromes during pregnancy.

Desensitization to ASA and NSAIDs has been performed to provide cardiac protection and anti-inflammatory treatment in intolerant patients with no alternative medications. Desensitization was initiated in 1927 by Widal[55] with the administration of small daily doses of ASA to ASA-intolerant asthmatic patients until toleration was achieved (**Table 4**). A refractory period was initially observed after a respiratory reaction induced by indomethacin, and tolerance to ASA was induced after a positive oral aspirin challenge.[56] Although the mechanism of desensitization is unknown, desensitized patients tolerate ASA and NSAIDs at pharmacologic doses, and prolonged desensitization can be achieved by daily administration of ASA or NSAIDs.[57] Protocols for ASA and NSAID desensitization are based on the controlled progressive administration of incremental doses starting at 30 mg of ASA and progressing to 60 mg, 100 mg, 150 mg, 325 mg, and 650 mg at 90-minute intervals, as described in the recent Practice parameters.[58] Respiratory responses are measured by forced expiratory volume in 1 second, and a decline of 15% is considered a positive challenge. The dose is then repeated until no reaction occurs and the patient continues until reaching 325 mg or 650 mg. Cross-desensitization is universal for all NSAIDs once desensitization has been achieved at therapeutic levels.[59] Patients who have severe gastrointestinal intolerance to ASA and NSAIDs have been challenge with lysil-aspirin, either nasally or bronchially.[60] Desensitization has been less successful for intolerant patients with cutaneous reactions.[61] Twenty-two patients with urticarial reactions induced by ASA and NSAIDs were desensitized to ASA and tolerated other NSAIDs after ASA desensitization was maintained with daily doses of 325 mg. A study of 11 cardiac patients with a history of acute urticaria/angioedema after ASA and NSAIDs indicated that 9 were able to be desensitized with a fast protocol using incremental ASA doses at 15 to 30 minute intervals (**Table 5**).[62] Similar protocols have been used to desensitized cardiac patients undergoing stent placements.[63]

Long-term ASA Desensitization

Sixty-five ASA-sensitive patients with asthma were desensitized from 1988 to 1994.[64] Increasing oral doses of ASA, up to 650 mg, were administered and daily doses

Table 4	
Desensitization to aspirin in an asthmatic patient	
Time (min)	**Dose (mg)**
0	4
90	40
180	81
240	162
330	325
420	650

Aspirin to be continued at 650 mg by mouth twice daily.
Data from White AA, Stevenson DD, Simon RA. The blocking effect of essential controller medications during aspirin challenges in patients with aspirin-exacerbated respiratory disease. Ann Allergy Asthma Immunol 2005;95(4):330–5.

Table 5
Desensitization to aspirin in a patient with aspirin-related urticaria-angioedema

Time (min)	Dose (mg)
0	0.1
20	0.3
40	1
60	3
80	10
100	30
120	40
140	81
160	162

Aspirin to be continued at 162 mg once per day.
Data from Wong JT, Nagy CS, Krinzman SJ, et al. Rapid oral challenge-desensitization for patients with aspirin-related urticaria-angioedema. J Allergy Clin Immunol 2000;105(5):997–1001.

ranging from 350 mg to 1,950 mg, with a mean of 1,214 mg, were used for 1 to 6 years. These patients presented a significant reduction in the number of sinus infections and asthma hospitalizations, an improvement in the sense of smell, and a decrease in prednisone treatments. A significant reduction in the number of sinus and polyp operations and the use of nasal corticosteroids was also found. Desensitization and maintenance of daily ASA is recommended in patients who have failed medical treatment and have undergone multiple surgeries for polyps or sinusitis.[65] The administration of leukotriene inhibitors during desensitization helps shift the response to the upper respiratory tract without blunting the response.[66] Four pregnant woman with antiphospholipid syndrome were desensitized orally to aspirin with few side effects and were maintained several months on aspirin.[67]

DESENSITIZATION TO CHEMOTHERAPY AND MONOCLONALS

All chemotherapy agents can cause hypersensitivity reactions[68] and those reactions have limited the used of critical drugs in very sick patients for fear of inducing a more severe reaction and possibly death.[69] The choice of an alternative chemotherapy regimen is often limited by tumor sensitivity and, because of the increasing number of cancer survivors, patients are exposed to multiple courses of the same or similar chemotherapy agents. Increased exposures lead to sensitization and to hypersensitivity reactions in an increasing patient population.[70] One-third of the patients exposed to seven or more cycles of carboplatin develop hypersensitivity reactions, including anaphylaxis, and deaths have been reported with re-exposure (**Fig. 1**).[71,72] The need to offer first-line therapy after cancer recurrence and to overcome hypersensitivity reactions has been at the core of the desensitization research and clinical developments.[73]

Desensitization to Chemotherapy Drugs Including Taxenes and Platins

Protocols for the desensitization of hypersensitivity reactions to chemotherapy drugs have been used with success,[19,74–79] but side effects have been prominent and no outcome measurements have been available. Based on in vitro and in vivo data generated in the author's division,[16] a standardized three-solution, 12-step protocol was

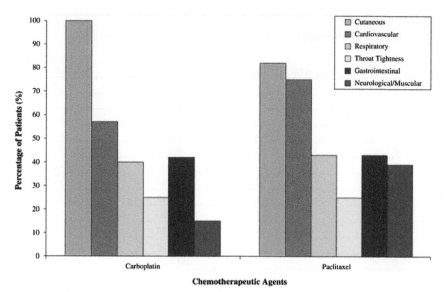

Fig. 1. Frequency of symptoms and signs during initial hypersensitivity reactions. (*From* Castells MC, Tennant NM, Sloane DE, et al. Hypersensitivity reactions to chemotherapy: outcomes and safety of rapid desensitization in 413 cases. J Allergy Clin Immunol 2008;122(3):578; with permission.)

generated that allowed for gradual increases in the infusion rate and drug concentration, infusing the target dose over 5.8 hours, as seen in **Tables 6** and **7**. Three solutions—A, B, and C, containing X/100 mg, X/10 mg, and X mg, respectively, diluted in 250 mL of D5 water—were used in sequence of increasing concentrations. The concentration of solutions A, B, and C were (X/100)/250, (X/10)/250, and (X)/250 mg/mL, respectively. Solution A was used for steps 1 to 4, Solution B for steps 5 to 8, and Solution C for steps 9 to 12. The rate of the infusion was changed every 15 minutes, with each step delivering approximately twice the dose of the previous step. The final step 12 maintained a constant rate of infusion to deliver the remainder of the total dose. One-on-one care (nurse/patient ratio) was provided for each desensitization, and nurses were trained by the allergy team on how to administer the protocol and how to recognize the symptoms of hypersensitivity reactions.

Table 6
Standard desensitization protocol using a total dose of 500 mg as an example

Total Dose	500 mg	Solution Concentration	Total Dose in Each Solution (mg)
Solution A	250 mL	0.02 mg/mL	5.0[a]
Solution B	250 mL	0.20 mg/mL	50.0[a]
Solution C	250 mL	2.00 mg/mL	500.0[a]

[a] The sum of the doses in Solutions A, B, and C equals 555 mg. Total dose infused is 500 mg.
  Data from Lee CW, Matulonis UA, Castells MC. Carboplatin hypersensitivity: a 6-h 12-step protocol effective in 35 desensitizations in patients with gynecological malignancies and mast cell/IgE-mediated reactions. Gynecol Oncol 2004;95(2):370–6.

Table 7 Steps for protocol used in Table 6					
Step	Solution	Rate (ml/h)	Time (min)	Administered Dose (mg)	Cumulative Dose Infused (mg)
1	A	2	15	0.010	0.010
2	A	5	15	0.025	0.035
3	A	10	15	0.050	0.085
4	A	20	15	0.100	0.185
5	B	5	15	0.250	0.435
6	B	10	15	0.500	0.935
7	B	20	15	1.000	1.935
8	B	40	15	2.000	3.935
9	C	10	15	5.000	8.935
10	C	20	15	10.000	18.935
11	C	40	15	20.000	38.935
12	C	75	184.4	461.065	500.000
			Total time = 5.82 h		Total dose infused = 500 mg

Data from Lee CW, Matulonis UA, Castells MC. Carboplatin hypersensitivity: a 6-h 12-step protocol effective in 35 desensitizations in patients with gynecological malignancies and mast cell/IgE-mediated reactions. Gynecol Oncol 2004;95(2):370–6.

Once a patient completed a successful course of desensitization, all subsequent repeated courses of chemotherapy were given in the out-patient facility with a desensitization-trained chemotherapy nurse in one-to-one attendance. The volumes of the bags were adjusted for time constraints to100 mL of D5 water.

Rapid Desensitization for Hypersentivity Reactions to Taxenes

Paclitaxel is a widely used antineoplastic agent with activity against ovarian, breast, and other solid tumors. It was initially isolated from the bark of the Pacific yew tree (Taxus brevifolia) in the 1970s, and its antimitotic activity is a result of the bundling of microtubules, which arrests cell division. Docetaxel is a semisynthetic taxane originally extracted from the needles of the European yew tree (Taxus baccata), whose antimitotic activity is similar to that of paclitaxel.[80]

A high incidence of hypersensitivity reactions (HSRs) were observed with paclitaxel in early clinical trials, involving flushing, hemodynamic changes, dyspnea, musculoskeletal pain, paresthesias, and gastrointestinal symptoms, with fatalities reported. Symptoms frequently occurred during the first course of therapy, within seconds to minutes of beginning the infusion, indicating a lack of need for prior sensitization.[13] Slower infusion rates and premedication with H1, H2 antihistamine receptor antagonists, and corticosteroids have decreased the incidence of HSRs to less than 10%.[81] Despite those interventions, there is a subset of patients with taxene-responsive cancers who present HSRs, in whom rapid desensitization is indicated.[80] Attempts at using docetaxel in patients with paclitaxel HSRs have not proven universally successful.[49] HSRs to taxenes resemble anaphylactic reactions induced by the acute release of mast cell/basophil mediators, but skin tests have been negative, indicating that the diluent cremophor or the generation of reactive metabolites capable of activating complement or directly mast cells/basophils may be responsible.[29]

The author used a standard desensitization protocol developed at the Brigham and Women's Hospital to desensitize 40 patients who presented a hypersensitivity reaction after the first or second infusion of paclitaxel or docetaxel for a total of 176 desensitizations.[7,49,82] The limited infusion times avoids neutropenia. The most prominent presenting symptoms of hypersensitivity to taxenes included flushing, pruritus, urticaria, chest pain, hypotension and hypertension, loss of consciousness, gastrointestinal symptoms, musculoskeletal pain, and dyspnea with O_2 desaturation. The initial HSR reactions in those patients were immediate (less than 10 seconds) to a maximum of 15 minutes, with one patient reporting urticaria during 2 weeks following her initial HSR. Readministration at a slow infusion rate, after additional antihistamines and corticosteroids, failed in four patients. One patient, switched to docetaxel, developed a similar HSR, indicating that the vehicle for paclitaxel, cremophor, was not responsible for the HSR reaction. The solutions and protocols for the desensitization protocol are described in **Tables 6** and **7**.

Administration time for all desensitizations ranged from 4 to 8 hours. All 40 patients were successfully desensitized and had repeated desensitizations, completing their chemotherapy cycles. Breakthrough reactions occurred in 12% of the desensitizations and the reactions were less severe than the initial reaction and did not preclude the completion of any treatment course. We noted that the incidence of allergic disease (seasonal allergic rhinitis, asthma, allergy to other drugs, venom sensitivity) was 57%, which far exceeds the 15% to 20% reported for the general population.[83] An earlier review of 19 patients with paclitaxel-induced HSRs found a statistically significant difference in the rate of hymenoptera venom sensitivity, but not other types of allergy, in patients with HSRs when compared with control patients.[84] Patients with allergic conditions seem to be at higher risk for HSRs to taxanes.

Rapid Desensitization for HSRs to Platins

Carboplatin is an effective and well-tolerated cytotoxic agent used as standard front-line chemotherapy for ovarian cancer.[85] Many patients achieve a clinical complete remission with the platinum-based regimen but later develop recurrent disease within 3 years of diagnosis. For patients with platinum-sensitive recurrent cancer, disease relapsing after at least a 6-month disease-free interval, platinum-based chemotherapy remains the most active regimen. In addition to its clinical effectiveness, carboplatin has a low incidence of toxicity and limited nausea or vomiting with anti-emetic therapy.[86] Therefore, the ability to administer carboplatin safely as front-line therapy and in the relapse setting provides a significant clinical benefit to the patient. Patients treated with multiple courses of carboplatin experience increased incidence of HSRs; these reactions are uncommon during the initial courses, but the incidence of reactions increases to 27% in patients receiving more than seven cycles of carboplatin.[87,88] Thus, most cases of carboplatin HSR are observed during the retreatment for relapsed disease. Symptoms of HSR vary from cutaneous reactions, such as flushing and urticaria, to life-threatening respiratory and cardiovascular compromise, including bronchospasm, chest pain, and hypotension, with more than 50% of patients developing at least moderately severe symptoms (see **Fig. 1**).

HSRs to carboplatin are thought to be mast cell/IgE mediated because skin tests performed on the volar surface of the forearm with a drop of a nonirritating concentration of carboplatin at 1 mg/mL to 10 mg/mL is positive in over 80% of reactive patients.[71,89] Eliminating carboplatin as a treatment option presents a significant disadvantage, but death from reintroduction of platinums has been described.[69] Several protocols for reintroduction of carboplatin and other platinums have been developed.[90,91] The author and colleagues treated 54 patient for 162 desensitization

Table 8
Characteristics of initial hypersensitivity reactions to chemotherapy

Symptoms	Carboplatin 31 pts n (%)	Paclitaxel 22 pts n (%)	Docetaxel 1 pt n (%)	Trastuzumab 1 pt n (%)	Doxorubicin 1 pt n (%)	Uromitexa 1 pt n (%)
Cutaneous						
Flushing	17 (54.8)	19 (86.4)	1 (100)	—	1 (100)	—
Pruritus	24 (77.4)	1 (4.5)	—	1 (100)	1 (100)	—
Urticaria	9 (29)	1 (4.5)	—	1 (100)	—	1 (100)
Cardiovascular						
Chest pain	8 (25.8)	15 (68.2)	1 (100)	—	—	1 (100)
Tachy/bradycardia	2/1 (9.7)	2/0 (9.1)	—	—	—	—
Hyper/hypotension	2/2 (12.9)	5/1 (27.3)	—	—	—	—
Lightheadedness	4 (12.9)	4 (18.2)	—	—	—	—
Loss of consciousness	2 (6.5)	4 (18.2)	—	—	—	—
Pulmonary						
Dyspnea	12 (38.7)	10 (45.5)	—	1 (100)	1 (100)	1 (100)
Desaturation	5 (16.1)	7 (31.8)	—	—	—	1 (100)
Gastrointestinal						
Nausea/vomiting	6 (19.4)	1 (4.5)	—	—	—	—
Abdominal pain	5 (16.1)	6 (27.3)	—	—	—	—
Oropharynx						
Throat tightness	3 (9.7)	4 (18.2)	—	1 (100)	—	—
Musculoskeletal						
Back pain	1 (3.2)	10 (45.5)	—	—	—	—

Data from Lee CW, Matulonis UA, Castells MC. Rapid inpatient/outpatient desensitization for chemotherapy hypersensitivity: standard protocol effective in 57 patients for 255 courses. Gynecol Oncol 2005;99(2):393–9.

Table 9
Characteristics of breakthrough reactions occurring during desensitization

	Carboplatin (11 pts)	Paclitaxel (6 pts)	Trastuzumab (1 pt)
Cutaneous			
Flushinig	4	3	1
Pruritus	7	1	1
Urticaria	3	1	1
Cardiovascular			
Chest pain	1	2	—
Tachy/bradycardia	20	1/10	—
Hyper/hypotension	2/1	1/1	—
Pulmonary			
Dyspnea	3	—	—
Desaturation	1	—	—
Gastrointestinal			
Abdominal pain	1	1	—
Oropharynx			
Throat tightness	1	—	1

Data from Lee CW, Matulonis UA, Castells MC. Rapid inpatient/outpatient desensitization for chemotherapy hypersensitivity: standard protocol effective in 57 patients for 255 courses. Gynecol Oncol 2005;99(2):393–9.

courses with the standardized desensitization protocol described in **Tables 6** and **7**, the same as for taxene desensitizations with three solutions for 6 hours and 12 steps.[7] Positive skin test for the initial patient series was positive in 80.8% of 21 initial patients. Patients received a median of eight courses before developing their initial hypersensitivity reaction. Most patients had reactions during their second-line therapy for recurrent cancer. Typically after recurrence of their disease, patients were re-exposed to carboplatin during the seventh cycle and develop reactions during the eighth cycle. This observation suggests that a prolonged period of sensitization is required before the onset of HSR. The reaction profile was consistent with type I HSRs (see **Fig. 1**) and included flushing, pruritus, urticaria, nausea, dyspnea, tachycardia, hypertension or

Table 10
Effect of desensitization on skin test reactivity: wheal/flare (mm) response for patient 10

	Controls		Carboplatin	
	Histamine (Prick)	Diluent (Intradermal)	10 mg/mL (Intradermal)	Wheal Ratio[a]
Before desensitization	Positive (5/15)	Negative (4/0)	Positive (8/15)	1.6
After desensitization	Positive (4/13)	Negative (4/0)	Negative (4/1)	1

[a] Wheal produced by carboplatin (intradermal) versus wheal produced by histamine (prick).
Data from Lee CW, Matulonis UA, Castells MC. Carboplatin hypersensitivity: a 6-h 12-step protocol effective in 35 desensitizations in patients with gynecological malignancies and mast cell/IgE-mediated reactions. Gynecol Oncol 2004;95(2):370–6.

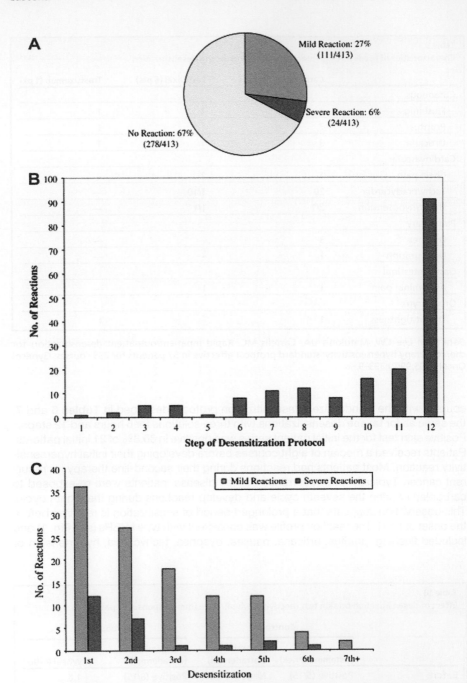

Fig. 2. (A) Number and severity of reactions during desensitization. A mild reaction was defined as absence of chest pain, changes in blood pressure, dyspnea, oxygen, desaturation, or throat tightness. A severe reaction included one of these. (B) Desensitization step at which reactions occurred (total number of reactions = 180). (C) Desensitization course at which reactions recurred (total number of reactions = 135, of which 111 were mild and 24 were severe). (From Castells MC, Tennant NM, Sloane DE, et al. Hypersensitivity reactions to chemotherapy: outcomes and safety of rapid desensitization in 413 cases. J Allergy Clin Immunol 2008;122(3):579; with permission.)

hypotension, and chest pain. Most patients had their initial HSR during the infusion, with six patients experiencing symptoms within 15 minutes of infusion, but no delayed reactions were observed. Cutaneous manifestations were present in 96% of the patients and extracutaneous symptoms were present in 77% of the patients, including hypotension and loss of consciousness (**Table 8**). In contrast, with patients presenting reactions to paclitaxel, there was a low incidence of musculoskeletal pain, including back pain (3% versus 45%, see **Table 8**). All patients successfully received all planned courses of carboplatin though the desensitization program. Breakthrough reactions occurred in 12% of the desensitizations, with mild reactions, none of which resulted in cardiovascular collapse or death (**Table 9**). To determine the effect of desensitization on cutaneous mast cell reactivity, a skin test was performed before and after desensitization. The result of the skin test to carboplatin was positive before desensitization but became negative after the infusion (**Table 10**), demonstrating the inhibition of cutaneous mast cell reactivity, consistent with other studies (**Fig. 2**).[71]

Rapid Desensitization for Biologic Agents and Monoclonal Antibodies

HSRs to humanized monoclonal antibodies are rare but their frequency is increasing as increased cancer and rheumatologic patients are exposed to multiple courses. Patients with HSR to rituximab (Rituxan) have been described to trastuzumab (Herceptin), and to anti-TNFα monoclonal antibodies.[92–95] In patients with reactions compatible with a hypersensitivity type I, in whom an IgE/mast cell mechanism can be demonstrated, desensitizations have been reported for humanized monoclonal antibodies.[96] The author and colleagues used the protocol described in **Tables 11** and **12** to desensitize patients to rituximab and trastazumab.[7,8] The initial reaction was severe in both cases and included anaphylaxis. An IgE mechanism was demonstrated by positive skin test to nonirritant concentrations of the drugs. Breakthrough symptoms were less severe than the initial reaction and allowed the patients to complete their courses. Patients received their first desensitization in the intensive care setting and for repeated desensitizations were transitioned to the out-patient clinics with one-on-one nurse support. One patient desensitized to trastazumab presented side effects during the first two initial desensitizations and was later transitioned to the out-patient setting, where she underwent eight more courses without side effects, with a modified protocol.

Outcomes of Desensitizations and Cancer Progression

The author and colleagues did a safety study in the largest series of chemotherapy and monoclonal antibodies desensitizations, providing safety data for 413 cases. Drugs included carboplatin, cisplatin oxaliplatin, paclitaxel, liposomal doxorubicin, and rituximab. Of the subjects in the study, 94% presented mild or no reactions and only 6%

Table 11			
Desensitization protocol for rituximab IV (851 mg): solution preparation			
	Volume (mL)	Concentration (mg/mL)	Total Amount of Drug in Each Solution (mg)
Solution 1	250	0.034	8.510
Solution 2	250	0.340	85.100
Solution 3	250	3.377	844.303

Amount of drug prepared exceeds dose of drug delivered during desensitization because solutions 1 and 2 are not completely infused. A full dose is 851 mg of rituximab.

Table 12
Desensitization protocol for rituximab IV (851 mg): protocol for administration

Step no.	Solution no.	Rate (mL/h)	Time (min)	Volume Infused Per Step (mL)	Administered Dose (mg)	Cumulative Dose (mg)
1	1	2.0	15	0.50	0.0170	0.0170
2	1	5.0	15	1.25	0.0426	0.0596
3	1	10.0	15	2.50	0.0851	0.1447
4	1	20.0	15	5.00	0.1702	0.3149
5	2	5.0	15	1.25	0.4255	0.7404
6	2	10.0	15	2.50	0.8510	1.5914
7	2	20.0	15	5.00	1.7020	3.2934
8	2	40.0	15	10.00	3.4040	6.6974
9	3	10.0	15	2.50	8.4430	15.1404
10	3	20.0	15	5.00	16.8861	32.0264
11	3	40.0	15	10.00	33.7721	65.7986
12	3	75.0	186	232.50	785.2014	851.0000

Total time = 351 minutes (5.85 hours).

presented reactions that required antihistamines or steroids. No epinephrine was used in any case and no deaths occurred. All patients received their treatment courses after the initial desensitization. The majority of the reactions occurred during step 12, when patients were receiving the drug at the maximal rate and full concentration. When desensitizations were repeated, the side effects were less frequent and less severe, because of additional steps added before the step at which the patient reacted or was given additional antihistamines. The addition of antileukotriene therapy and prostaglandin blockade with aspirin seems to improve the side effects over the use of steroids.[97]

Whether chemotherapy desensitizations are effective at tumor killing or control needs to be defined. In a small population of 26 patients receiving carboplatin desensitization for recurrent cancer, 10 (38.5%) had a radiographic response (partial or complete response) or a greater than 50% drop of initial CA125 value, 11 (42.3%) had stable disease radiographically or CA125 response (<50% drop), and 5 (19.2%) had progressive disease after 1 to 2 cycles of carboplatin. Of the three patients receiving paclitaxel desensitization for recurrent cancer, one had clinical response to therapy, one had stable disease, and one had progressive disease. Of 16 patients receiving paclitaxel desensitization for newly diagnosed cancer, 16 patients (100%) achieved clinical remission. Those are the expected rates for cancer patient populations not receiving chemotherapy desensitizations.

SUMMARY

Rapid desensitization protocols are available to patients who present with IgE and non-IgE-dependent hypersensitivity to drugs, including anaphylaxis to antibiotics, chemotherapy, monoclonals, aspirin, and other drugs. Typical hypersensitivity symptoms include pruritus, flushing, urticaria, angioedema, respiratory and gastrointestinal distress, and changes in blood pressure, including hypotension and shock. Associated musculoskeletal symptoms and back pain can be present in patients reacting to taxenes and monoclonal antibodies. During rapid desensitization, drug antigens are reintroduced in an incremental fashion, allowing for full therapeutic doses to be delivered with minor or no side effects. Temporary toleration is achieved in hours and can be maintained if drug antigens are administered at regular intervals, depending on pharmacokinetic parameters. Desensitization should only be done in settings with one-on-one nurse-patient care and where resuscitation personnel and resources are readily available. After a successful desensitization, repeated desensitizations can be done in outpatient or inpatient settings with similar conditions for patients on chemotherapy of monoclonal therapies. This provides flexibility and allows patients to remain in clinical studies. Breakthrough symptoms during desensitization are less severe than the initial HSR and deaths have not been reported in the last 5 years. Managing breakthrough symptoms with antihistamines and steroids and decelerating the dose escalation with intermediate infusion steps successfully improves the tolerability of desensitization protocols. Blocking leukotrienes and prostaglandins has improved side effects. Reactions occurring days to weeks after drug treatment, such as serum sickness, erythema multiforme, Stevens-Johnson syndrome, and toxic epidermal necrolysis may not be considered for desensitization protocols.

Education of nurses, pharmacists, and oncology and allergy specialists will lead to the judicious use of desensitization protocols for patients with hypersensitivity reactions in need of first-line therapy. Basic research is needed to uncover the cellular and molecular mechanisms underlying the temporary toleration induced by desensitization, so that pharmacologic interventions can improve its safety and efficacy. From the outcomes and safety data gathered, it appears that a flexible 12-step protocol could be universally used for all drug desensitizations.

REFERENCES

1. Lazarou J, Pomeranz BH, Corey PN. Incidence of adverse drug reactions in hospitalized patients. JAMA 1998;259:1200–5.
2. Van Der Klauw MM, Wilson JHP, Stricker B. Drug-assocaited anaphylaxis: 20 years of reporting in The Netherlands (1974–1994) and review of the literature. 1996;26:1355–66.
3. Gruchalla RS. Acute drug desensitization. Clin Exp Allergy 1998;28(Suppl 4): 63–4.
4. Gruchalla RS. 10. Drug allergy. J Allergy Clin Immunol 2003;111(Suppl 2): S548–807.
5. Wong JT, Nagy CS, Krinzman SJ, et al. Rapid oral challenge-desensitization for patients with aspirin-related urticaria-angioedema. J Allergy Clin Immunol 2000; 105(5):997–1001.
6. Moyes V, Driver R, Croom A, et al. Insulin allergy in a patient with Type 2 diabetes successfully treated with continuous subcutaneous insulin infusion. Diabet Med 2006;23(2):204–6.
7. Lee CW, Matulonis UA, Castells MC. Rapid inpatient/outpatient desensitization for chemotherapy hypersensitivity: standard protocol effective in 57 patients for 255 courses. Gynecol Oncol 2005;99(2):393–9.
8. Castells MC, Tennant NM, Sloane DE, et al. Hypersensitivity reactions to chemotherapy: outcomes and safety of rapid desensitization in 413 cases. J Allergy Clin Immunol 2008;122(3):574–80.
9. O'Donovan WJ, Klorfajn I. Sensitivity to penicillin: anaphylaxis and desensitization. Lancet 1946;444–6.
10. Wendel GD, Stark BJ, Jamison RB, et al. Penicillin allergy and desensitization in serious infections during pregnancy. N Engl J Med 1985;312(19):1229–32.

11. Borish L, Tamir R, Rosenwasser LJ. Intravenous desensitization to beta-lactam antibiotics. J Allergy Clin Immunol 1987;80(3 Pt 1):314–9.

12. Lee CW, Matulonis UA, Castells MC. Carboplatin hypersensitivity: a 6-h 12-step protocol effective in 35 desensitizations in patients with gynecological malignancies and mast cell/IgE-mediated reactions. Gynecol Oncol 2004;95(2):370–6.

13. Markman M, Kennedy A, Webster K, et al. Paclitaxel-associated hypersensitivity reactions: experience of the gynecologic oncology program of the Cleveland Clinic Cancer Center. J Clin Oncol 2000;18(1):102–5.

14. Puchner TC, Kugathasan S, Kelly KJ, et al. Successful desensitization and therapeutic use of infliximab in adult and pediatric Crohn's disease patients with prior anaphylactic reaction. Inflamm Bowel Dis 2001;7(1):34–7.

15. Kepley CL. Antigen-induced reduction in mast cell and basophil functional responses due to reduced Syk protein levels. Int Arch Allergy Immunol 2005; 138(1):29–39.

16. Morales AR, Shah N, Castells M. Antigen-IgE desensitization in signal transducer and activator of transcription 6-deficient mast cells by suboptimal doses of antigen. Ann Allergy Asthma Immunol 2005;94(5):575–80.

17. Solensky R. Drug hypersensitivity. Med Clin North Am 2006;90(1):233–60.

18. Zhao Y, Qiao H. Detection of specific IgE antibodies to major and minor antigenic determinants in sera of penicillin allergic patients. Chin Med J (Engl) 2003; 116(12):1904–10.

19. Meyer L, Zuberbier T, Worm M, et al. Hypersensitivity reactions to oxaliplatin: cross-reactivity to carboplatin and the introduction of a desensitization schedule. J Clin Oncol 2002;20(4):1146–7.

20. Cristaudo A, Sera F, Severino V, et al. Occupational hypersensitivity to metal salts, including platinum, in the secondary industry. Allergy 2005;60(2):159–64.

21. Castells M. Update on mast cells and mast cell precursors and hypersensitivity responses. Allergy Asthma Proc 1997;18(5):287–92.

22. Simons FE. 9. Anaphylaxis. J Allergy Clin Immunol 2008;121(Suppl 2): S402–1168.

23. Schwartz LB, Metcalfe DD, Miller JS, et al. Tryptase levels as an indicator of mast-cell activation in systemic anaphylaxis and mastocytosis. N Engl J Med 1987; 316(26):1622–6.

24. Torres MJ, Blanca M, Fernandez J, et al. Selective allergic reaction to oral cloxacillin. Clin Exp Allergy 1996;26(1):108–11.

25. Pichichero ME, Pichichero DM. Diagnosis of penicillin, amoxicillin, and cephalosporin allergy: reliability of examination assessed by skin testing and oral challenge. J Pediatr 1998;132(1):137–43.

26. Findlay SR, Kagey-Sobotka A, Lichtenstein LM. In vitro basophil histamine release induced by mannitol in a patient with mannitol-induced anaphylactoid reaction. 1984;73:578–83.

27. Shepherd GM. Hypersensitivity reactions to chemotherapeutic drugs. Clin Rev Allergy Immunol 2003;24(3):253–62.

28. Luskin AT, Luskin SS. Anaphylaxis and anaphylactoid reactions: diagnosis and management. Am J Ther 1996;3(7):515–20.

29. Szebeni J, Muggia FM, Alving CR. Complement activation by Cremophor EL as a possible contributor to hypersensitivity to paclitaxel: an in vitro study. J Natl Cancer Inst 1998;90(4):300–6.

30. Ying S, Meng Q, Scadding G, et al. Aspirin-sensitive rhinosinusitis is associated with reduced E-prostanoid 2 receptor expression on nasal mucosal inflammatory cells. J Allergy Clin Immunol 2006;117(2):312–8.

31. Szczeklik A, Stevenson DD. Aspirin-induced asthma: advances in pathogenesis and management. J Allergy Clin Immunol 1999;104(1):5–13.
32. Sanak M, Sampson AP. Biosynthesis of cysteinyl-leucotrienes in aspirin-intolerant asthma. 1999;29:306–311.
33. Pruzansky JJ, Patterson R. Desensitization of human basophils with suboptimal concentrations of agonist. Evidence for reversible and irreversible desensitization. Immunology 1988;443–7.
34. Paolini R, Numerof R, Kinet JP. Phosphorylation/dephosphorylation of high affinity IgE receptors: a mechanism for coupling/uncoupling a large signaling complex. 1992;89:10733–7.
35. Pienkowski MM, Kazmier WJ, Adkinson NF Jr. Basophil histamine release remains unaffected by clinical desensitization to penicillin. J Allergy Clin Immunol 1988;82(2):171–8.
36. Macglashan D, Miura K. Loss of syk kinase during IgE-mediated stimulation of human basophils. J Allergy Clin Immunol 2004;114(6):1317–24.
37. Odom S, Gomez G, Kovarova M, et al. Negative regulation of immunoglobulin E-dependent allergic responses by Lyn kinase. J Exp Med 2004;199(11): 1491–502.
38. Malaviya R, Uckun FM. Role of STAT6 in IgE receptor/FcepsilonRI-mediated late phase allergic responses of mast cells. J Immunol 2002;168(1):421–6.
39. Kelkar PS, Li JT. Cephalosporin allergy. N Engl J Med 2001;345(11):804–9.
40. Romano A, Mayorga C, Torres MJ, et al. Immediate allergic reactions to cephalosporins: cross-reactivity and selective responses. J Allergy Clin Immunol 2000;106(6):1177–83.
41. Romano A, Viola M, Gueant-Rodriguez RM, et al. Imipenem in patients with immediate hypersensitivity to penicillins. N Engl J Med 2006;354(26): 2835–7.
42. Burrows JA, Toon M, Bell SC. Antibiotic desensitization in adults with cystic fibrosis. Respirology 2003;8(3):359–64.
43. Turvey SE, Cronin B, Arnold AD, et al. Antibiotic desensitization for the allergic patient: 5 years of experience and practice. Ann Allergy Asthma Immunol 2004;92(4):426–32.
44. Madaan A, Li JT. Cephalosporin allergy. Immunol Allergy Clin North Am 2004; 24(3):463–76, vii.
45. Ghosal S, Taylor CJ. Intravenous desensitization to ceftazidime in cystic fibrosis patients. J Antimicrob Chemother 1997;39(4):556–7.
46. Papakonstantinou G, Bogner JR, Hofmeister F, et al. Cefotaxime desensitization. Clin Investig 1993;71(2):165–7.
47. Poston SA, Jennings HR, Poe KL. Cefazolin tolerance does not predict ceftriaxone hypersensitivity: unique side chains precipitate anaphylaxis. Pharmacotherapy 2004;24(5):668–72.
48. Gorman SK, Zed PJ, Dhingra VK, et al. Rapid imipenem/cilastatin desensitization for multidrug-resistant Acinetobacter pneumonia. Ann Pharmacother 2003;37(4): 513–6.
49. Feldweg AM, Lee CW, Matulonis UA, et al. Rapid desensitization for hypersensitivity reactions to paclitaxel and docetaxel: a new standard protocol used in 77 successful treatments. Gynecol Oncol 2005;96(3):824–9.
50. Castells M. Desensitization for drug allergy. Curr Opin Allergy Clin Immunol 2006; 6(6):476–81.
51. Lin RY. Desensitization in the management of vancomycin hypersensitivity. Arch Intern Med 1990;150(10):2197–8.

52. Wong JT, Ripple RE, Maclean JA, et al. Vancomycin hypersensitivity: synergism with narcotics and "desensitization" by a rapid continuous intravenous protocol. J Allergy Clin Immunol 1994;94(2 Pt 1):189–94.
53. Gea-Banacloche JC, Metcalfe DD. Ciprofloxacin desensitization. J Allergy Clin Immunol 1996;97(6):1426–7.
54. Berges-Gimeno MP, Stevenson DD. Nonsteroidal anti-inflammatory drug-induced reactions and desensitization. J Asthma 2004;41(4):375–84.
55. Widal MF, Abrami P, Lermeyez J. Anaphylaxie et idiosyncrasie. Presse Med 1922;189–92 [in French].
56. Lumry WR, Curd JG, Zeiger RS, et al. Aspirin-sensitive rhinosinusitis: the clinical syndrome and effects of aspirin administration. J Allergy Clin Immunol 1983; 71(6):580–7.
57. Berges-Gimeno MP, Simon RA, Stevenson DD. Long-term treatment with aspirin desensitization in asthmatic patients with aspirin-exacerbated respiratory disease. J Allergy Clin Immunol 2003;111(1):180–6.
58. Macy E, Bernstein JA, Castells MC, et al. Aspirin challenge and desensitization for aspirin-exacerbated respiratory disease: a practice paper. Ann Allergy Asthma Immunol 2007;98(2):172–4.
59. Berges-Gimeno MP, Simon RA, Stevenson DD. Early effects of aspirin desensitization treatment in asthmatic patients with aspirin-exacerbated respiratory disease. Ann Allergy Asthma Immunol 2003;90(3):338–41.
60. Patriarca G, Nucera E, Di Rienzo V. Nasal provocation test with lysine acetylsalicylate (LAS) in aspirin sensitive patients. Ann Allergy 1991;67:60–2.
61. Grzelewska-Rzymowska I, Roznlecki J, Szmidt M. Aspirin desensitization in patients with aspirin-induced urticaria and angioedema. Allergol Immunopathol 1988;16:305–8.
62. Silberman S, Neukirch-Stoop C, Steg PG. Rapid desensitization procedure for patients with aspirin hypersensitivity undergoing coronary stenting. Am J Cardiol 2005;95(4):509–10.
63. Pfaar O, Klimek L. Aspirin desensitization in aspirin intolerance: update on current standards and recent improvements. Curr Opin Allergy Clin Immunol 2006;6(3):161–6.
64. Lee JY, Simon RA. Does it make sense to "desens"? Aspirin desensitization in the treatment of chronic rhinosinusitis. Curr Allergy Asthma Rep 2006;6(3): 183–4.
65. White AA, Stevenson DD, Simon RA. The blocking effect of essential controller medications during aspirin challenges in patients with aspirin-exacerbated respiratory disease. Ann Allergy Asthma Immunol 2005;95(4):330–5.
66. White A, Ludington E, Mehra P, et al. Effect of leukotriene modifier drugs on the safety of oral aspirin challenges. Ann Allergy Asthma Immunol 2006;97(5): 688–93.
67. Alijotas-Reig J, Miguel-Moncin M, Cistero-Bahima A. Aspirin desensitization in the treatment of antiphospholipid syndrome during pregnancy in ASA-sensitive patients. Am J Reprod Immunol 2006;55(1):45–50.
68. Weiss RB, Bruno S. Hypersensitivity reactions to cancer chemotherapeutic agents. Ann Intern Med 1981;94(1):66–72.
69. Zweizig S, Roman LD, Muderspach LI. Death from anaphylaxis to cisplatin: a case report. Gynecol Oncol 1994;53(1):121–2.
70. Sood AK, Gelder MS, Huang SW, et al. Anaphylaxis to carboplatin following multiple previous uncomplicated courses. Gynecol Oncol 1995;57(1): 131–2.

71. Markman M, Zanotti K, Peterson G, et al. Expanded experience with an intradermal skin test to predict for the presence or absence of carboplatin hypersensitivity. J Clin Oncol 2003;21(24):4611–4.
72. Markman M. Toxicities of the platinum antineoplastic agents. Expert Opin Drug Saf 2003;2(6):597–607.
73. Morgan M, Bowers DC, Gruchalla RS, et al. Safety and efficacy of repeated monthly carboplatin desensitization. J Allergy Clin Immunol 2004;114(4):974–5.
74. Essayan DM, Kagey-Sobotka A, Colarusso PJ, et al. Successful parenteral desensitization to paclitaxel. J Allergy Clin Immunol 1996;97(1 Pt 1):42–6.
75. Choi J, Harnett P, Fulcher DA. Carboplatin desensitization. Ann Allergy Asthma Immunol 2004;93(2):137–41.
76. Robinson JB, Singh D, Bodurka-Bevers DC, et al. Hypersensitivity reactions and the utility of oral and intravenous desensitization in patients with gynecologic malignancies. Gynecol Oncol 2001;82(3):550–8.
77. Moreno-Ancillo A, Dominguez-Noche C, Gil-Adrados AC, et al. Anaphylactoid reaction to carboplatin: successful "desensitization". Allergol Immunopathol (Madr) 2003;31(6):342–4.
78. Gammon D, Bhargava P, McCormick MJ. Hypersensitivity reactions to oxaliplatin and the application of a desensitization protocol. Oncologist 2004;9(5):546–9.
79. Wrzesinski SH, McGurk ML, Donovan CT, et al. Successful desensitization to oxaliplatin with incorporation of calcium gluconate and magnesium sulfate. Anticancer Drugs 2007;18(6):721–4.
80. Weiss RB, Donehower RC, Wiernik PH, et al. Hypersensitivity reactions from taxol. J Clin Oncol 1990;8(7):1263–8.
81. Walker FE. Paclitaxel (TAXOL): side effects and patient education issues. Semin Oncol Nurs 1993;9(Suppl 2):6–10.
82. Price KS, Castells MC. Taxol reactions. Allergy Asthma Proc 2002;23(3):205–8.
83. Markman M, Zanotti K, Kulp B, et al. Relationship between a history of systemic allergic reactions and risk of subsequent carboplatin hypersensitivity. Gynecol Oncol 2003;89(3):514–6.
84. Grosen E, Siitari E, Larrison E, et al. Paclitaxel hypersensitivity reactions related to bee-sting allergy. Lancet 2000;355(9200):288–9.
85. Dizon DS, Dupont J, Anderson S, et al. Treatment of recurrent ovarian cancer: a retrospective analysis of women treated with single-agent carboplatin originally treated with carboplatin and paclitaxel. The Memorial Sloan-Kettering Cancer Center experience. Gynecol Oncol 2003;91(3):584–90.
86. Bookman MA, Greer BE, Ozols RF. Optimal therapy of advanced ovarian cancer: carboplatin and paclitaxel vs. cisplatin and paclitaxel (GOG 158) and an update on GOG0 182-ICON5. Int J Gynecol Cancer 2003;13(6):735–40.
87. Markman M, Kennedy A, Webster K, et al. Clinical features of hypersensitivity reactions to carboplatin. J Clin Oncol 1999;17(4):1141.
88. Kook H, Kim KM, Choi SH, et al. Life-threatening carboplatin hypersensitivity during conditioning for autologous PBSC transplantation: successful rechallenge after desensitization. Bone Marrow Transplant 1998;21(7):727–9.
89. Zanotti KM, Rybicki LA, Kennedy AW, et al. Carboplatin skin testing: a skin-testing protocol for predicting hypersensitivity to carboplatin chemotherapy. J Clin Oncol 2001;19(12):3126–9.
90. Goldberg A, Confino-Cohen R, Fishman A, et al. A modified, prolonged desensitization protocol in carboplatin allergy. J Allergy Clin Immunol 1996;98(4):841–3.
91. Confino-Cohen R, Fishman A, Altaras M, et al. Successful carboplatin desensitization in patients with proven carboplatin allergy. Cancer 2005;104(3):640–3.

92. Wolbink GJ, Vis M, Lems W, et al. Development of antiinfliximab antibodies and relationship to clinical response in patients with rheumatoid arthritis. Arthritis Rheum 2006;54(3):711–5.
93. Hellerstedt B, Ahmed A. Delayed-type hypersensitivity reaction or serum sickness after rituximab treatment. Ann Oncol 2003;14(12):1792.
94. Tada K, Ito Y, Hatake K, et al. Severe infusion reaction induced by trastuzumab: a case report. Breast Cancer 2003;10(2):167–9.
95. Nikas SN, Voulgari PV, Drosos AA. Urticaria and angiedema-like skin reactions in a patient treated with adalimumab. Clin Rheumatol 2006;1–2.
96. Alexander S, Hopewell S, Hunter S, et al. Rituximab and desensitization for a patient with severe factor IX deficiency, inhibitors, and history of anaphylaxis. J Pediatr Hematol Oncol 2008;30(1):93–5.
97. Breslow RG, Caiado J, Castells MC. Acetylsalicylic acid and montelukast block mast cell mediator-related symptoms during rapid desensitization. Ann Allergy Asthma Immunol 2009;102(2):155–60.

Index

Note: Page numbers of article titles are in **boldface** type.

A

Acetaminophen, skin tests for, 523
Acetylsalicylic acid
   desensitization to, 590–592
   provocation test for, 575
   skin tests for, 520
Acute generalized exanthematous pustulosis, 409–410, 524–525
Acyclovir, skin tests for, 518, 520
Alcuronium, anaphylaxis to, 433
Alfentanil, skin tests for, 442
Allergologic investigations, 413–414
Allopurinol, DIHS/DRESS due to, 486, 492–493
Allylisopropylacetylurea, skin tests for, 520
Aminoglycosides, skin tests for, 511
5-Aminosalicylic acid, skin tests for, 520
Amoxicillin
   basophil activation test for, 560
   provocation test for, 575
   skin tests for, 508–511, 520
Ampicillin, skin tests for, 508–511
Anaphylaxis. *See also specific substances.*
   in skin testing, 507–508
   perioperative. *See* Perioperative anaphylaxis.
   to pholcodine, **419–427,** 432
   to radiocontrast media, 455–456
Anemia, hemolytic, 410
Anesthesia, anaphylaxis during. *See* Perioperative anaphylaxis.
Antibiotics
   anaphylaxis to, 433–434
   basophil activation test for, 560–561
   desensitization to, 588–590
   skin tests for, 508–511, 520–523, 526
Anticonvulsants, DIHS/DRESS due to, 485–492
Antihistamines, for hypersensitivity prevention
   perioperative agents, 444–445
   radiocontrast media, 463
Aprotinin, anaphylaxis to, 435–436
Argatroban, as heparin alternative, 477
Aspirin
   basophil activation test for, 560–562
   desensitization to, 590–592

Immunol Allergy Clin N Am 29 (2009) 607–620
doi:10.1016/S0889-8561(09)00046-0
0889-8561/09/$ – see front matter © 2009 Elsevier Inc. All rights reserved.

immunology.theclinics.com

Printed and bound by CPI Group (UK) Ltd, Croydon, CR0 4YY

03/10/2024

01040452-0005